Contemporary Surgical Clerkships

Series Editor

Adam E. M. Eltorai, Marlborough, USA

AF167445

This series of specialty-specific books will serve as high-yield, quick-reference reviews specifically for the numerous third- and fourth-year medical students rotating on surgical clerkships. Edited by experts in the field, each book includes concise review content from a senior resident or fellow and an established academic physician. Students can read the text from cover to cover to gain a general foundation of knowledge that can be built upon when they begin their rotation, or they can use specific chapters to review a subspecialty before starting a new rotation or seeing a patient with a subspecialty attending.

These books will be the ideal, on-the-spot references for medical students and practitioners seeking fast facts on diagnosis and management. Their bullet-pointed format, including user-friendly figures, tables and algorithms, make them the perfect quick-reference. Their content breadth covers the most commonly encountered problems in practice, focusing on the fundamental principles of diagnosis and management. Carry them in your white coat for convenient access to the answers you need, when you need them.

Tejal S. Brahmbhatt • Dane R. Scantling
Editors

Trauma Surgery Clerkship

A Guide for Senior Medical Students

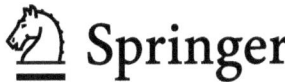 Springer

Editors
Tejal S. Brahmbhatt
Division of Acute Care Surgery
(Trauma, Emergency General Surgery
Surgical Critical Care)
Cedars-Sinai Medical Center
Los Angeles, CA, USA

Dane R. Scantling
Division of Acute Care Surgery
Boston Medical Center/Boston University
Chobanian and Avedisian
School of Medicine
Boston, MA, USA

ISSN 2730-941X   ISSN 2730-9428   (electronic)
Contemporary Surgical Clerkships
ISBN 978-3-032-01411-5   ISBN 978-3-032-01412-2   (eBook)
https://doi.org/10.1007/978-3-032-01412-2

Editorial Contact: Jessica Chio
This Springer imprint is published by the registered company Springer Nature Switzerland AG
The registered company address is: Gewerbestrasse 11, 6330 Cham, Switzerland

If disposing of this product, please recycle the paper.

Contents

Chapter 1
The Social Determinants of Health and the Goal of Health Equity

Olivia A. Sacks and Tracey Dechert

Overview

- According to the CDC, social determinants of health (SDOH) are "the conditions in the environments where people are born, live, work, play, worship, and age that affect a range of health, functioning, and quality-of-life outcomes and risks."
- The SDOH fits within a larger context of structural determinants which include governmental and economic policies which set priorities and allocate resources within society.
- SDOH includes the social and community context, educational opportunities, economic opportunities, a person's physical environment, and their ability to access health and healthcare (Fig. 1.1).
- SDOH affects everyone, it is not something one can have or not have. It is not positive or negative. However, under-resourced populations have more adverse events in relation to their SDOH.
- Health equity is the goal of attaining the highest health for all people. It is the responsibility of physicians (and students) to understand the factors which impact their patients to improve the health of their society.

O. A. Sacks · T. Dechert (✉)
Department of Surgery, Boston University Chobanian & Avedisian School of Medicine, Boston, MA, USA
e-mail: Olivia.sacks@bmc.org; Tracey.Dechert@bmc.org

© The Author(s), under exclusive license to Springer Nature Switzerland AG 2025
T. S. Brahmbhatt, D. R. Scantling (eds.), *Trauma Surgery Clerkship*, Contemporary Surgical Clerkships, https://doi.org/10.1007/978-3-032-01412-2_1

1

Fig. 1.1 Domains of the social determinants of health

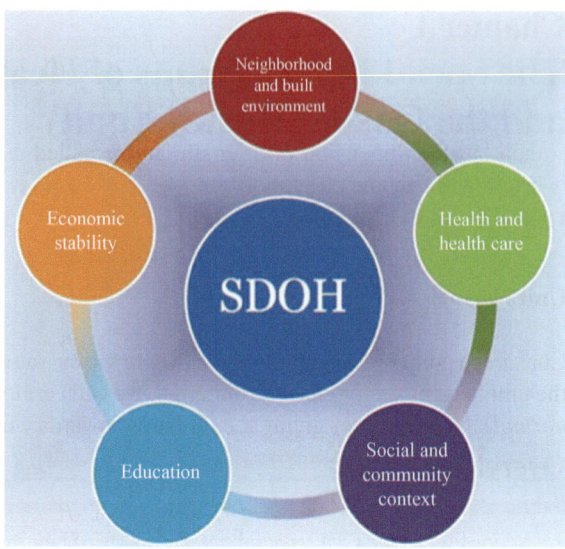

Fig. 1.2 Factors contributing to disease and health. (Source: Institute for Clinical Systems Improvement, Going Beyond Clinical Walls Solving Complex Problems (October 2014))

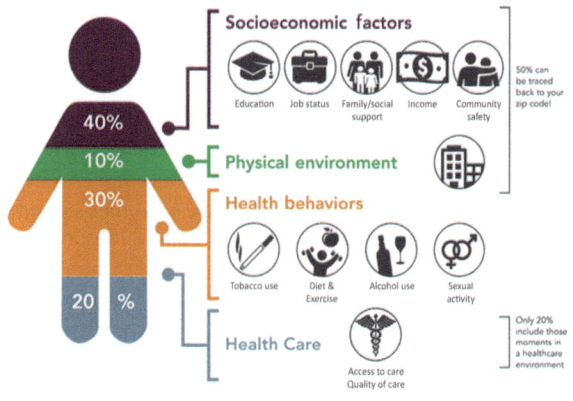

Background

- While we tend to think of health in terms of whether a person has a disease, 80% of an individual's health is actually determined by their social/environmental milieu (Fig. 1.2).
- Health behaviors are influenced by our SDOH. For example, diet and exercise is influenced by the constraints of a person's physical environment.
- Other examples are education, housing, income, and access to food and clean water.

Neighborhood and Built Environment

- A person's built environment can have a large impact on their health and wellbeing.
- For example, access to clean water and air has a large effect on the health and wellbeing of both children and adults [1].
- Experiencing neighborhood crime and violence can increase the rate of post-traumatic stress disorder. In a recent study in Chicago, a decrease in volent crime at the community level was associated with decreased cardiovascular and coronary artery disease mortality rates [2].

Health and Healthcare

- Not all US citizens have access to timely, high-quality acute care and preventative care.
- As of 2018, one in ten people in our country did not have health insurance [3].
- In the United States, over 30 million people do not have access to a level 1 or level 2 trauma center within 1 h of being injured, which can have a significant impact on the natural course of their illness or injury [4].

Social and Community Context

- Social connection and community engagement can be protective factors in people's health [5].
- On the other end of the spectrum, there are clear links between bullying victimization and suicide attempts. Bullying perpetration is also associated with poor health-related outcomes, such as violent behavior, suicidality, substance use, and unemployment [6].

Education

- Education level is associated with better health and longer life.
- In a recent longitudinal study of trauma patients, having a high-school education or lower was associated with the poorest functional, physical, and mental health outcomes [7].

Economic Stability

- Economic stability is woven into all of the prior domains. Economic status informs what neighborhood a person can live in, whether they are housed, where they get their healthcare and education.
- Nearly 1 in 14 people in the United States experiences one bout of homelessness in their lifetime.
- People of lower socioeconomic status have higher injury rates and mortality across many mechanisms [8].
- Poverty has a major adverse effect on health in general after controlling for health-related behaviors.

Redlining and Structural Racism

- Redlining practices of the 1930s created maps that assigned different levels of risk to urban areas, defining which areas would qualify for federally backed loans [9].
- Areas with a high percentage of Black residents were considered "hazardous" and did not qualify for these loans.
- These racist practices have significant downstream effects that endure today including a profound wealth gap between white and Black residents.
- Recent studies in Philadelphia and Boston show that redlined areas have higher rates of firearm violence.
- Addressing the structural determinants of health within these neighborhoods, such as poverty and lack of homeownership, may decrease firearm violence in those neighborhoods.

Trauma-Informed Care (TIC)

- TIC is the proactive framework that is grounded in an understanding of and responsiveness to the impact of trauma.
- Each person's experiences shape the way they interact with the system they are in and each other.
- A trauma-informed provider has an amazing opportunity to change the trajectory of the healthcare experience for their patients.
- There are four R's of TIC [10]:

    - *R*ealize the widespread nature of trauma.
    - *R*ecognize the signs and symptoms of trauma.
    - *R*espond by fully integrating TIC into practices, including hospital policy.
    - *R*esist the act of retraumatizing our patients by prioritizing their interests.

- TIC has six core principles:

  - Safety: Ensure a safe environment both physically and emotionally for patients;
  - Trustworthiness and Transparency: Create a space for human connection through up front communication;
  - Peer Support: Integrate credible messengers;
  - Collaboration and Mutuality: Create a model for respect and equitable care;
  - Empowerment and Choice: Ensure survivors play a critical role in medical decision making and healing;
  - Awareness: Address cultural, historical, and gender biases [10].

- TIC is relevant to students and physicians in all specialties, but should especially frame the way we approach patients and vulnerable communities [11].

Considering Health Equity

- While equality is about sameness and equal access, equity is about fairness and proportional representation in opportunities (Fig. 1.3).
- The association between low socioeconomic status and poor health is well understood, but the mechanisms to improve it are lacking.
- Recognizing disparities helps identify problems, but this exercise is only useful if surgeons work to address these deeply unfair problems.
- If we lived in an equitable society, the people most impacted would be most assisted.

Fig. 1.3 Equality versus equity

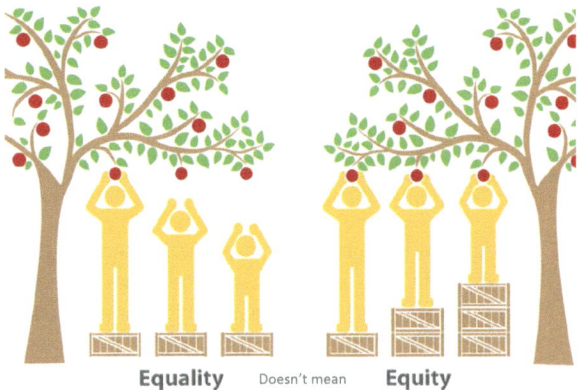

Equality Doesn't mean **Equity**

Fig. 1.4 Example of how
to translate data into action

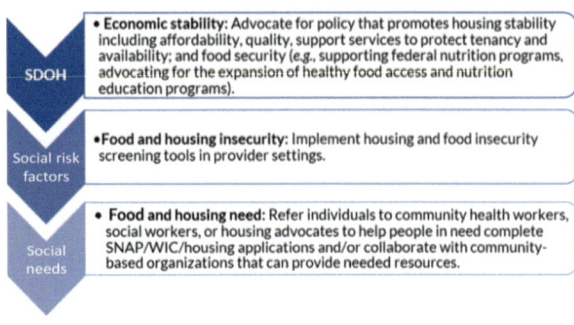

Advocacy in Trauma Surgery

- Translating data into action remains one of the most important and challenging pieces of trauma care.
- Surgeons can improve the health of trauma patients by screening for social risk factors, such as housing, food security, firearm safety, interpersonal violence, and substance use disorders.
- Putting advocacy into practice includes practicing trauma informed care, partnering with community organizations to improve patient care, and advocating at a policy level (Fig. 1.4).
- Using knowledge of the social milieu of patients, we can engage social services and community resources to tailor care.
- While many of our efforts in trauma are focused on tertiary prevention, more work on SDOH can address primary and secondary prevention to decrease the number of traumatic injuries overall.
- The American Medical Association's Declaration of Professional Responsibility includes that physicians should "advocate for social, economic, educational, and political changes that ameliorate suffering and contribute to human wellbeing."

How to Get Involved

- Medical students can play an important part in the care of trauma patients.
- Get to know your patients: visit patients who have recently undergone emergency surgery and screen patients for social risk factors that may impact their recovery [12].
- Start a Socially Responsible Surgery (SRS) chapter at your school (Fig. 1.5). SRS aims to bridge the gap between public health and surgery through advocacy, education, research, and service.

Fig. 1.5 Socially
Responsible Surgery logo

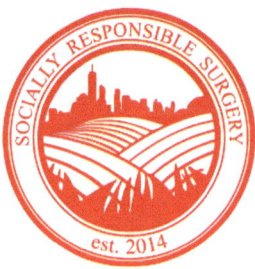

Conclusion

- No matter what type of physician you choose to become, it is important to remember the ways in which physicians can reach beyond themselves and effect important change for local communities and people.
- The goal of understanding the social determinants of health and intervening on modifiable risk factors is to move toward a world where no support or accommodations are needed.
- In this vision of the world, the system is changed (Fig. 1.6). Society is equitable and all members are socially, physically, and psychologically safe, our basic economic needs are met, and we are able to exercise our right to basic human dignity.

Fig. 1.6 Social justice

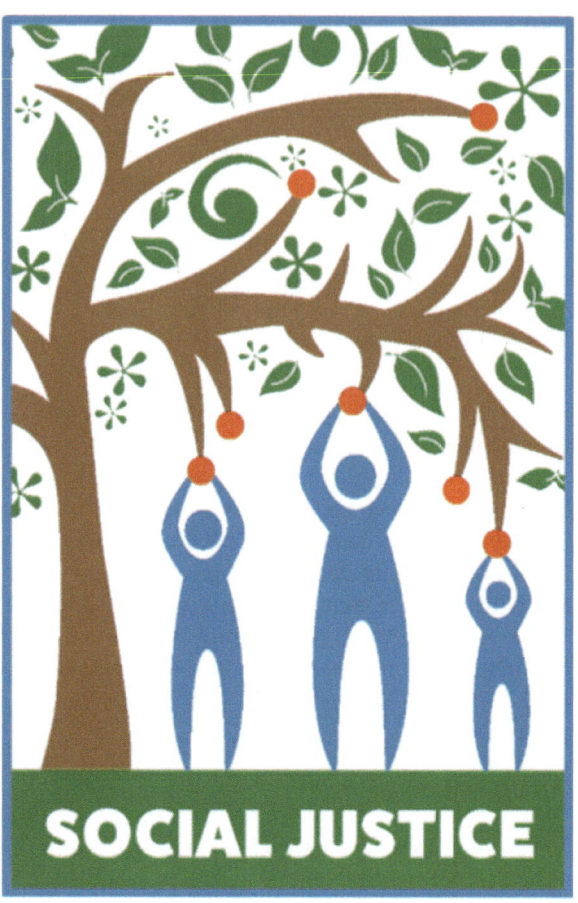

References

1. Ruckart PZ, Ettinger AS, Hanna-Attisha M, Jones N, Davis SI, Breysse PN. The Flint water crisis: a coordinated public health emergency response and recovery initiative. J Public Health Manag Pract. 2019;25(Suppl 1, Lead Poisoning Prevention):S84–90.
2. Eberly LA, Julien H, South EC, et al. Association between community-level violent crime and cardiovascular mortality in Chicago: a longitudinal analysis. J Am Heart Assoc. 2022;11(14):e025168.
3. Berchick ER, Barnett JC. Health insurance coverage in the United States: 2017. United States Census Bureau; 2018.
4. Carr BG, Bowman AJ, Wolff CS, et al. Disparities in access to trauma care in the United States: a population-based analysis. Injury. 2017;48(2):332–8.
5. Holt-Lunstad J. Why social relationships are important for physical health: a systems approach to understanding and modifying risk and protection. Annu Rev Psychol. 2018;69(1):437–58.
6. Serafini G, Aguglia A, Amerio A, et al. The relationship between bullying victimization and perpetration and non-suicidal self-injury: a systematic review. Child Psychiatry Hum Dev. 2023;54(1):154–75.

7. Haider AH, Herrera-Escobar JP, Al Rafai SS, et al. Factors associated with long-term outcomes after injury: results of the functional outcomes and recovery after trauma emergencies (FORTE) multicenter cohort study. Ann Surg. 2020;271(6):1165–73.
8. Frencher SK Jr, Benedicto CM, Kendig TD, Herman D, Barlow B, Pressley JC. A comparative analysis of serious injury and illness among homeless and housed low income residents of New York City. J Trauma. 2010;69(4 Suppl):S191–9.
9. Poulson M, Neufeld MY, Dechert T, Allee L, Kenzik KM. Historic redlining, structural racism, and firearm violence: a structural equation modeling approach. Lancet Reg Health Am. 2021;3:100052.
10. SAMHSA's Trauma and Justice Strategic Initiative. SAMHSA's concept of trauma and guidance for a trauma-informed approach. 2014.
11. Portelli Tremont JN, Klausner B, Udekwu PO. Embracing a trauma-informed approach to patient care—in with the new. JAMA Surg. 2021;156(12):1083–4.
12. Bedi NS, LaRaja A. Beyond the walls of a hospital: empowering students & surgeons to incorporate the social determinants of health into clinical care. Ann Surg. 2023;277:e494–5.

Chapter 2
Trauma Epidemiology and Prevention

Olivia A. Sacks and Lisa C. Allee

Overview

- Trauma is the physical damage that results when a human body is exposed to an amount of energy (kinetic, thermal, chemical, electrical, or radiant) that surpasses the body's physiological tolerance [1].
- Trauma surgeons are like the quarterbacks of care for the trauma patient. They work closely with many different teams to care for trauma patients in a holistic way:

  - Surgical subspecialties (i.e., orthopedic; ear, nose, and throat; oral maxillofacial; vascular; neurosurgery)
  - Physical and occupational therapists
  - Speech language pathologists
  - Addiction medicine
  - Social work and violence prevention teams

- In this specialty, injury is approached as a disease rather than accidents or incidents. For example, when discussing motor vehicle-related injury, traumatologists prefer the term "motor vehicle collision," avoiding the term accident. Motor vehicle collisions have measurable incidence, prevalence, and severity much like a disease such as hypertension. They are not accidents.
- Injuries are preventable and costly.
- Violence and injury have long-term impacts on people's overall functioning both physically and emotionally.

O. A. Sacks · L. C. Allee (✉)
Boston University Chobanian & Avedisian School of Medicine, Boston Medical Center, Boston, MA, USA
e-mail: Olivia.sacks@bmc.org; liallee@bu.edu

T. S. Brahmbhatt, D. R. Scantling (eds.), *Trauma Surgery Clerkship*, Contemporary Surgical Clerkships,
https://doi.org/10.1007/978-3-032-01412-2_2

- There are racial and ethnic disparities in injury and violence rates.
- Trauma centers have an obligation to participate in injury and violence prevention efforts.

Background

According to the National Safety Council, an American is accidentally injured every second and killed every 3 min by a preventable event, like a vehicle crash, fall, drowning, or another preventable incident.

Fatal Injuries

Injuries are the leading cause of death for people ages 1–44 in the United States (US) (https://www.cdc.gov/injury/wisqars/leadingcauses.html). In 2020, 278,345 persons died of an injury, and this number has significantly increased in the last decade [2].

Most deaths secondary to trauma occur within minutes of the injury. Many do not make it to the hospital, and of those that do, many die within the first hours of care. These deaths are generally the result of massive hemorrhage or severe neurologic injury [3].

Non-Fatal Injuries

There are an even higher number of US citizens affected by non-fatal trauma than fatal trauma. In 2020, there were nearly 23 million visits to the emergency department after a traumatic injury. The leading causes of non-fatal injury in 2020 were fall and struck by/against (Fig. 2.1).

The cost of these injuries in the United States exceeds 4.2 trillion, which includes spending on health care, lost work productivity, and estimates of cost for lost quality of life and death [4]. The cost to individuals, family, and society is even greater and more difficult to quantify.

Fig. 2.1 Leading cause of non-fatal injury overall in the United States

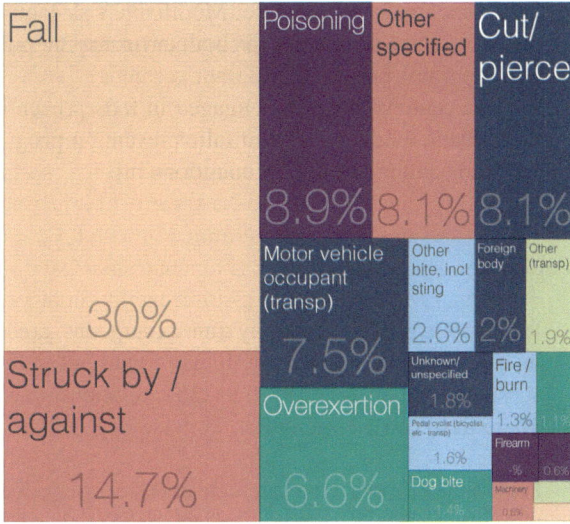

Epidemiology and Prevention of Trauma by Mechanism

The mechanism of a trauma refers to the agent or mode by which the patient was injured. It can be interpersonal, intrapersonal, or unintentional. The following are not all encompassing but include the top mechanisms of injury seen at trauma centers.

Falls

- Falls were the most common cause of non-fatal injury in the United States between 2010 and 2020 across all age groups.
- Every second an older adult 65+ suffers a fall in the United States, with approximately 36 million falls and 32,000 fall-related deaths each year [4].
- It is estimated that by 2030, older adults will outnumber young adults for the first time in history, making fall prevention that much more important.
- One-third of injury-related hospitalizations are fall-related, resulting in significant burden on hospitals [4].
- Falls are an example of the need for multidisciplinary trauma care. These injuries often include the need for different subspeciality surgeons, internal medicine physicians, physical and occupational therapy, social work, and nutritionists.
- One in five falls causes a fracture or head injury. Over 95% of hip fractures are caused by falling, and falls are the most common cause of traumatic brain injuries [5].
- If fall death rates continue to rise as they have in the past two decades, we can anticipate seven fall deaths for older adults every hour by 2030 [6].

- Falls are largely preventable. Modifiable risk factors for falls include physical activity and rehabilitation, the built environment, polypharmacy, and fall prevention programs [7].
- Trauma centers should be engaged in falls prevention activities, including risk assessment, evidenced-based falls prevention programs, and collaboration with statewide and regional falls coalitions [8].

Poisoning

- While not typically treated by trauma surgeons, poisoning is a priority of trauma/injury prevention nationally. It is a requirement for trauma centers to address substance use disorder given its close relationship to traumatic injury.
- There has been a large uptick in poisoning deaths since the onset of the opioid epidemic.
- Poisoning eclipsed motor vehicle collision as the leading cause of injury-related mortality in 2011 secondary to the opioid crisis.
- Efforts to combat the opioid crisis focus on harm reduction, which includes needle exchanges, naloxone distribution and training, improving access to treatment, and changing prescribing practices [3].
- Trauma center's engagement in screening, brief intervention, and referral to treatment (SBIRT) efforts is mandatory to aid with prevention of poisoning related to all substance use disorders [9].

Motor Vehicle Collisions and Traffic-Related Injury

- The third most common cause of injury-related death in 2020 was motor vehicle collisions.
- Injury patterns for this mechanism are diverse, dependent on the mechanism of injury as well as whether the victim was restrained.
- Concomitant drug and alcohol use is a major factor in fatal motor vehicle collisions. Around 26% of women and 43% of men who died of a motor vehicle collision of all ages had elevated blood alcohol content [3].
- Over 7000 pedestrians were killed as a result of an MVC in 2020 [10].
- Approx. 1000 bicyclists die and over 130,000 are injured in crashes in the United States yearly, the estimated costs associated with these exceed $23 billion. [10]
- Mandatory seatbelt laws have improved compliance with seat belting which has reduced morbidity, but the United States continues to have lower compliance with seatbelt use than other developed countries [11].
- Screening, brief intervention, and referral to treatment (SBIRT) efforts specific to impaired driving are an essential component of trauma prevention activities [9].

Firearms and Intimate Partner Violence

- In 2020, more people in the United States died of firearm-related causes than any other year on record. This includes both homicide and suicide.
- Proportional to the population, the rate of firearm-related deaths has been steadily increasing in the past 30 years, but is still well beneath the high in 1974 [12].
- In the last few years, firearm violence surpassed motor vehicle collisions as the leading cause of death children (<18) in the United States (Fig. 2.2).
- In 2020, 54% of firearm-related deaths were suicides, while 43% were homicides (Fig. 2.3). Firearm-related mortality disproportionally affects males, people of Black race, and younger people.
- Homicide composes two-thirds of deaths in this population, but the number of deaths caused by suicide is also rising dramatically.
- Children of Black race are most likely to die of firearm-related homicide and boys of white race are most likely to die by suicide [2].
- Twenty-five percent, or one in four women, report experiencing some form of IPV [2].
- Sexual violence over half of women have experienced sexual violence and one in three men. The estimated lifetime cost of rape is over $122,000 per victim [2].
- Physical violence—one in five homicide victims are killed by an intimate partner (IP) [2].
- Stalking/dating violence—this impacts millions of teens each year, 14% of women and 5% men report having been stalked by an IP [2].
- Having a hospital-based violence intervention program (HVIP) can support victims of violence and their family members and prevent subsequent violence-related injuries and long-term mental health sequelae [13].
- Advocacy efforts to support strong firearm legislation promoting safe access and storage should be part of every trauma center's mission [9].

Drowning

- Drowning is the second leading cause of death for children ages 1–14.

Fig. 2.2 Gun-related deaths, United States, 2020

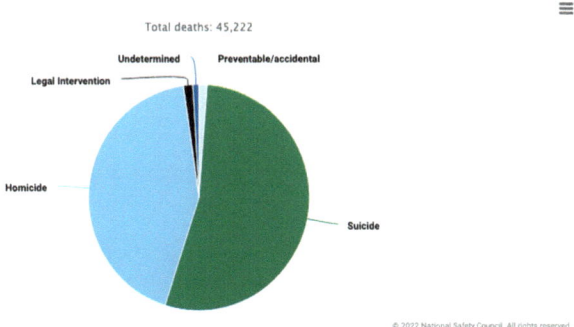

Total deaths: 45,222

Fig. 2.3 Leading causes of death in children, 1999–2020

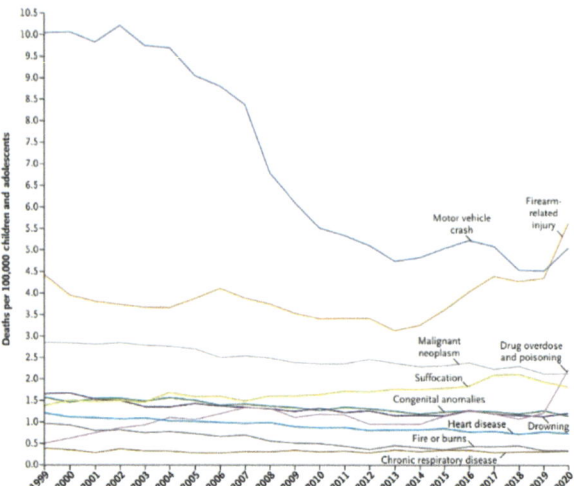

- In swimming pools, Black children ages 10–14 years drown at rates 7.6 times higher than white children.
- In natural water, American Indian and Alaskan Native people have rates 2.7 times higher than white people [4].
- Drowning prevention includes formal swimming lessons, fencing of pools, life jacket use, and supervision. Trauma centers can encourage these activities through education and community partnerships [14].

Prevention

- We can consider the ways we can help through the lens of primary, secondary, and tertiary prevention (Fig. 2.4).

  - *Primary prevention*: intervening before health effects occur
  - *Secondary prevention*: screening to identify and control diseases at early stages
  - *Tertiary prevention*: managing disease post diagnosis to slow progression

- In addition, there is *primordial prevention*: risk factor reduction targeted toward an entire population through a focus on social and environmental conditions (social determinants) which will be covered in the next chapter.

Fig. 2.4 Primary, secondary, tertiary prevention

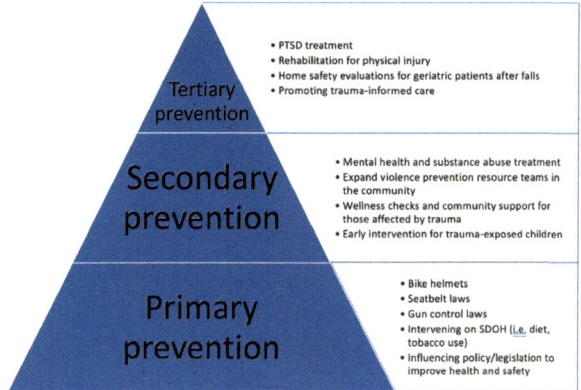

References

1. Neira J. A call for action to declare trauma as a disease. InterAcademy Partnership; 2019.
2. Centers for Disease Control and Prevention. Key injury and violence data. https://www-cdc-gov.ezproxy.bu.edu/injury/wisqars/overview/key_data.html. Accessed 22 Dec 2022.
3. Meagher AZB. Trauma. In: Feliciano DV, Mattox KL, Moore EE, editors. Trauma, vol. 9E. McGraw Hill; 2021.
4. Centers for Disease Control and Prevention. Cost of injury data. https://www-cdc-gov.ezproxy.bu.edu/injury/wisqars/cost/index.html. Accessed 22 Dec 2022.
5. Falls in older persons. 2022. Accessed 3 Jan 2023. https://www.cdc.gov/falls/data-research/facts-stats/index.html.
6. Centers for Disease Control and Prevention. Facts about falls. https://www.cdc.gov/falls/facts.html. Accessed 21 Dec 2022.
7. Hoffman G, Franco N, Perloff J, Lynn J, Okoye S, Min L. Incidence of and county variation in fall injuries in US residents aged 65 years or older, 2016-2019. JAMA Netw Open. 2022;5(2):e2148007.
8. ACS COT. Statement on older adult falls and falls prevention. Updated 2019. https://www.facs.org/about-acs/statements/older-adult-falls-and-falls-prevention/.
9. American College of Surgeons. Resources for the Optimal Care of the Injured Patient 2022 standards. https://www.facs.org/quality-programs/trauma/quality/verification-review-and-consultation-program/standards/.
10. National Highway Traffic Safety Administration. Traffic safety facts, 2019 data—bicyclists and other cyclists. Washington, DC: US Department of Transportation; 2021. (Publication no. DOT HS 813 197).
11. Centers for Disease Control and Prevention. Motor vehicle crash deaths. https://www.cdc.gov/vitalsigns/motor-vehicle-safety/index.html. Accessed 21 Dec 2022.
12. Kaufman EJ, Wiebe DJ, Xiong RA, Morrison CN, Seamon MJ, Delgado MK. Epidemiologic trends in fatal and nonfatal firearm injuries in the US, 2009-2017. JAMA Intern Med. 2021;181(2):237–44.
13. National Network of Hospital-based Violence Intervention Programs. NNHVIP policy white paper—hospital-based violence intervention: practices and policies to end the cycle of violence. 2023. https://www.thehavi.org.
14. Centers for Disease Control and Prevention. Drowning prevention. https://www.cdc.gov/drowning/prevention/index.html.

Chapter 3
Trauma Systems

Forrest B. Fernandez

Introduction

Trauma care has improved dramatically over the last 70 years. Improved surgical technique and resuscitative strategies account for a significant portion of this improvement. The ability to provide the injured patient immediate access to experienced providers, equipped with the required resources to provide life-saving interventions in patients with time-dependent injury, remains the primary aim of the modern trauma system. A wealth of data now demonstrates that when timely care is accessible through a well-coordinated, all-inclusive trauma system, significant reductions in both mortality and morbidity (9–25%) inevitably result [3–10].

Goals of a Trauma System

Primary Goals

- Ensure immediate access to time life-saving therapies in patients with time-dependent injury regardless of point of injury within the region.

F. B. Fernandez (✉)
Perelman School of Medicine, Philadelphia, PA, USA
e-mail: forrest.fernandez@pennmedicine.upenn.edu

© The Author(s), under exclusive license to Springer Nature
Switzerland AG 2025
T. S. Brahmbhatt, D. R. Scantling (eds.), *Trauma Surgery Clerkship*,
Contemporary Surgical Clerkships,
https://doi.org/10.1007/978-3-032-01412-2_3

Secondary Goals

- Ensure effective triage criteria and strategy unique to the challenges of the region.
- Minimize transport times for patients requiring definitive care.
- Ensure critical resources are deployed at verified/accredited trauma centers.
- Ensure strategically effective placement of trauma centers.
- Ensure availability of post-acute rehabilitation services.
- Injury prevention interventions to reduce injury occurrence.
- Provide advocacy to regional policy making organizations facilitating improved access and quality of care.
- Provide trauma registry data in order to optimize outcomes.
- Provide a framework in which the region can effectively respond to local and regional mass casualty threats.

Trauma Systems History

Modern civilian trauma systems draw their origins from lessons learned during military conflict. The challenges of battlefield medicine can differ from civilian settings in severity, wounding mechanism, and prevalence of multiple patient scenarios. Nonetheless, military conflicts have proven to be an effective laboratory from which major improvements in civilian trauma care have been discovered. Key challenges faced in combat casualty care include all of the following:

- Austere environs at the point of injury
- Point of injury may occur far from available treatment facilities
- Limited ability to mobilize trained pre-hospital providers to the scene
- Local conditions on the ground which challenge timely transport for definitive care (ongoing hostilities, terrain, weather, time of day)
- Sustainment challenges (decreased demand for resources during peacetime, lack of funding, lack of public awareness)
- Historical lack of robust registries documenting care

One does not have to be particularly imaginative to see the similarities to challenges faced in civilian settings, particularly rural regions which account for 25% of the current US population.

Improvements in combat casualty care have been most dramatic in the last century, beginning with the advent of World War II (WWII). Improved surgical techniques (i.e., colostomy diversion of colonic injuries, vascular bypass and repair techniques), better resuscitative capabilities (blood and plasma transfusion), and improved casualty evacuation all contributed to markedly improved outcomes for the injured. For this conflict, 50 in 100 injured combatants receiving treatment for injuries would survive—a most dramatic improvement over the WWI era (4/100) [11].

The advent of the helicopter and its use for casualty evacuation would prove to be a vital advancement improving overall quality of care. Although helicopter technology existed in the WWII era, its arrival to production did not occur until the end of the war, greatly limiting its impact. The Korean and Vietnam conflicts were the first conflicts where helicopter use in casualty evacuation was wide spread. By the time of the Vietnam conflict, improved surgical capabilities in the theater of conflict in combination with much improved casualty evacuation brought the died of wounds rate down to 15.8%. Still, in both the Korean and Vietnam conflicts, the time from injury to evacuation to arrival at a tertiary facility in the US mainland typically took about 6 weeks.

The more recent US conflicts (Operation Enduring Freedom/Operation Iraqi Freedom) have seen the lowest death rates after injury ever recorded at just 9.4%. The long duration of these conflicts allowed a steady buildup of trauma system capabilities within the theater of operations which at its peak enabled rapid transport (60–90 min) of injured casualties to forward surgical units capable of performing immediate life and limb saving (damage control) surgery. Well-coordinated helicopter and fixed wing assets assisted by artificial intelligence decision-making systems greatly reduced time from injury to evacuation as well as evacuation to higher levels of care. Transport time to tertiary and quaternary facilities in Germany and US mainland was reduced often to a matter of 2–3 days in most cases. Simultaneously, availability of a full-fledged trauma registry combined with much improved communications network provided real-time access of surgeons in the battlespace to their counterparts in Level IV treatments facilities, thereby facilitating optimal decision-making for the individual patient and overall surveillance of care by the performance improvement process.

History of American Civilian Trauma Systems

As in previous conflicts, practitioners returning from WWII immediately brought lessons learned and translated them into civilian practice. However, it took almost 20 years for those lessons to transition into state and federal policies which could provide a financial foundation to a developing US civilian trauma system. The first modern civilian trauma centers originated in urban environs in the mid-60s and 70s but were not integrated into formal trauma systems. Cook County Hospital was one of the nation's first trauma centers in Chicago, Illinois. The Emergency Medical Services Systems (EMS) Act of 1973 provided some of the first federal funding to establish EMS systems. This bill provided four million dollars to the state of Illinois to develop a trauma system integrating Cook County hospital with some 40 other Illinois hospitals. Over the subsequent 8 years, over 300 million dollars in federal grants helped establish 304 regional EMS systems. Unfortunately, by the 1980s, some of the initial public enthusiasm for developing a robust national trauma system had waned. The Omnibus Budget Reconciliation Act of 1981, brought significant reductions in available federal funding for trauma. Responsibility for funding of systems had fallen to the states with some states continuing to thrive but others stalling in their progress to develop modern trauma systems. By 1995, only 20 states had state-wide trauma systems; only 5 of which were fully functional. Fortunately, in the last 30 years, a wealth of evidence has mounted, demonstrating much improved injury outcomes with the deployment of all-inclusive trauma systems. Today, most states have a well-developed trauma system with varying degrees of reliance on air transport depending on the unique demographic and geographic factors in play within their regions.

The Critical Role of the American College of Surgeon in US Trauma System Development

The American College of Surgeons Committee on Trauma (ACS-COT) has played a critical leadership role in the development of the US trauma system since its inception in 1922. In 1976, ACS-COT published its first edition of "Optimal Hospital Resources for the Care of the Injured Patient." This document helped define key resource requirements for hospitals aspiring to become trauma centers. Key requisites for the highest level designations (Level I and II) were as follows:

- In-house trauma surgeons with a responding team.
- 24/7 OR availability
- Subspecialty availability (neurosurgery, orthopedics, plastics, thoracic, and vascular surgery being the most critical).

Many updates have been made to the Optimal Resources Document, now in its seventh edition. The ACS-COT now performs the primary role of on-site verification for the majority of states with the remaining states having their own independent verification or accreditation authority. Some states have dual accrediting authorities utilizing both ACS verification as well as state accrediting authorities. Regardless of the regulating authority, most states have adopted a surveillance methodology for trauma centers that follows the Optimal Resource Document recommendations, utilizing on-site interviews of physician, nursing, and ancillary providers supporting the trauma service line. Additionally, a selected review of treatment rendered in actual cases obtained through the center's trauma registry is typical. Survey cycles most commonly occur at 3-year intervals for mature trauma centers. The frequency of surveys can be shortened to 1–2-year cycles where critical significant issues are identified. In cases where a surveyed center fails to resolve an ongoing critical significant issue(s), trauma center designation may be revoked.

The ACS-COT has also fostered a host of educational resources which have been critical to standardization of care across the modern US trauma system. These include all of the following:

- *Advanced Trauma Life Support*: Now the industry standard in evidence-based resuscitative trauma care. Developed nationally by the ACS-COT beginning in

1980, after initial pilot courses as early as 1977, pioneered by Dr. James Styner, the course has been updated multiple times over the last 40 years. Now in its tenth edition, the course remains the industry standard in basic resuscitative trauma care and is a requirement for all trauma providers to maintain through the trauma center verification process.

- *Advanced Trauma Operative Management Course (ATOM)*: Teaching surgical techniques for penetrating trauma to surgical providers in live porcine model.
- *Advanced Surgical Skills for Exposure in Trauma (ASSET)*: Cadaver-based course teaching operative exposures and skills required for life- and limb-threatening injury.
- *Basic Endovascular Skills for Trauma (BEST)*: Hands-on course teaching endovascular techniques such as Resuscitative Endovascular Balloon Occlusion of the aorta (REBOA) for life-threating trauma.
- *Disaster Management and Emergency Preparedness (DMEP)*: Teaches core competencies required for effective response to mass casualty situations.
- *Rural Trauma Team Development Course (RTTDC)*: Collaborative team-based course designed to improve rural trauma care through collaborative training with trauma centers in their region.
- *Stop the Bleed*: A course instructing lay providers the rudimentary skills required to stop hemorrhage at the point of injury before first responders arrive to the scene now has over 2.4 million trained.
- *Trauma Quality Improvement Project (TQIP) Best Practice Guidelines*: Currently the college has published seven different evidence-based best practice guidelines written after in-depth review of available evidence by leading experts in their respective fields. These guidelines cover commonly encountered entities such as geriatric trauma, traumatic brain injury, massive transfusion, and are released almost annually with the primary goal of improving overall care by reducing unnecessary variation from current evidence-based best practice.

Finally, ACS-COT has played a critical role in advocating for an increasingly powerful national trauma registry. In 2008, Trauma Quality Improvement Project (TQIP) was introduced—a marked advancement over the National Trauma Databank (NTDB). For the first time, robust, risk-adjusted data monitoring of trauma center outcomes was available to the individual trauma center. This powerful tool provides a much clearer picture of how trauma centers perform compared to other centers in similar patients (risk-adjusted). TQIP has received wide acceptance across the country and currently over 875 centers participate. Risk-adjusted trauma system outcomes are now available through the TQIP collaboratives, which are increasingly prevalent and allow trauma center collaboration and sharing of best practice to improve care across state and regional areas of interest.

Recent National Initiatives and Unanswered Questions

Important recent national federal initiatives in trauma continue to harness resources of both the military and civilian sectors. In 2016, the National Academies of Science, Engineering, and Medicine along with the Committee on Military Trauma Care's Learning Health System and Its Translation to the Civilian Sector, and representatives of the Boards of Health Sciences Policy, Health of Select Populations, and Health and Medicine Division convened a large group of the nation's leading civilian and military trauma experts to review the current state of the US trauma system and identify opportunities to translate lessons learned from the recent conflicts into the civilian trauma system. It is estimated that there currently exists an excess mortality as high as 20% which is due to unnecessary variation in care, among and within, trauma centers nationwide. This initiative has the intent of eliminating this excess mortality (zero preventable deaths after injury). It also identified a critical strategic goal of developing military-civilian partnerships to ensure that the providers and resources are appropriately sustained, enabling the nation to respond appropriately to large scale disasters and military conflicts that will inevitably arise in the future [12].

Recently, there has been a rapid uptick in the number of trauma centers nationwide. Improving reimbursement of trauma care has provided some fiscal incentives to trauma center designation, but not always expanding the care opportunities in rural and underserved regions. Trauma center volume has been shown to equate with outcome and currently a minimum volume of 600–650 major trauma patients per year is considered critical to maintaining optimal patient outcomes [13]. New centers starting within the catchment areas of existing legacy centers have, in some cases, reduced patient volume to the extent that it has negatively affected outcomes or hampered the ability of Level I teaching centers to meet minimum case requirements for new trainees. The ACS-COT and many of the state accrediting authorities are now beginning to look at policy initiatives to regulate the placement of new trauma center and ensure that the negative impact on legacy centers is minimized.

Finally, the last several years have seen an increasing focus on long-term outcomes (>1 year) in an effort to better understand the ultimate impact of injury on patient function. Research efforts are increasingly looking for the ideal longer-term markers of outcome in an effort to guide deployment of valuable resources to the areas that will have the most beneficial long-term impact on patient recovery of function.

Global Trauma Challenge

An abundance of literature now exists associating establishment of an effective trauma system with improved outcomes both in developed and underdeveloped countries [3–10, 14–16]. Despite this, there continues to be wide variation in the extent of trauma system development even in some highly developed countries. Currently it is estimated that five million people die each year due to traumatic injury with 90% of these lethal injuries occurring in middle- or low-income countries [17]. Experts estimate that improvements in the trauma systems within these countries would prevent as much as 1/3 of these deaths. In low-income countries, a major trauma patient may have as much as a 6× risk of death when compared to countries with highly developed trauma systems such as the United States [18]. The majority of these deaths occur outside the hospital where transport times remain long.

ACS-COT has identified prehospital and hospital provider education, adequate system resources, and an organized system as critical elements to optimal trauma care. In many underdeveloped countries, all three of these categories are underdeveloped largely due to scarce funding sources. Just as in the United States, unfunded initiatives invariably fall short of their true potential to improve care.

Conclusions

Trauma systems are integral to reliable treatment outcomes across a region. Effective trauma systems facilitate value-based care by triaging the patient severity to the right local or regional institution with available services matching the patient's need. The ability of the modern trauma system to achieve its goals is continuously under review through outcomes data generated from registry data, as well as ongoing research trials evaluating care delivery methodologies.

The return on investment for resources will always be rich for efforts to improve our modern, all-inclusive trauma system, as the prevalence of injury remains high and its impact on our society immense. Moreover, the gains associated with improved trauma infrastructure will inevitably have the added collateral benefit of improving outcomes in other hospital service lines.

References

1. Centers for Disease Control and Prevention. National Center for Injury Prevention and Control. Web-based Injury Statistics Query and Reporting System (WISQARS) fatal injury data. 2019. https://wisqars.cdc.gov/.
2. Centers for Disease Control and Prevention. The economics of injury and violence prevention. https://www.cdc.gov/injury/features/health-econ-cost-of-injury/index.html.
3. Brian C, Joseph T, Barbara LO, Etienne P, Linda P, Lawrence L, et al. A systematic review and meta-analysis comparing outcome of severely injured patients treated in trauma centers following the establishment of trauma systems. J Trauma. 2006;60(2):371–8.
4. Nathens AB, Jurkovich GJ, Rivara FP, Maier RV. Effectiveness of state trauma systems in reducing injury-related mortality: a national evaluation. J Trauma. 2000;48(1):25–30.
5. Kobi P, Limor AD, Michael S, Yoram K, Moshe M, Avraham R, et al. Increased survival among severe trauma patients: the impact of a national trauma system. Arch Surg. 2004;139(11):1231–6.

6. Pierre B, Ageron FX, Julien B, Albrice L, Marion B, Elisabeth R, et al. A regional trauma system to optimize the pre-hospital triage of trauma patients. Crit Care. 2015;19(1):111.

7. Belinda JG, Pam MS, Ann MS, Rory W, Mark CF, Rodney J, et al. Improved functional outcomes for major trauma patients in a regionalized, inclusive trauma system. Ann Surg. 2012;255(6):1009–15.

8. Glen HT, James FR 3rd, Ross M, Edward LA 3rd, Steven M, Mary SJ. Delaware's inclusive trauma system: impact on mortality. J Trauma. 2010;69(2):245–52.

9. Ellen JM, Frederick PR, Gregory JJ, Avery BN, Katherine PF, Brian LE, et al. A national evaluation of the effect of trauma-center care on mortality. N Engl J Med. 2006;354(4):366–78.

10. Cales RH. Trauma mortality in Orange County: the effect of implementation of a regional trauma system. Ann Emerg Med. 1984;13(1):1–10.

11. The History-And Future-of Combat Care, MAJ GEN George Alexander, MD. US Army Retired. 2018. https://www.ausa.org/articles/history%E2%80%94and-future%E2%80%94-combat-care.

12. National Academies of Sciences, Engineering, and Medicine. A national trauma care system: integrating military and civilian trauma systems to achieve zero preventable deaths after injury. Washington, DC: The National Academies Press; 2016.

13. Nathens AB, Jurkovich GJ, Rivara FP, et al. Effectiveness of state trauma systems in reducing injury-related mortality: a national evaluation. J Trauma. 2000;48:25–30; discussion 30–31.

14. Zhou J, Wang T, Belenkiy I, Hardcastle TC, Rouby J-J, Jiang B, for the International Trauma Rescue & Treatment Association (ITRTA) Study Group. Management of severe trauma worldwide: implementation of trauma systems in emerging countries: China, Russia and South Africa. Crit Care. 2021;25:286. https://doi.org/10.1186/s13054-021-03681-8.

15. Causes of Death Collaborators. Global, regional, and national age-sex-specific mortality for 282 causes of death in 195 countries and territories, 1980–2017: a systematic analysis for the Global Burden of Disease Study 2017. Lancet. 2018;392(10159):1736–88.

16. Twijnstra MJ, Moons KG, Simmermacher RK, Leenen LP. Regional trauma system reduces mortality and changes admission rates: a before and after study. Ann Surg. 2010;251(2):339–43.

17. Mock C, Joshipura M, Arreola-Risa C, Quansah R. An estimate of the number of lives that could be saved through improvements in trauma care globally. World J Surg. 2012;36(5):959–63.

18. Mock CN, Adzotor KE, Conklin E, Denno DM, Jurkovich GJ. Trauma outcomes in the rural developing world: comparison with an urban level I trauma center. J Trauma. 1993;35(4):518–23.

Chapter 4
Trauma Team Activation and Response

Mirjana Jovanovic and Daniel Holena

Overview

- Trauma team activation is a process of care that occurs at trauma centers to prepare for the arrival of an injured patient.
- The decision to transport an injured patient to a trauma center vs. non-trauma center from the prehospital setting is typically based on prespecified triage criteria including physiology, anatomy, mechanism of injury, and other patient factors.
- The decision to activate the trauma team within a trauma center is typically based on similar factors but may vary from institution to institution.
- Additionally, some centers have tiered responses that seek to match the resources necessary for resuscitation to the expected needs of the incoming patient.
- The nomenclature for these responses is also variable from center to center but may be numerical (Trauma Level 1 vs. Trauma Level 2) or categorical (Trauma Alert vs. Trauma Response). The composition of the trauma team may therefore vary by the level of activation.

M. Jovanovic
Medical College of Wisconsin, Milwaukee, WI, USA
e-mail: mjovanovic@mcw.edu

D. Holena (✉)
Division of Acute Care Surgery, Medical University of South Carolina, Charleston, USA
e-mail: holena@musc.edu

Prehospital Trauma Triage

The decision to transport a patient to a trauma center vs. a non-trauma center is based on prehospital trauma triage criteria and has been shown to improve the outcomes of injured patients. The effectiveness of field triage is assessed using metrics termed *undertriage* and *overtriage*. Undertriage is defined as transporting patients with severe injuries to non-trauma hospitals, which is associated with increased mortality in adults and children. Overtriage is defined as transporting patients with minor to moderate injuries to trauma centers instead of non-trauma centers, which may result in overuse of limited resources and impact the care of other patients. Because the consequences of undertriage are generally more severe than overtriage, the trauma system is designed to keep undertriage at a minimum at the cost of higher rates of overtriage.

Although there is not a national prehospital triage protocol for injured patients, the American College of Surgeons Committee on Trauma provides background resources to guide field triage decisions for local adaption and is based on four domains: physiology, anatomy, mechanism, and patient factors. It is important to note that the activation criteria of the receiving trauma center itself may not always align with local prehospital guidelines for activation as there is local variation in both arenas.

- **Step 1**: *Physiologic Criteria*: Allows for rapid identification of critically injured patients through focus on vital signs and mental status, as measured by Glasgow Coma Scale (GCS) (Fig. 4.1).
- Vital sign criteria demonstrate a high predictive value for severe injury. Systolic blood pressure (SBP) <90 mmHg and a respiratory rate (RR) <10 or >29 are significant predictors of severe injury and the need for a high level of trauma care.
- Recommendation for transport to the highest-level trauma center available within the geographic constraints of the regional trauma system if any of the following are identified (Fig. 4.3):

  - GCS ≤13, or
  - SBP of <90 mmHg, or
  - RR of <10 or >29 breaths per minute (<20 in infant aged <1 year) or need for ventilatory support

- **Step 2**: *Anatomic Criteria*: Patients may initially have normal prehospital physiology but have an anatomic injury that will require the highest level of care.
- Recommendation for transport to the highest-level trauma center available within the geographic constraints of the regional trauma system if any of the following are identified:

  - All penetrating injuries to head, neck, torso, and extremities proximal to elbow or knee
  - Chest wall instability or deformity (e.g., flail chest)
  - Two or more proximal long-bone fractures

Fig. 4.1 Components of
the Glasgow Coma Score
(GCS)

Glasgow Coma Score

Eye opening	
Spontaneous	4
Open to verbal command	3
Open to pain	2
No eye opening	1
Verbal response	
Oriented	5
Confused	4
Inappropriate words	3
Incomprehensible sounds	2
No verbal response	1
Motor response	
Follows commands	6
Localizes to pain	5
Withdrawals from pain	4
Flexes to pain	3
Extends to pain	2
No Movement	1
Total score	3–15

- Rushed, degloved, mangled, or pulseless extremity
- Amputation proximal to wrist or ankle
- Pelvic fractures
- Open or depressed skull fractures
- Paralysis

Important Considerations

- *Tourniquet Use*

  - The use of tourniquets among EMS systems varies; inclusion of tourniquet use as a criterion could lead to overuse of tourniquets instead of basic hemorrhage control methods and thus potentially result in overtriage; and the "crushed, degloved, mangled, or pulseless extremity," "all penetrating injuries to head, neck, torso, and extremities proximal to elbow or knee," and "amputation proximal to wrist or ankle" criteria were as likely to identify severely injured patients regardless of tourniquet use.

- *Pelvic Fractures*

  - Patients with pelvic fractures should receive rapid and specialized care because of the possibility of internal hemorrhage and other associated injuries.

- **Step 3**: *Mechanism of Injury*: An injured patient who does not meet Step 1 or Step 2 criteria should be evaluated in terms of mechanism of injury (MOI) to determine if the injury might be severe. Evaluation of MOI will help to determine if the patient should be transported to a trauma center.

  - Recommendation for transport to the highest-level trauma center available within the geographic constraints of the regional trauma system if any of the following are identified:
  - Falls

    - Adults: >20 feet (one story = 10 feet)
    - Children: >10 feet or two to three times the height of the child

  - High-risk motor vehicle collision

    - Intrusion, including roof: >12 inches driver side; >18 inches any site
    - Ejection (partial or complete) from automobile
    - Death in same passenger compartment
    - Vehicle telemetry data consistent with a high risk for injury

  - Automobile versus pedestrian/bicyclist thrown, run over, or with significant (>20 mph) impact
  - Motorcycle collision >20 mph

- **Step 4**: *Special Considerations*: Injured patients with comorbid conditions who do not meet physiologic, anatomic, or mechanism of injury triage criteria may still benefit from transport to a trauma center.

  - Special consideration for transport to the highest-level trauma center available within the geographic constraints of the regional trauma system for patients who meet the following criteria:

- Older adults
    - Risk for injury/death increases after age 55 years
    - SBP <110 might represent shock after age 65 years
    - Low impact mechanisms (e.g., ground-level falls) might result in severe injury
- Children
    - Should be triaged preferentially to pediatric capable trauma centers
- Anticoagulants and bleeding disorders
    - Patients with head injury are at high risk for rapid deterioration
- Burns
    - Without other trauma mechanism: triage to burn facility
    - With trauma mechanism: triage to trauma center
- Pregnancy >20 weeks

Who Is the Trauma Team?

The composition of the trauma team may vary by institution and by level of trauma activation, but most typically consists of a multidisciplinary team that may include surgeons, emergency medicine physicians, respiratory therapists, nurses, advanced practitioners, pharmacists, anesthesiologists, radiology technicians, and social workers (Fig. 4.2).

- The trauma team leader serves as a dedicated team leader and is usually an emergency medicine physician or trauma surgeon. The training level of the team leader may range from resident to attendings.
- The primary surveyor performs a targeted physical examination focused on identifying pathology that poses an immediate threat to life or limb. This provider may be of varying background (medical student, resident physician, advanced practitioners). See the primary survey.
- Trauma nurses play a critical role on the team by attaching the patient to monitoring devices, obtaining intravenous access, infusing fluids and blood products, and administering medications as indicated.
- Radiology technicians provide early imaging studies as adjuncts to the primary survey, including chest and pelvic radiographs.
- Pharmacists may be present to assist with the preparation and dosing of medications.
- A physician capable of endotracheal intubation (usually either trained in emergency medicine or anesthesia) may support the airway needs of the patient and may not respond to lower tiers of activation where it is unlikely the patient will require intubation.

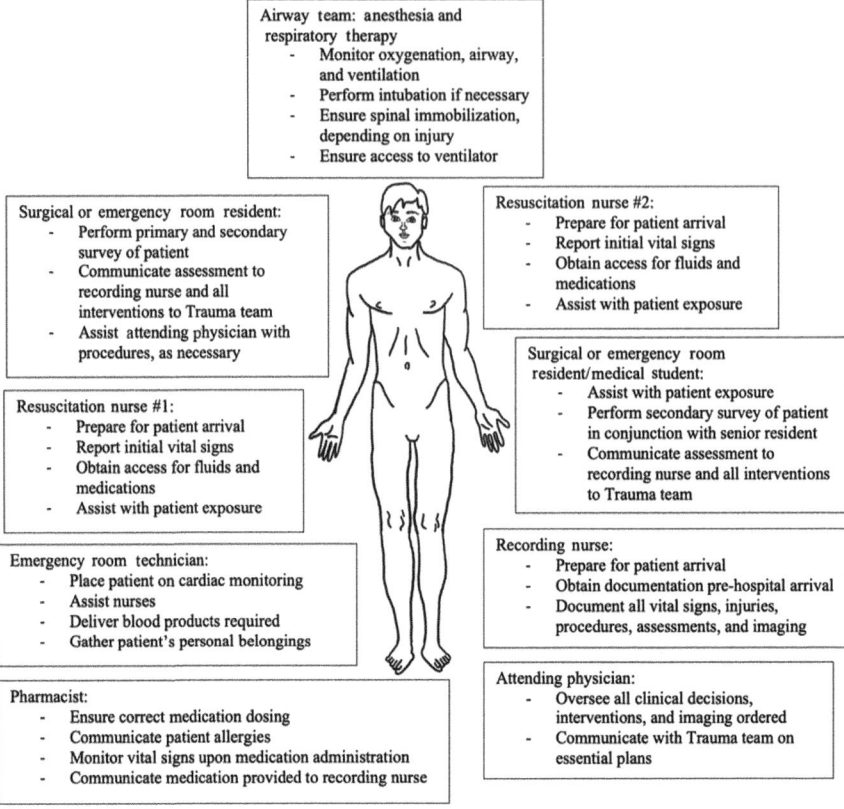

Fig. 4.2 A typical depiction of the locations and roles of team providers during a trauma resuscitation

- Social workers assist in identification of unknown patients and establishing communication with family members.
- A medical scribe, often a nurse or medical assistant, may be present to ensure accurate documentation of the resuscitation in a timely manner.
- At some institutions, chaplaincy may be a part of the team to administer to the spiritual needs of the patient and their family.

Trauma Time-out

At many centers prior to patient arrival, the trauma team summarizes the patient's pre-reported injuries, treatments in the field, and vital signs that were received from the prehospital setting. Additionally, the team familiarizes themselves with one another so that communication during the resuscitation is more effective. Depending on the estimated time arrival of the patient, if time permits, the trauma team also discusses possible interventions, imaging, and procedures that will be necessary to stabilize the patient.

EMS Handoff

Upon arrival to the trauma bay, the EMS handoff is critical for accurate management of the patient (Fig. 4.3). Many systems of handoff are available, but among the most widely used is the mnemonic "*IMIST-AMBO*":

Moderate risk injury requiring trauma center care	
Mechanism of injury	High risk patients

w Pedestrian or bicycle rider thrown, run over, or with significant impact.
w Fall from height >10 feet at any age
w High-risk automobile crash
    - Partial or complete ejection
    - Significant intrusion (>12 inches on occupant side or >18 inches on any site or need for extrication
    - Child (Age 0–9) unrestrained or in unsecured child safety seat
	w Older adults >55 years
	w Ground level fall in children <5 years or adults >65 years
	w Anticoagulant use or with history of bleeding disorder
	w Child abuse suspicion
	w Pregnant patients >20 weeks
	w Suspected head injury
	w Burn patients due to trauma mechanism

High risk for serious injury Any of the following criteria requires immediate transport to highest-level trauma center.	
Injury patterns	Mental status & vital signs

w Penetrating injuries to head, neck, torso, and extremities proximal to elbow or knee
w Chest wall instability or deformity (e.g., flail chest)
w Two or more proximal long-bone fractures
w Crushed, degloved, pulseless extremity
w Pelvic fracture
w Amputation proximal to wrist or ankle
w Open or depressed skull fracture
w Paralysis
	All patients
	  w GCS < 13
	  w Systolic blood pressure <90 mmHg
	  w Respiratory rate <10 or >29 breaths per minute
	  w Respiratory support requirement
	  w Pulse oximetry <90%

Fig. 4.3 Physiologic, anatomic, mechanistic, and patient characteristics mandating prehospital transport to a specialized trauma center

- *I*—Identification of the patient
- *M*—Mechanism of injury/medical complaint
- *I*—Injuries and physical findings on Inspection from head to toe
- *S*—Vital signs patient physiology
- *T*—treatments administered in the prehospital setting and the patient's response to those treatments
- *A*—Allergies
- *M*—Medications the patient takes regularly
- *B*—Background medical history
- *O*—Other information, including social and scene information

The handoff between EMS and the trauma team should ideally occur before the primary survey begins to prevent loss of information from competing verbal communications.

Bibliography

1. Dumas RP, Vella MA, Hatchimonji JS, Ma L, Maher Z, Holena DN. Trauma video review utilization: a survey of practice in the United States. Am J Surg. 2020;219(1):49–53. https://doi.org/10.1016/j.amjsurg.2019.08.025. Epub 2019 Sept 10. PMID: 31537325; PMCID: PMC8428979.
2. Kostiuk M, Burns B. Trauma assessment. [Updated 2022 May 29]. In: StatPearls [Internet]. Treasure Island: StatPearls Publishing; 2022. [Figure, Glasgow Coma Scale (GCS). Created by Michael Kostiuk, DO] Available from: https://www.ncbi.nlm.nih.gov/books/NBK555913/figure/article-30531.image.f1/.
3. Maddry JK, Arana AA, Clemons MA, Medellin KL, Shults NM, Perez CA, Savell SC, Gutierrez XE, Reeves LK, Mora AG, Bebarta VS. Impact of a standardized EMS handoff tool on inpatient medical record documentation at a level I trauma center. Prehosp Emerg Care. 2021;25(5):656–63. https://doi.org/10.1080/10903127.2020.1824050. Epub 2020 Oct 9.
4. Newgard CD, Fischer PE, Gestring M, Michaels HN, Jurkovich GJ, Lerner EB, Fallat ME, Delbridge TR, Brown JB, Bulger EM, the Writing Group for the 2021 National Expert Panel on Field Triage. National guideline for the field triage of injured patients: recommendations of the National Expert Panel on Field Triage, 2021. J Trauma Acute Care Surg. 2022;93(2):e49–60. https://doi.org/10.1097/TA.0000000000003627.
5. Wandling MW, Nathens AB, Shapiro MB, Haut ER. Police transport versus ground EMS: a trauma system-level evaluation of prehospital care policies and their effect on clinical outcomes. J Trauma Acute Care Surg. 2016;81(5):931–5. https://doi.org/10.1097/TA.0000000000001228. PMID: 27537514.

Chapter 5
Disasters and Mass Casualty Incidents

Grace Niziolek and Lewis J. Kaplan

Introduction

Disasters or crises may be naturally occurring or man-made (Fig. 5.1) [1]. Both disasters and crises overwhelm existing resources and threaten the normal operation of a healthcare system or facility [2]. Therefore, it is essential for healthcare facilities and their staff to prepare for disasters or crises whether they are external to the facility (hurricane) or internal (fire that destroys the electrical system). Given the wide range of potential etiologies (Fig. 5.1), an all-hazards approach (i.e., not specific for a single etiology) is ideal and avoids needing to train for multiple different kinds of scenarios or approaches [3]. Recent violent extremism events, both abroad and at home, have highlighted mass shootings (more than four victims) as well as the "E" aspect of CBRNE (chemical, biologic, radiation, nuclear, and explosive) events including those from improvised explosive devices (2013 Boston Marathon bombing) as major threats [4, 5]. Collectively, these kinds of threats underscore that preparation must include agencies beyond the healthcare facility as well as the public who may act in a bystander responder fashion (1 October 2017 Las Vegas, NV mass shooting) [6]. Preparation to render care during a disaster is a basic skill that should be present in every healthcare facility worker.

G. Niziolek · L. J. Kaplan (✉)
Division of Trauma, Surgical Critical Care and Emergency Surgery, Perelman School of Medicine, University of Pennsylvania, Philadelphia, PA, USA
e-mail: Lewis.Kaplan@pennmedicine.upenn.edu

Fig. 5.1 Natural versus manmade disaster or crisis examples. Legend: This figure demonstrates some examples of natural compared to manmade disasters or crises. Note that wildfires may be naturally occurring but may also be the result of human error or deliberate action. Similarly, vehicle collisions may be multiple vehicles involved in a road traffic accident, or a vehicle that impacts pedestrians, especially during public gatherings. CBRNE = chemical, biologic, radiologic, nuclear, or explosive (including improvised explosive devices)

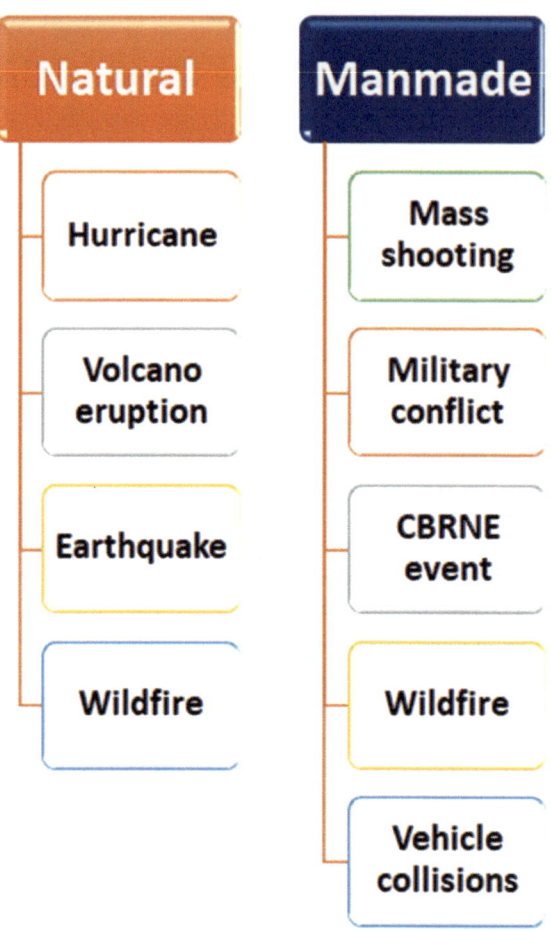

Situational Awareness

Multiple avenues of information flow may alert a facility to an external disaster including local television or radio news, Internet-based news, social media (SoMe), and emergency communication channels. The American Red Cross in particular monitors SoMe for disaster-based information. Since SoMe provides a forum for some who may be planning violent acts within the facility or toward healthcare workers at a particular facility, monitoring may provide clues to the potential for an internal disaster, including firearm-based violence [7]. Once such clues are identified, a coordinated approach with law enforcement is ideal to prevent disaster occurrence. Unsurprisingly, most facilities focus on receiving patients from an external disaster rather than caring for or evacuating patients in the event of an internal disaster. Both scenarios must be anticipated, and preparation should assess skills and equipment and therapeutics required for success.

Disaster Preparation

Each team member deployed during a disaster has a specific role that is readily identifiable and understandable—and therefore trainable—within an Incident Command Structure (ICS) [8]. The facility is led by an Incident Commander within the framework of a multilevel communication and action structure that is well described and taught by the Federal Emergency Management Agency (FEMA). Preparation within the facility, as well as for external agency members (Emergency Medical Services (EMS), etc.), requires education, training, and then practice. Disaster simulation may occur on a table-top to review coordination of elements but must also utilize live-action drills. Since disaster preparation includes partners, practice with those partners is equally essential [9].

Key partners include law enforcement, emergency medical services, public health services, and local government; engagement with regional, state, and federal agencies and assets should also be planned, evaluated, and drilled. It is this kind of preparation that underpinned the successful mobilization and activation of resources to care for victims of the 2016 Florida Pulse nightclub mass shooting [10]. These partners are essential to control patient flow to and into the facility, provide security for healthcare workers and patients as well as to mobilize resources including personnel, emergency supplies, and therapeutics should the duration of the disaster be extended. Most disasters that acutely overwhelm acute care facility resources are short-lived but of high intensity. This is why planning for equitable distribution of patients is essential when there are several facilities in the same general space (aka "load balancing") [11]. Longer duration disaster management, such as after Hurricane Katrina, mobilized resources in a sustained fashion as flood waters left destroyed infrastructure in the wake of their recession, derailing power, communication, waste management, and shelter [12]. When the facility remains operational, the kind of care that is renderable reflects the degree of resource stress that exists.

Disaster Response

Once a disaster is identified, each facility should establish a command post, activate incident command individuals, and disaster response team members [13]. An effective and regularly tested communication approach to alert team members (in-hospital and out-of-hospital) to a disaster should be activated as well to enable disaster response roles (for which they have been trained) and to bring additional staff to the facility. Elective procedures should be postponed, and ongoing procedures completed as rapidly as possible. Rapid discharge of suitable patients may be required to increase available beds. Non-critically ill or injured patients should be evacuated from the emergency department in anticipation of patient surge. Visitation should be suspended during the initial patient surge phase. A security cordon may be necessary to stop family, friends, or others from rapidly entering the facility in

search of specific individuals. Of course, that security cordon may also stop a potential attacker from turning the facility into a secondary disaster site as well. In the
case of an internal disaster, preparation for patient and staff evacuation are also
imperative and require appropriate equipment for power loss [14]. Those concerns
include managing invasive mechanical ventilation, vasoactive infusions, and transport of patients from above ground-level floors through stairs to reach a safe location for care while awaiting transport to another care facility. Clearly both internal
and external disasters carry the potential to overwhelm a facility's capacity to render care.

Facility Level of Operation and Care Goals

Three tiers of operation may be broadly defined for healthcare facilities: conventional (usual), contingency, and crisis [15]. Under normal operations, the goal is the
best care for the individual in a first-come, first-served fashion; facilities may
accommodate up to a 20% increase in usual patient volume. Local resources are
commonly engaged. Under contingency operation (up to a 100% increase in patient
volume), the care goal remains essentially unchanged but the resources available to
render that care may be more limited than usual; standard of care is initially maintained but as patient volume increases, that standard is no longer able to be met and
regional resources are activated. Under crisis standards (200% or more of usual
patient volume), the goal is to render the best care for the greatest number of people;
national resources are commonly triggered to help support care. This standard
requires patients to be evaluated within the context of likely survivability, the
resources required to potentiate survivability, and the resources that are available.
This process is termed triage and occurs in two sites—the disaster site and the
healthcare facility [16].

Disaster Triage

Field triage at the site of a disaster generally identifies several discrete classes of
victims: uninjured but present, minimally injured ("walking wounded"), moderately injured, severely injured, and dead. Each of these classes map to a prioritization scheme for evacuation to a care center as opposed to care on site. Several
approaches have been utilized to identify injured individuals and their priority evaluation. Perhaps the most simple and most common is known as START (simple
triage and rapid treatment) and is color-based: black = dead/expected to rapidly die;
red = high risk of death and in need of immediate therapy; yellow = injured but not
at risk of rapid death; green = minimally injured and may potentially be treated on
site [17]. A related approach is termed SALT (sort, assess, lifesaving interventions,
treatment/transport) and is endorsed by the American College of Surgeons and the

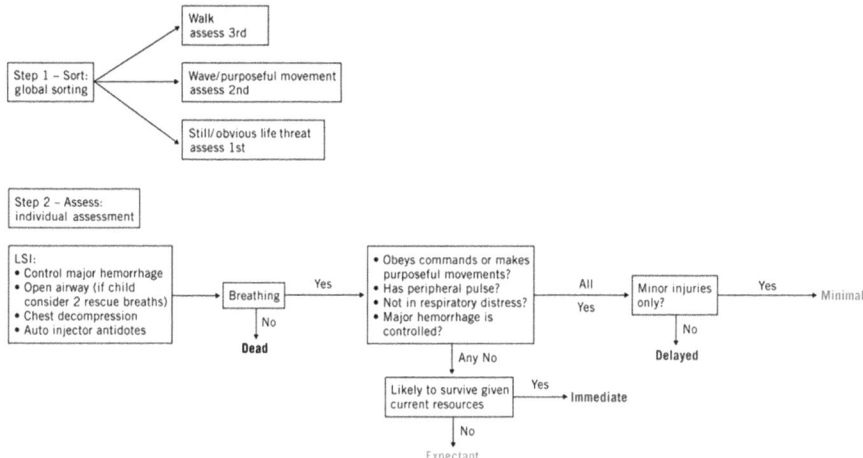

Fig. 5.2 SALT triage approach. Legend: This graphic demonstrates the SALT (sort, assess, life-saving intervention (LSI), treatment/transport) approach to mass casualty or disaster triage. (Reproduced with permission from: Lerner et al. [18])

American College of Emergency Physicians [18, 19] (Fig. 5.2). At present, SALT appears to be more accurate for the immediate and delayed groups in the field. While both of these approaches help guide EMS transport to the nearest appropriate facility, specific note is made of bystander transport for patients who are unlikely to have undergone triage [20]. This practice may readily overwhelm the closest facility and highlights the need for hospital-based triage as well.

Hospital-based triage helps align patients who present via private vehicle, police, or EMS with required care. Therefore, clinicians should be trained to perform triage in a way consistent with available resources including but not limited to emergency physicians, surgeons, anesthesiologists, operating rooms, nurses, technicians, ED and critical care beds, and blood components at a minimum. Triage may ideally occur outside of the ED and benefits from security or law enforcement aid. Multiple triage tools may be used including SALT and START without one approach demonstrating superiority; often the selected tool reflects local conditions or a national approach [21, 22]. Accordingly, the tool that may perform the best is the one that is familiar to all and regularly practiced.

Ethics

When operating under crisis standards, decisions may need to be made regarding the allocation of scarce resources such as ICU beds, invasive mechanical ventilation, or therapeutic agents. All of these were highlighted during the early waves of the SARS-CoV-2 pandemic [23]. There are a variety of approaches that one may take in order to decide who receives a scare resource. Regardless of which one is selected for use, the tool should be transparent and readily reviewable by the public. Indeed, multi-professional input should drive tool creation and ideally includes representatives from the public. It is important to recognize that there are criticisms of all existing approaches and no single one has emerged as superior. Elements such as age, chronic medical conditions, acute physiology, organ failure scores, community role, and more are found in different proposed or utilized tools raising concerns regarding bias and equity in those tools [24, 25]. One aspect is universally embraced—that the individual(s) rendering the decision regarding the allocation of scarce resources is at a remove from direct patient care. The clinician-patient interaction and relationship introduces a powerful bias that makes unbiased decision-making challenging at best.

Service Animals

Disaster care may bring patients who are accompanied by a service animal. The Americans with Disabilities Act (ADA) encode legal facility access for such animals other than into sterile areas or those that require isolation [26]. Note that this act does not require a facility to permit access for emotional support animals. All US service animals are either dogs or miniature horses. Moreover, the service animal must perform a specific task for their dyad partner. Healthcare clinicians are allowed to ask if the animal is a service animal, but the animal should be wearing a harness that identifies them as such. Clinicians are also allowed to ask what task the animal performs. Currently, the human acute care facility is not required to provide medical or surgical aid to an injured service animal who accompanies an injured patient. Additionally, the facility is also not required to provide routine care (feeding, watering, toileting aid) to the service animal—those duties fall to a family member but may be at times provided by a related service animal organization [27].

Disaster Resolution and Clinician Impact

As the disaster is resolving, the flow of patients also lessens, providing a clear signal for the facility that resolution is pending. This serves as a signal to prepare to return to normal operations once the influx of patients and the care they require has decreased to manageable volumes. While there is typically substantial desire to rapidly resume normal operations at the usual pace, it is essential to pause and assess the impact of the disaster on frontline healthcare personnel. Load-leveling across different facilities in a region distributes patients to help avoid a single facility becoming overwhelmed. This approach may bring patients to a facility for which they are not typically prepared or are inadequately resourced to address at that rate or volume. As a result, disasters bring substantial stress at points of access such as the ED and to nursing staff in particular [28]. The facility should have a coordinated and preplanned method to assess for untoward consequences in their clinicians. Debriefings are well received as a form of communal outreach and support; some will benefit from counselling to reengage in their normal work [29]. Mass casualty incidents from firearm violence may be a particularly virulent driver of clinician stress and disability in the wake of a man-made disaster. Clinician preparation for disasters and mass casualty incidents benefits from focused training and resource deployment—both are supported by a variety of professional organizations invested in disaster preparation, training, and leadership (Table 5.1).

Table 5.1 Key agencies for disaster training and education resources

Federal Emergency Management Agency (FEMA)	Disaster planning resources CBRNE threat guide Disaster information sharing Incident command and role training Grant funding www.FEMA.gov
Centers for Disease Control (CDC)	CBRN threat guide Bioterrorism medical countermeasures Disaster management mobile device APP www.cdc.gov/disasters/index.html
Biomedical Advanced Research Development Authority (BARDA)	CBRN threat guide Medical countermeasures Private-public partnerships Grant funding www.medicalcountermeasures.gov/BARDA
American Red Cross (ARC)	Unique resources for weather-related disasters Disaster management mobile device APP Relief resource provider including shelter Major provider of blood components including whole blood www.redcross.org/about-us/our-work/disaster-relief.html
American College of Surgeons (ACS)	Disaster Management and Emergency Preparedness course Acute bleeding control training (STOP THE BLEED) Trauma center verification program www.facs.org/quality-programs/trauma/education
Society of Critical Care Medicine (SCCM)	Fundamental Disaster Management course Fundamentals of Critical Care-Resource Limited course Disaster Response Relief program www.sccm.org/disaster
Office of the Assistant Secretary for Preparedness and Response (ASPR)	Disaster management tools and Disaster Available Supplies in Hospitals interactive tool (dashtool.org) https://ASPR.hhs.gov

Conclusion

Disasters or crises may be natural or man-made and include mass casualty incidents from a variety of etiologies, of which firearm violence is characteristic. Public, clinician, and facility preparation for disasters should adopt an all-hazards approach to train broad preparation and role adoption. Facilities must prepare for external and internal disasters and should do so with local, regional, state, and national partners. Since disasters can alter the capacity to deliver the prevailing standard of care, facilities should articulate how they plan to allocate scarce resources when operating under crisis standards. Disasters may adversely impact the mental health and balance of frontline clinicians. Routine inquiry regarding mental health and untoward impacts of disaster care are essential in preserving the capabilities and integrity of frontline healthcare workers. Disaster care defines a role for every worker in the facility and benefits from routine training, reinforcement, and practice.

References

1. Gillespie DF, Streeter CL. Conceptualizating and measuring disaster preparedness. Int J Mass Emerg Disasters. 1987;5(2):155–76.
2. Melmer P, Carlin M, Castater CA, et al. Mass casualty shootings and emergency preparedness: a multidisciplinary approach for an unpredictable event. J Multidiscip Healthc. 2019;12:1013.
3. Collander B, Green B, Millo Y, et al. Development of an "all-hazards" hospital disaster preparedness training course utilizing multi-modality teaching. Prehosp Disaster Med. 2008;23(1):63–7.
4. Razak S, Hignett S, Barnes J. Emergency department response to chemical, biological, radiological, nuclear, and explosive events: a systematic review. Prehosp Disaster Med. 2018;33(5):543–9.
5. Gates JD, Arabian S, Biddinger P, et al. The initial response to the Boston marathon bombing: lessons learned to prepare for the next disaster. Ann Surg. 2014;260(6):960.
6. Haider AH, Haut ER, Velmahos GC. Converting bystanders to immediate responders: we need to start in high school or before. JAMA Surg. 2017;152(10):909–10.
7. Pelzer R. Policing of terrorism using data from social media. Eur J Secur Res. 2018;3(2):163–79.
8. Chang HH. A literature review and analysis of the incident command system. Int J Emerg Manag. 2017;13(1):50–67.
9. Djalali A, Carenzo L, Ragazzoni L, et al. Does hospital disaster preparedness predict response performance during a full-scale exercise? A pilot study. Prehosp Disaster Med. 2014;29(5):441–7.
10. Smith CP, Cheatham ML, et al. Injury characteristics of the Pulse Nightclub shooting: lessons for mass casualty incident preparation. J Trauma Acute Care Surg. 2020;88(3):372–8.
11. Dichter JR, Devereaux AV, Sprung CL, et al. Mass critical care surge response during COVID-19: implementation of contingency strategies–a preliminary report of findings from the Task Force for Mass Critical Care. Chest. 2022;161(2):429–47.
12. Zorn CR, Shamseldin AY. Post-disaster infrastructure restoration: a comparison of events for future planning. Int J Disaster Risk Reduct. 2015;13:158–66.
13. Verheul ML, Dückers ML. Defining and operationalizing disaster preparedness in hospitals: a systematic literature review. Prehosp Disaster Med. 2020;35(1):61–8.

14. King MA, Dorfman MV, Einav S, et al. Evacuation of intensive care units during disaster: learning from the Hurricane Sandy experience. Disaster Med Public Health Prep. 2016;10:20–7.
15. Hick JL, Einav S, Hanfling D, et al. Surge capacity principles: care of the critically ill and injured during pandemics and disasters: CHEST consensus statement. Chest. 2014;146(4):e1S–6S.
16. Ryan K, George D, Liu J, et al. The use of field triage in disaster and mass casualty incidents: a survey of current practices by EMS personnel. Prehosp Emerg Care. 2018;22(4):520–6.
17. Douglas N, Leverett J, Paul J, et al. Performance of first aid trained staff using a modified START triage tool at achieving appropriate triage compared to a physiology-based triage strategy at Australian mass gatherings. Prehosp Disaster Med. 2020;35(2):184–8.
18. Lerner EB, Cone DC, Weinstein ES, et al. Mass casualty triage: an evaluation of the science and refinement of a national guideline. Disaster Med Public Health Prep. 2011;5(2):129–37.
19. Lerner EB, Schwartz RB, Coule PL, et al. Mass casualty triage: an evaluation of the data and development of a proposed national guideline. Disaster Med Public Health Prep. 2008;2(S1):S25–34.
20. Heard CL, Pearce JM, Rogers MB. Mapping the public first-aid training landscape: uptake, knowledge, confidence and willingness to deliver first aid in disasters/emergencies–a scoping review. Disasters. 2018;44:205.
21. Bazyar J, Farrokhi M, Khankeh H. Triage systems in mass casualty incidents and disasters: a review study with a worldwide approach. Open Access Maced J Med Sci. 2019;7(3):482.
22. Bazyar J, Farrokhi M, Salari A, et al. Accuracy of triage systems in disasters and mass casualty incidents; a systematic review. Arch Acad Emerg Med. 2022;10(1):e32.
23. Riviello ED, Dechen T, O'Donoghue AL, et al. Assessment of a crisis standards of care scoring system for resource prioritization and estimated excess mortality by race, ethnicity, and socially vulnerable area during a regional surge in COVID-19. JAMA Netw Open. 2022;5(3):e221744.
24. Sanchez-Pinto LN, Parker WF, Mayampurath A, et al. Evaluation of organ dysfunction scores for allocation of scarce resources in critically ill children and adults during a healthcare crisis. Crit Care Med. 2021;49(2):271–81.
25. Farrell TW, Ferrante LE, Brown T, et al. AGS position statement: resource allocation strategies and age-related considerations in the COVID-19 era and beyond. J Am Geriatr Soc. 2020;68(6):1136–42.
26. U.S. Department of Labor. Americans with Disabilities Act. www.dol.gov/general/topic/disability/ada. Accessed 20 Aug 2022.
27. Martin ND, Pascual JL, Julie Hirsch CV, et al. Excluded but not forgotten: veterinary emergency care during emergencies and disasters. Am J Disaster Med. 2020;15(1):25–31.
28. Naushad VA, Bierens JJ, Nishan KP, et al. A systematic review of the impact of disaster on the mental health of medical responders. Prehosp Disaster Med. 2019;34(6):632–43.
29. Brooks SK, Dunn R, Amlôt R, et al. Training and post-disaster interventions for the psychological impacts on disaster-exposed employees: a systematic review. J Ment Health. 2018:1–25. https://doi.org/10.1080/09638237.2018.1437610.

Chapter 6
Physiologic Response to Injury and Shock

W. Andrew Smedley and Avi Bhavaraju

Overview

- Shock is circulatory failure with impaired end-organ perfusion [1, 2]

  - Decreased oxygen (O_2) delivery, increased O_2 consumption, and/or inadequate O_2 utilization → cellular and tissue hypoxia → cell death and organ dysfunction
  - Effects are reversible with early intervention
  - Delay in treatment leads to irreversible shock
  - Tissue hypoxia → normal aerobic metabolism shifts to anaerobic metabolism → lactic acidosis

- Types of shock—Four broad categories [1–4]

  - Hypovolemic—Decreased intravascular volume leading to impaired cardiac output (CO) and end-organ perfusion

    - Hemorrhagic
    - Non-hemorrhagic

W. A. Smedley
Department of Surgery, University of Arkansas for Medical Sciences (UAMS),
Little Rock, AR, USA
e-mail: WASmedley@uams.edu

A. Bhavaraju (✉)
Department of Surgery, Division of Trauma & Acute Care Surgery, University of Arkansas
for Medical Sciences (UAMS), Little Rock, AR, USA

© The Author(s), under exclusive license to Springer Nature
Switzerland AG 2025
T. S. Brahmbhatt, D. R. Scantling (eds.), *Trauma Surgery Clerkship*,
Contemporary Surgical Clerkships,
https://doi.org/10.1007/978-3-032-01412-2_6

– Distributive—Peripheral vasodilation and decreased systemic vascular resistance (SVR) → impaired venous return, decreased CO, and poor end-organ perfusion.

  • Septic—Systemic response to infection due to inflammation and toxin-induced endothelial damage and capillary permeability
  • Neurogenic—Disruption of the autonomic nervous system → loss of sympathetic tone → unopposed parasympathetic response (vagus nerve mediated)
  • Anaphylactic—Increased capillary permeability, peripheral vasodilation, and cardiovascular collapse due to an adverse allergen antibody reaction

– Cardiogenic—Inadequate CO due to impaired ventricular function

  • Cardiomyopathies (including Takotsubo in trauma patients)
  • Arrhythmias
  • Mechanical (valvular pathology)

– Obstructive—Inadequate cardiac output

  • Pulmonary vascular—significant pulmonary embolism, severe pulmonary hypertension
  • Mechanical—extrinsic compression of the right heart causing impaired filling (e.g., tension pneumothorax [PTX], diaphragmatic hernia, cardiac tamponade)

• Shock in the traumatically injured patient

– Hemorrhagic/hypovolemic until proven otherwise

  • Exsanguinating hemorrhage

    – Chest
    – Abdomen
    – Pelvis
    – Retroperitoneum
    – Long bone fractures
    – Externally (e.g., lacerations, wounds, open fractures, amputations)

  • Hypovolemic without hemorrhage

    – Insensible losses/exposure
    – Open body cavities

– Obstructive—Immediately life threatening in the critically injured

  • Cardiac tamponade or tension PTX
  • Should be identified during the primary survey
  • Maintain high index of suspicion with penetrating injuries to the cardiac box or chest

- If high clinical suspicion → finger thoracostomy or pericardial window/pericardiocentesis to prevent cardiovascular collapse

- Cardiogenic—Blunt cardiac injury/cardiac contusion

  - Usually seen with high energy mechanism chest injuries
  - Clinical picture: signs of chest trauma (ecchymosis, crepitus, rib/sternal fractures) + arrhythmia + shock state (cool, clammy skin, cyanosis)

    - Arrythmia on tele + EKG
    - Cardiac dysmotility on ECHO
    - Elevated cardiac enzymes (+/−)

- Neurogenic—Spinal cord injuries (more common with cervical spine injuries) [5] and severe TBI

  - Should be considered with the constellation of bradycardia, hypotension, and neurological deficits or decreased mental status on exam

- Anaphylactic—Usually seen with IV contrast or commonly used medications (analgesics, antibiotics)

  - Classically associated with a rash, but rash is not required for diagnosis

Background

In 1978, the American College of Surgeons Committee on Trauma introduced the Advanced Trauma Life Support (ATLS) course [6]. This course provided a systematic framework for practitioners to approach treating critically injured patients. ATLS highlighted the importance of rapid identification of the shock state and immediate intervention through a regimented system [7]. Once the patient has been identified to be in shock, the focus should be on delineating hypovolemic/hemorrhagic versus non-hemorrhagic shock.

One should approach this with the knowledge that hemorrhagic shock is overwhelmingly the most common type of shock in trauma patients. It should be immediately identified, controlled, and resuscitation initiated during the primary survey.

Further understanding the physiologic response to hemorrhage and the shock state is critical to understanding how to appropriately resuscitate a traumatically injured patient.

ATLS organizes hemorrhagic shock into four classes.

Class I hemorrhage is loss of 15% of total blood volume or approximately 750 mL. The patient may be anxious, but should have stable vital signs (normotensive, HR < 100 bpm, not tachypneic). You may observe slightly decreased UOP in these patients (30 mL/h) [4].

Class II hemorrhage is 15–30% blood volume loss (750–1500 mL). Similar to Class I, these patients will be normotensive; however, tachycardia, narrow pulse pressure, tachypnea, and further decreasing urine output (20–30 mL/h) may be observed. Both Class I and II hemorrhage have historically been treated with crystalloid resuscitation with close monitoring for response, but more contemporary trauma resuscitation strategies focus on blood product replacement rather than crystalloid.

Advancing to class III hemorrhage (30–40% blood volume loss, approximately 1.5–2 L), hemodynamic derangements become more apparent. Confusion, hypotension, tachycardia (>120 bpm), narrow pulse pressure, tachypnea (30–40 breaths/min), and poor UOP (5–15 mL/h) all become common. These are the typical physiologic manifestations of impaired organ perfusion (confusion = impaired brain perfusion; hypotension + tachycardia = volume loss with compensatory HR increase to improve CO and O_2 delivery to tissues; narrow pulse pressure = decreased CO with increased peripheral vascular resistance to maintain peripheral flow; tachypnea = physiologic response to lower CO by trying to improve oxygenation and increase O_2 delivery; low UOP = impaired renal perfusion).

In class IV hemorrhage (>2 L or >40% blood loss), patients may become lethargic, their tachycardia worsens (>140 bpm), and urinary output is minimal. As steps are taken to control hemorrhage, simultaneous balanced blood product resuscitation should be initiated in class III and IV hemorrhagic shock [4].

Despite the benefits of this classification system, calculating total blood loss in the traumatically injured is difficult and inaccurate [8].

To address the challenges of the ATLS classification system, a physiologic classification of shock has been proposed by Bonanmo et al. [5] Starting with two 500 mL boluses of crystalloid, this classification of shock guides the practitioner through clinical responses to the stage of shock and recommended interventions.

The physiologic classification is divided into four groups: table compensated (Stage I and II), severe unstable (Stage III), critical/impending cardiac arrest (Stage IV), and cardiac arrest by exsanguination (Stage V) [8]. In stable compensated hemorrhagic shock (HS), the patient will present with tachycardia and external "skin signs" of shock (cool, pale, clammy) (Stage I) and be responsive to a fluid bolus (Stage II). Severe unstable shock (Stage III) is characterized by absent response to fluid bolus or a transient response to product resuscitation for less than 20–30 min. Critical HS or impending cardiac arrest (Stage IV) shows signs of heart and brain ischemia (e.g., encephalopathy, arrythmia, decreased contractility), is refractory to fluid resuscitation, and ultimately leads to cardiac arrest due to exsanguination (Stage V).

As the body progresses into hemorrhagic shock, physiologic changes can be observed at a cellular level. The initial insult causes both humoral (B cell) and cellular (T cell) lymphocyte response. This leads to cytokine production of both pro-inflammatory (IL-1, IL-6, TNF-α) and anti-inflammatory cytokines (IL-4, IL-10, IL-13) [1]. In ideal conditions, these processes self-regulate and promote healing and recovery; however, in severe trauma this feedback loop can be disrupted leading to systemic inflammatory response syndrome (SIRS). SIRS is associated with muscle weakness, immunosuppression, malaise, and capillary permeability [1]. This can progress to sepsis, septic shock, DIC, multi-organ dysfunction, and ultimately death.

The lethal triad in trauma is a feedback loop of coagulopathy, acidosis, and hypothermia. Trauma-induced coagulopathy (TIC), part of the lethal triad, is a major contributor to mortality and morbidity in hemorrhagic shock.

- In the shock state, tissue hypoperfusion leads to tissue hypoxia, anaerobic metabolism, and subsequent lactic acidosis. Exposure and large volume fluid resuscitation lead to hypothermia. Hypothermia combined with acidosis then promotes TIC. As the patient's pH and temperature drop, the coagulation protease activity declines impairing the coagulation cascade and subsequent clot formation (hypocoagulability) [9].
- Tissue hypoperfusion and direct tissue injury lead to derangements in fibrinolysis, endothelial function, and platelet dysfunction [10]. Hyperfibrinolysis is driven by release of tPA due to endothelial hypoperfusion and thrombin-generated negative feedback. Endothelial dysfunction occurs by degradation of the endothelial glycocalyx. This impairs endothelial signaling and barrier permeability.
- Tissue hypoperfusion also leads to epinephrine and pro-inflammatory cytokine release (hypercoagulability). Direct tissue injury also leads to hyper- and hypocoagulable states. When direct tissue injury occurs, it initiates the coagulation cascade via tissue factor (TF), a transmembrane protein on endothelial cells that, when exposed, interacts with factor VIIa, leading to clot propagation [9]. Further, clotting factor and platelet consumption during the formation of clot at the site of tissue injury leads to a hypocoagulable state.

Trauma-induced coagulopathy is a complex, multifactorial process that is the focus of much research. In the clinical setting, viscoelastic hemostatic assays (VHAs) have been developed to help inform the clinician on the patient's coagulation status and help guide resuscitation.

- Thromboelastography (TEG) and rotational thromboelastometry (ROTEM) are currently the two most popular VHAs. A sample of the patient's blood is heated to 37 °C (normothermia), placed in a cup, and a pin inserted into the blood. Then either the cup (TEG) or pin (ROTEM) oscillates, and clot formation, rate, strength, and stability are measured. The results are represented on a graph with the X-axis representing time and Y-axis representing clot amplitude.
- These results are used to guide the order of blood product resuscitation and not the initiation of resuscitation: FFP for extended clotting time, cryoprecipitate for impaired clot rate, platelets for decreased clot strength, and tranexamic acid may be indicated for low clot stability (increased lysis) [6]. This provides the patient

with resuscitation that promotes return to physiologic coagulation and minimizes hemodilution that can lead to worsening coagulopathy.

With the increasing prevalence of VHA-guided resuscitation and a growing body of literature on traumatic coagulopathy, focus has been placed on balanced blood product resuscitation. Blood products should be administered in a balanced fashion and as rapidly as possible once massive hemorrhage becomes apparent. Further administration of crystalloid should be avoided in hemorrhagic shock as it can promote hemodilution, hypothermia, and ultimately worsen coagulopathy [9].

Common ratios used at trauma centers throughout the United States include 1:1:1 resuscitation consisting of plasma, platelets, and RBCs and 1:2 plasma to RBCs [9]. Recently, the benefits of whole blood have been demonstrated in the literature [11, 12] and is slowly becoming available at major trauma centers throughout the United States

Whole blood and balanced product resuscitation is critical in the traumatically injured as it decreases morbidity and mortality while minimizing product transfusion requirements, hemodilution, and transfusion-induced coagulopathy.

As the body recovers from hemorrhagic shock after appropriate hemorrhage control and resuscitation, the physiologic derangements will begin to normalize.

When adequate tissue perfusion is restored, the body will no longer rely heavily on anaerobic metabolism. Thus, serum lactate levels will trend toward normal, base deficit (a marker of serum lactate and tissue oxygen utilization [13]) will improve, and UOP will increase as end-organ perfusion improves.

This will be accompanied by improved mentation, urine output, and hemodynamic stability. These markers of end-organ perfusion all indicate the patient is recovering from their shock state, and the physiologic response to injury and shock is resolving.

Current State

- Physiologic response to injury and shock is a complex mechanism that originates from cytokine and catecholamine release due to tissue hypoperfusion and direct tissue injury.
- The inflammatory cascade leading to tissue injury and acidosis is well described.
- Individual factors in trauma-induced coagulopathy (platelet dysfunction, fibrinolysis, endothelial dysfunction) are thoroughly detailed in the literature.
- There is limited understanding of the interactions between the hypo- and hypercoagulable state of the injured patient.
- Widespread use of viscoelastic hemostatic assays (TEG and ROTEM) has improved our response to hemorrhagic shock while minimizing resuscitation-induced injury.

Take-Home Points

- Shock is tissue hypoperfusion leading to end-organ dysfunction.
- There are four broad categories of shock: hypovolemic, distributive, cardiogenic, and obstructive.
- Traumatic shock is hemorrhagic/hypovolemic until proven otherwise.
- Rapid identification and reversal of the shock state is imperative to maximizing patient outcomes.
- The degree of hemorrhagic shock is notoriously difficult to quantify in the acute setting.
- The lethal triad of coagulopathy, hypothermia, and acidosis is a positive feedback loop that must be immediately addressed to prevent mortality.
- Both tissue hypoperfusion and direct tissue injury play a significant role in the physiologic response to traumatic injury.

References

1. van Aswegen H. Physiological response to trauma. Thoracic Key. 2016.
2. Haseer Koya H, Paul M. Shock. [Updated 2022 Jul 25]. In: StatPearls [Internet]. Treasure Island: StatPearls Publishing; 2022.
3. Dave S, Cho JJ. Neurogenic shock. [Updated 2022 Feb 10]. In: StatPearls [Internet]. Treasure Island: StatPearls Publishing; 2022. Available from: https://www.ncbi.nlm.nih.gov/books/NBK459361/.
4. Gaieski DF, Mikkelsen ME. Definition, classification, etiology, and pathophysiology of shock in adults. In: Post TW, editor. UpToDate. Waltham: UpToDate; 2022. Accessed on 30 Nov 2022. Available from: https://www.wolterskluwer.com/en/solutions/uptodate.
5. Ruiz IA, Squair JW, Phillips AA, Lukac CD, Huang D, Oxciano P, et al. Incidence and natural progression of neurogenic shock after traumatic spinal cord injury. J Neurotrauma. 2018;35(3):461–6.
6. Kortbeek JB, Al Turki SA, Ali J, Antoine JA, Bouillon B, Brasel K, et al. Advanced trauma life support, 8th edition, the evidence for change. J Trauma. 2008;64(6):1638–50.
7. ATLS Subcommittee; American College of Surgeons Committee on Trauma. Advanced trauma life support (ATLS®). J Trauma Acute Care Surg. 2013;74(5):1363–6.
8. Bonanno FG. The need for a physiological classification of hemorrhagic shock. J Emerg Trauma Shock. 2020;13(3):177.
9. Moore EE, Moore HB, Kornblith LZ, Neal MD, Hoffman M, Mutch NJ, et al. Trauma-induced coagulopathy. Nat Rev Dis Primers. 2021;7(1):30.
10. Kutcher M, Cohen M. Coagulopathy in trauma patients. In: Post TW, editor. UpToDate. Waltham: UpToDate; 2022. Accessed on 26 Nov 2022. Available from: https://www.wolterskluwer.com/en/solutions/uptodate
11. Spinella PC. Warm fresh whole blood transfusion for severe hemorrhage: U.S. military and potential civilian applications. Crit Care Med. 2008;36(Suppl):S340–5.
12. Spinella PC, Cap AP. Whole blood. Curr Opin Hematol. 2016;23(6):536–42.
13. Paydar S, Fazelzadeh A, Abbasi H, Bolandparvaz S. Base deficit: a better indicator for diagnosis and treatment of shock in trauma patients. J Trauma. 2011;70(6):1580–1.

Chapter 7
Initial Resuscitation of the Trauma Patient

Anthony Loria and Michael A. Vella

Introduction

- This chapter discusses aspects of the initial management of the trauma patient, from emergency medical service (EMS) triage to obtaining vascular access.
- We specifically focus on EMS and in-hospital triage, the concept of the golden hour and the importance of early resuscitation/definitive management, obtaining rapid vascular access, prevention of the lethal diamond, EMS hand-off, and general trauma bay design.

Treatment as Quickly as Possible (The Golden Hour)

- Trauma-related deaths occur in three peaks (Fig. 7.1). The first peak is immediately after injury and is often related to traumatic brain injury, spinal cord transection, and major cardiac/vascular injuries.
- Colloquially referred to as "the golden hour," the 60 min following injury historically represents the time period during which rapid resuscitation and operative intervention may prevent death. The deaths beyond the immediate period are often related to hemorrhage and thoracic injuries (i.e., tension pneumothorax). Late deaths (third peak) are often due to infection and multi-organ failure.
- Mortality remains high (approximately 40%) in the subset of patients presenting with hypotension and occurs early after injury (within 30 min). Delays in operative intervention and blood product resuscitation are associated with increased

A. Loria · M. A. Vella (✉)
Department of Surgery, University of Rochester Medical Center, Rochester, NY, USA
e-mail: Michael_Vella@URMC.Rochester.edu

© The Author(s), under exclusive license to Springer Nature Switzerland AG 2025
T. S. Brahmbhatt, D. R. Scantling (eds.), *Trauma Surgery Clerkship*, Contemporary Surgical Clerkships,
https://doi.org/10.1007/978-3-032-01412-2_7

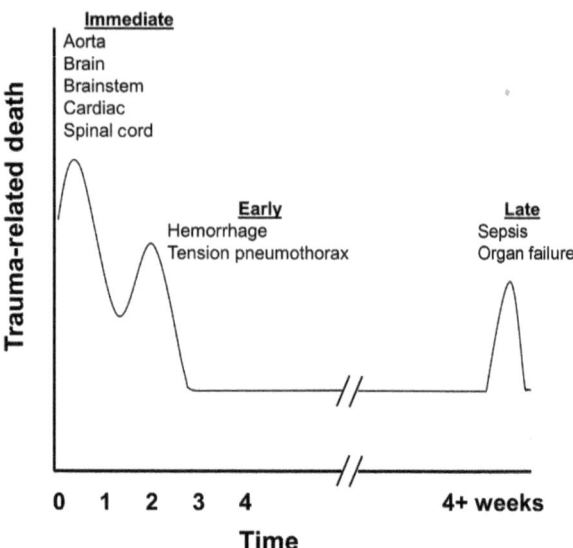

Fig. 7.1 Classical teaching on the distribution of trauma-related mortalities. The three peaks of trauma-related mortality

mortality and many preventable deaths occur far faster [1]. Thus, the concept of the "golden hour," or definitive treatment within 60 min, has ultimately been replaced by the dictum "as soon as possible." The ultimate goal is to prevent all potentially preventable deaths.

- Rapid transfer to definitive care is paramount. Minimizing prehospital procedures (and associated delays in transfer), especially in patients with penetrating injuries (gunshot and stab wounds) may improve outcomes [2].
- It is important to understand that the physiology, injury patterns, and management of blunt and penetrating injuries can vary and may dictate what interventions are required in the prehospital and immediate in-hospital settings.

Lethal Diamond

- Trauma and hemorrhagic shock induce complex physiologic derangements, culminating in the "lethal" or "bloody vicious" triad of (1) hypothermia, (2) acidosis, and (3) coagulopathy. More recently, the addition of hypocalcemia prompted the term "lethal diamond" (Fig. 7.2) [3].
- One can start anywhere on the diamond, as each physiological derangement exacerbates the next. For example, major hemorrhage leads to coagulopathy, which leads to further bleeding and acidosis, which lead to hypothermia, which, in turn, leads to further bleeding. Ongoing hemorrhage combined with citrate contained in blood products can cause hypocalcemia, which is associated with increased mortality in trauma patients.

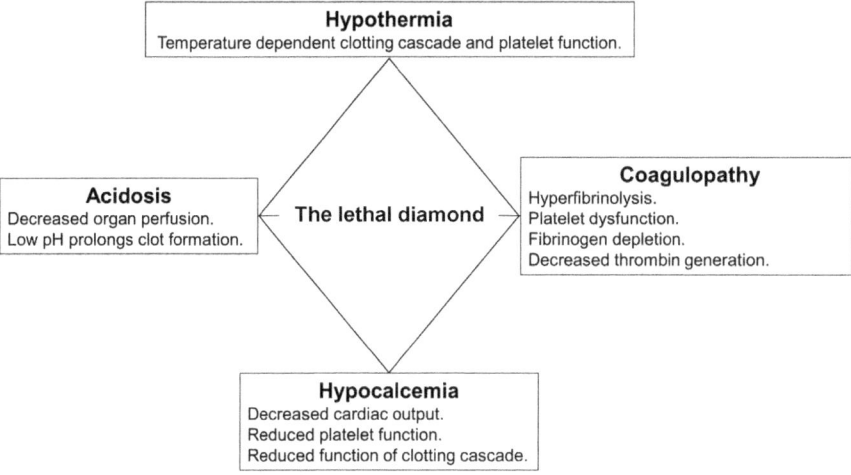

Fig. 7.2 The lethal diamond, adapted from Ditzel et al. [3]

- Failure to quickly correct these underlying physiologic derangements often leads to patient death, even if major hemorrhage is controlled.
- Prevention of the lethal diamond forms the basis of damage control resuscitation and damage control operative techniques. Damage control resuscitation in hemorrhaging patients refers to the minimization of crystalloid fluid in favor of a balanced resuscitation with a 1:1:1 ratio of packed red blood cells: fresh frozen plasma: platelets and/or the use of whole blood while definitive hemorrhage control occurs. A damage control operation refers to an abbreviated procedure in which bleeding and contamination are controlled, the cavity(ies) left open for re-exploration, and the patient returned to the intensive care unit for ongoing resuscitation and warming. These concepts are discussed in more depth elsewhere.

Patient Triage

- Not all hospitals are equipped to handle seriously injured patients, and, by extension, not all hospitals are "trauma centers." In the United States, trauma centers are generally *designated* by governmental agencies and *verified* by either a state or by the American College of Surgeons, depending on locale. Designation generally depends on need, whereas verification is based upon meeting strict standards [4]. Level I trauma centers represent the highest level of care and are *generally* able to manage all traumatic injuries without need for transfer.
- The goal of trauma triage is to match a patient's needs to the medical facility equipped to provide definitive care. Triage can be thought of as occurring in two distinct yet related parts: (1) triaging patients to the appropriate facility from the

scene or referring center and (2) determining the appropriate in-hospital trauma team response at the referral trauma center.

- *Field Triage*: National field triage guidelines have recently been established to match patient needs with institutional capabilities within the confines of a local/regional trauma system.[4] Emergency medical service (EMS) personnel assess injured patients to determine the severity of injury and appropriate medical facility destination. Patients are stratified into high vs. moderate risk of serious injury based on (1) injury patterns, (2) mental status, and (3) vital signs (Table 7.1) [5]. At times, EMS may bypass a closer facility in favor of a more distant, but better equipped, trauma center. In other cases (e.g., need for urgent airway control),

Table 7.1 National Guideline for the Field Triage of Injured Patients

High risk	
Injury patterns	*Vital signs and mental status*
Penetrating injury to head, neck, torso, proximal extremity	Age 0–9 years
Skull deformity (suspected fracture)	SBP < 70 mmHg + (2*age in years)
Suspected spinal injury with new motor/sensory loss	Age 10–64
Chest wall instability (possible flail chest)	SBP < 90 mmHg *OR*
Suspected pelvic fracture	HR > SBP
Crushed, degloved, mangled, pulseless extremity	Age 65+
Amputation proximal to wrist/ankle	SBP < 110 mmHg *OR*
Active bleeding requiring tourniquet or packing with continuous pressure	HR > SBP
	All patients
	Unable to follow commands (motor GCS < 6)
	RR <10 or >29 breaths/min
	Respiratory distress or support
	Room-air pulse oximetry <90%
Patients meeting *any of the above criteria* should be transported to the *highest-level trauma center* available within the regional trauma system	
Moderate risk	
Mechanism of injury	*EMS judgement*
High risk auto crash	Consider risk factors including
Partial/complete ejection	Low-level fall child <5 years or adult >65 years with head impact
Significant intrusion	Anticoagulant use
Death in passenger compartment	Suspicion of child abuse
Unrestrained child or in unsecured child safety seat	Special/high resource healthcare needs
Vehicle data consistent with severe injury	Pregnancy >20 weeks
Rider separation	Burns + trauma
Pedestrian/bicycle rider thrown/run over	Children should be triaged to pediatric capable center
Fall >10 feet (any age)	If concerned take to trauma center
Patients meeting any of the criteria in the yellow criteria *who do not meet red (high risk) criteria* should be *transported to a trauma center as available* (does not need to be the highest level)	

Adapted from 2021 National Guideline for the Field Triage of Injured Patients [4]

EMS may transport a patient to a closer non-trauma center first for stabilization.

- *In-Hospital Trauma Response*: Once the decision to transport a patient to a trauma center occurs, the center must assess its level of response in order to ensure the highest level of care is immediately available while not over utilizing resources. This occurs in a tiered response, varying by the type of equipment and personal mobilized to the emergency department upon notification. The American College of Surgeons has established *minimum* criteria for the highest-level activation (hospitals may elect to add to this list) [4]:

  - Systolic blood pressure <90 mmHg at any time in adults, pediatric age-specific hypotension.
  - Gunshot wound to neck, chest, abdomen.
  - Glasgow Coma Scale <9 (due to a mechanism of trauma).
  - Transfer from another hospital of a patient requiring ongoing blood transfusion.
  - Patient intubated in the field and directly transported to trauma center.
  - Patients with respiratory compromise or need emergent airway.
  - Transfer patients from ongoing hospital with respiratory compromise.
  - Emergency physician discretion.

- Other criteria are at the discretion of individual trauma centers and are generally based on (1) physiology, (2) identified injuries, and (3) mechanism of injury (Table 7.2).
- Some urban municipalizes in the United States allow transport of penetrating trauma patients by police officers, a practice that is *theoretically* faster than EMS transport has been shown in a recent multicenter observational trial to result in similar outcomes [6].
- For verification, trauma centers are required to monitor compliance with field and in-hospital triage guidelines and to determine under and over-triage rates. One would rather err on the side of overtriage, as undertriage (goal <5%) may delay appropriate care and negatively impact outcomes. However, overtriage does have financial and logistical implications. The Cribari Matrix and Need for Trauma Intervention (NFTI) are two methods used to evaluate appropriate triage [7].
- If a patient's injuries exceed a hospital's capacity, immediate transfer should be arranged. A complete workup and/or catalog of injuries are not a requirement for transfer and imaging and/or additional work-up should not be pursued at the referral facility if it will not change immediate management and/or will delay transfer.

Table 7.2 Representative trauma response guidelines adapted from the Kessler Trauma Center, University of Rochester Medical Center

Level I		Level II		Level III/consult	
Adult ≥16 years	Pediatrics ≤15 years	Adult ≥16 years	Pediatrics ≤15 years	Adult ≥16 years	Pediatrics ≤15 years
Confirmed blood pressure ≤90 mmHg any time	Age 0–9 = BP <70 + (2*age in years) Age 10+ same as adults	GSW to head, arm/leg proximal to elbow/ knee[a] Stab to head, neck, torso, groin[a] Active bleeding requiring tourniquet or wound packing[a] Suspected spinal injury with any neurologic changes Traumatic amputation proximal to wrist/ ankle Two or more suspected proximal bone fractures (including pelvic and open) Discretion of EM attending, triage nurse, or communication nurse		Significant head injury (skull fracture or hemorrhage) with torso or extremity trauma[a] Multiple rib fractures, flail chest[a] Pelvic fracture due to trauma[a] Pregnancy (>20 weeks) with abdominal trauma Significant injury with activity medical comorbidity or extremes of age Admission for care of acute injury related to known or suspected child physical abuse Discretion of EM attending, triage nurse, or communication nurse Single system injury with significant mechanism: (a) Partial or complete ejection, rollover vehicle (b) Fall >10 feet (c) Death in same passenger compartment (d) Pedestrian/bicycle rider thrown (e) History of high-speed crash with significant intrusion (f) Need for extrication for entrapped patient (g) Rider separated from vehicle with impact (motorcycle, ATV, horse, etc.) (h) Explosion/blast injury	
Gunshot to neck, torso, groin, buttock, junctional zone Respiratory compromise or pre-arrival intubation GCS ≤8 attributed to trauma Transfer patient receiving or has received blood transfusion CPR in progress or history of CPR after trauma Discretion of EM attending, triage nurse, or communication nurse					

[a]Not otherwise meeting a higher-level criterion

EMS Hand-Off

- Ideally, trauma teams have adequate pre-arrival notification from EMS in order to pre-brief and gather necessary equipment/personnel.
- Upon arrival, EMS must convey important information to the trauma team in the form of a hand-off. These concise summaries should ideally occur prior to transitioning the patient to the trauma bay gurney, otherwise important information can be missed. Previous work has shown that EMS hand-offs are frequently interrupted and that transfer of patients to the hospital gurney often occurs before hand-off completion [7]. In some cases (i.e., unstable airway), a more abbreviated report can occur.
- EMS agencies should be encouraged to use a standardized hand-off, and education should be provided on a regular basis. We encourage use of the MIST format (see below); more complete MIST reports have been associated with better trauma team function [8]:
  - *M*echanism of injury; *I*njuries identified; *S*igns (vital signs, best and worst GCS); *T*reatment rendered (vascular access, fluid/blood, medications, tourniquets, etc.)
- An example MIST report: "*20-year-old male, two gunshot wounds to left lower extremity. No other injuries identified. Lowest systolic blood pressure was 90, last blood pressure 95/60, heart rate 110, SpO2 94%, GCS 15. We placed a tourniquet on the left thigh which has stopped actively bleeding, placed a 16-Gauge IV in the right upper extremity, and gave 250 ml of crystalloid. Any questions?*"

Type and Route of Vascular Access

- Catheter diameters are measured in Gauge (varies inversely with diameter) and French (1 French unit = 0.33 mm).
- Flow through a catheter is directly related to catheter length and diameter through Poiseuille's Law:
  - $Q = \dfrac{\Delta P \pi r^4}{8 \eta l}$, (where Q = flow, P = pressure, r = catheter radius, l =
  - catheter length)
- Catheters that are short and wide have the highest flows. Doubling a catheter diameter increases the flow rate by 16-fold. Increasing catheter length decreases flow. This is why flow through a 14-Gauger peripheral IV (PIV) is faster than a standard triple lumen central venous catheter (CVC).
- Delays in hemorrhage control and resuscitation are associated with increased mortality, highlighting the need for rapid and successful vascular access [3].

- Large bore (14- or 16-Gauge) peripheral intravenous (PIV) catheters (generally in the upper extremity) are the recommended first line access strategy for the majority of trauma patients, providing flow rates of up to 400 ml/min [9].
- In patients who are hypotensive and/or in-extremis without existing access, or in those where IV access cannot be obtained quickly, we recommend proceeding with the intraosseous (IO) route as a bridge to more definitive access and while other access is being obtained. Although flow rates are slower (up to 125 ml/h), IO catheters have been shown to be faster than central venous catheters (CVC), twice as likely to be successful compared with PIV and CVC, and may lead to faster resuscitation [10, 11]. IO catheters can be placed in the tibial, humeral, and sternal locations, with faster flow rates noted at the humeral and sternal sites. In either case, blood and resuscitative medications can be infused rapidly. If possible, one should avoid placement of IO access in the tibial location if there is a concern for major vascular injury between the catheter site and the heart and in the humeral location in the event the ipsilateral arm is raised above the head (during thoracotomy, for example). In some instances, any location will suffice as a rapid means to begin the resuscitation process ("any port in a storm").
- Central venous access can be obtained in the jugular, subclavian, or femoral locations, with flow rates of 8.5 French introducer catheters reaching 600 ml/h [9]. However, we advise against CVC as the single first line strategy in critically injured patients without access due to the relatively low success rates and expected procedural duration [10]. In these circumstances, IO access can be obtained while CVC access is attempted.

Trauma Bay Design

- Poor design in healthcare can lead to improvised work-around solutions that create inefficacy and hazards to both patients and clinicians [12]. This is certainly true in the trauma bay, a general term used to describe the area in an emergency department in which major trauma patients are treated. Improperly placed monitoring equipment or supplies, for example, can hinder an otherwise smooth resuscitation.
- In general, trauma bays are equipped with monitors, airway devices (including video laryngoscopes and surgical airway equipment), procedural trays (thoracostomy and thoracotomy), arterial and central venous catheters, ultrasound machines, and hemorrhage control adjuncts (hemostatic dressings, pelvic binders, and tourniquets) to name a few (Fig. 7.3).
- Some trauma bays are equipped with timers to monitor resuscitation times, cameras and microphones to allow to audiovisual recording for teaching and performance improvement purposes (so-called trauma video review"), warming lights, procedural lights, and overhead X-ray equipment. In addition, some institutions utilize floor markings to denote where specific team members should stand during a resuscitation.

Fig. 7.3 Typical trauma
bay set-up as seen from
trauma video review
equipment

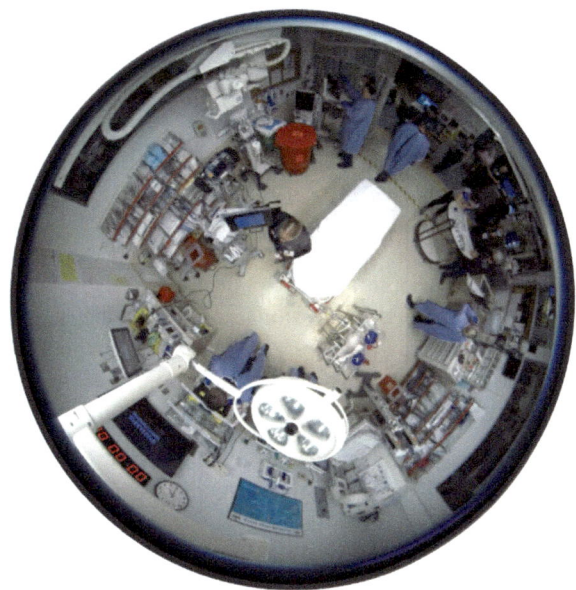

- Many trauma bays contain coolers or refrigerators to allow immediate access to blood products; if this is not the case, a mechanism is required to allow rapid transport from the blood bank.
- A trauma bay should be set up to allow for maximum efficiency as well as noise and crowd control. A clear line of sight between the trauma team and recording nurse is imperative to allow timely and accurate conveying of information.
- Resuscitation areas should generally be located in proximity to the CT scan and operating room.
- Trauma bay designs vary widely across institutions, but there are certain underlying principles we believe to be very important. Two of these are (1) standardization and (2) "just-in-time" stocking philosophy.
- Standardization: Trauma bays within a center should be identical or as close to identical as possible, meaning that equipment and location of personal should be consistent. This ensures, among other things, that team members are not frantically searching for needed equipment while a patient is decompensating.
- "Just-in-Time" philosophy: Borrowed from the automobile industry, the idea of "just-in-time" supply means that only the necessary equipment used for *most* resuscitations is located in the trauma bay at any given time [13]. Equipment that is less frequently used is located in a storage area close to but not in the trauma bay. This allows for improved efficiency and decreased clutter and is in opposition to the view of "just-in-case" supply, where any and all equipment is located in the immediate trauma resuscitation area. An example of "just-in-time" would be storing only 18-Gauge arterial lines in the trauma bay, with 20-Gauge located in an adjacent storage room [13].

- The use of simulation and trauma video review to identify latent safety threats and inefficiencies/opportunities in trauma bay set-up has been increasingly described [12].

Summary

- Trauma is a common cause of death and disability, and the care of injured patients involves medical professionals across a wide range of specialties.
- Efficient trauma bay design, appropriate triage, concise yet complete hand-offs, rapid vascular access with resuscitation, and prevention of the lethal diamond are critical in the management of severely injured patients.

References

1. Clarke JR, Trooskin SZ, Doshi PJ, et al. Time to laparotomy for intra-abdominal bleeding from trauma does affect survival for delays up to 90 minutes. J Trauma. 2002;52(3):420–5. https://doi.org/10.1097/00005373-200203000-00002.
2. Taghavi S, Maher Z, Goldberg AJ, et al. An Eastern Association for the Surgery of Trauma multicenter trial examining prehospital procedures in penetrating trauma patients. J Trauma Acute Care Surg. 2021;91(1):130–40. https://doi.org/10.1097/TA.0000000000003151.
3. Ditzel RM Jr, Anderson JL, Eisenhart WJ, et al. A review of transfusion- and trauma-induced hypocalcemia: is it time to change the lethal triad to the lethal diamond? J Trauma Acute Care Surg. 2020;88(3):434–9. https://doi.org/10.1097/TA.0000000000002570.
4. American College of Surgeons. Resources for optimal care of the injured patient. 2022. https://www.facs.org/quality-programs/trauma/quality/verification-review-and-consultation-program/standards. Accessed 19 Sept 2022.
5. Newgard CD, Fischer PE, Gestring M, et al. National guideline for the field triage of injured patients: recommendations of the National Expert Panel on Field Triage, 2021. J Trauma Acute Care Surg. 2022;93(2):e49–60. https://doi.org/10.1097/TA.0000000000003627.
6. Taghavi S, Maher Z, Goldberg AJ, et al. An analysis of police transport in an Eastern Association for the Surgery of Trauma multicenter trial examining prehospital procedures in penetrating trauma patients. J Trauma Acute Care Surg. 2022;93(2):265–72. https://doi.org/10.1097/TA.0000000000003563.
7. Harrell KN, Spain SJ, Whiteaker KA, et al. Modified need for trauma intervention criteria reduces Cribari trauma overtriage rate. J Trauma Nurs. 2020;27(4):195–9. https://doi.org/10.1097/JTN.0000000000000514.
8. Nagaraj MB, Lowe JE, Marinica AL, et al. Using trauma video review to assess EMS handoff and trauma team non-technical skills. Prehosp Emerg Care. 2021;27:10–7. https://doi.org/10.1080/10903127.2021.2000684.
9. Berman DJ, Schiavi A, Frank SM, et al. Factors that influence flow through intravascular catheters: the clinical relevance of Poiseuille's law. Transfusion. 2020;60(7):1410–7. https://doi.org/10.1111/trf.15898.
10. Dumas RP, Vella MA, Maiga AW, et al. Moving the needle on time to resuscitation: an EAST prospective multicenter study of vascular access in hypotensive injured patients using trauma video review. J Trauma Acute Care Surg. 2023;95(1):87–93.

11. Day MW. Intraosseous devices for intravascular access in adult trauma patients. Crit Care Nurse. 2011;31(2):76–90. https://doi.org/10.4037/ccn2011615.
12. Petrosoniak A, Hicks C. Design, build, train, excel: using simulation to create elite trauma systems. Int Anesthesiol Clin. 2021;59(2):58–66. https://doi.org/10.1097/AIA.0000000000000312.
13. Jenkins A. Just-in-time vs just-in-case: choosing the right strategy. 2021. https://www.net-suite.com/portal/resource/articles/inventory-management/just-in-time-vs-just-in-case.shtml. Accessed 28 Nov 2022.

Chapter 8
Blood Products and Transfusion

Yuqian Tian, Christopher D. Barrett, and Kevin M. Kemp

Background

Hemorrhagic shock is the second leading cause of early mortality in trauma and a leading cause of preventable death after injury. About 30–40% of trauma deaths are caused by hemorrhage and hemorrhagic shock, regardless of mechanism of injury. It accounts for approximately 50% of deaths during the prehospital period and is the number one cause of death during the first hour after patient arrives trauma center [1]. Control of hemorrhage is the priority when faced with an exsanguinating patient, but transfusion helps bridge the gap between the point of injury and definitive control of hemorrhage. Knowing which blood products are available along with their indications will ensure that the bleeding patient has the best opportunity for survival.

Damage Control Resuscitation: Preventing the Lethal Triad

Traditional trauma resuscitation has focused on the early administration of crystalloid solutions, followed by blood products. While crystalloids may have provided temporary expansion of the circulating plasma volume, numerous deleterious

Y. Tian
Department of Surgery, University of Nebraska Medical Center, Omaha, NE, USA
e-mail: ytian@unmc.edu

C. D. Barrett · K. M. Kemp (✉)
Division of Acute Care Surgery, Department of Surgery, University of Nebraska Medical Center, Omaha, NE, USA
e-mail: kevin.kemp@unmc.edu

© The Author(s), under exclusive license to Springer Nature Switzerland AG 2025
T. S. Brahmbhatt, D. R. Scantling (eds.), *Trauma Surgery Clerkship*, Contemporary Surgical Clerkships,
https://doi.org/10.1007/978-3-032-01412-2_8

effects have been observed. Trauma patients are at risk of experiencing the "lethal triad" of coagulopathy, acidosis, and hypothermia. Through a variety of mechanisms, crystalloids are known to contribute to all three aspects of the "lethal triad."

Massive hemorrhage leads to shock and hypoperfusion of organs, which causes hypothermia and acidosis. Acidosis and hypothermia inhibit coagulation resulting in impaired clot formation. Each factor in this triad closely interacts with each other and creates negative synergy that eventually leads to death from the inability of the blood to clot.

Damage control resuscitation (DCR) is the contemporary framework used to resuscitate patients experiencing life-threatening hemorrhage. The main principles of DCR are limiting administration of crystalloids, using balanced ratios of blood products for replacement of circulating volume, as well as correction of coagulopathy, and permissive hypotension.

The concept of balanced resuscitation is central to DCR. Two major studies set the foundation of today's balanced transfusion protocol, PROMMTT and PROPPR. PROMMTT was an observational study and concluded that increased ratio of plasma products to packed red blood cells (pRBCs) and platelets to pRBC ($\geq 1:1$) are independently associated with lower mortality in the first 6 h in trauma resuscitations [2]. These findings generated interest to further investigate the concept of balanced component transfusion. This led to the PROPPR trial in 2015, a multicenter, randomized controlled trial. pRBC, FFP, and platelets were transfused either in a ratio of 1:1:1 or 2:1:1. The former group did not show worse outcomes and instead achieved more hemostasis in the first 24 h [3]. This trial informed the modern resuscitation of hemorrhagic shock in trauma patients. Another more recent development in trauma resuscitation protocol is the introduction of low-titer O whole blood (LTOWB). The product contains physiologic amount of pRBC, platelets, and coagulation factors, which naturally provides a balanced resuscitation. There has been emerging literature including randomized control trials to demonstrate the feasibility, safety, and potential benefits of using LTOWB in military and civilian trauma settings [4, 5].

An important tool in helping to ensure the goals of damage control resuscitation are met is the massive transfusion protocol (MTP). Massive transfusion is most commonly defined as transfusion of more than 10 units of packed red blood cells in 24 h, though other definitions exist. Massive transfusion protocols rapidly bring blood products to the bedside of a bleeding patient to provide blood products in a fixed ratio to best approximate the losses from hemorrhage. A typical MTP pack might contain six units of packed red blood cells, six units of fresh frozen plasma, and a unit of apheresis platelets.

Measurement of Coagulopathy: The Role of Viscoelastic Assays

Viscoelastic assays, such as thromboelastography (TEG) and rotational thrombo-elastometry (ROTEM), are utilized in trauma to identify and quantify coagulopathy. These assays provide information about the mechanical properties of clot formation, propagation, and breakdown. Results from viscoelastic testing can demonstrate specific defects in coagulation pathways, guiding the administration of appropriate blood products. Point-of-care TEG study can be done with the first variable coming back within 5 min, allowing for immediate intervention. Compared to traditional laboratory assessments of coagulation, viscoelastic assays allow tailoring of therapy to the needs of the patient. It also provides information about both coagulation and fibrinolysis in one study, saving the time needed to collect multiple test results and piece information together [6]. Figure 8.1 is an example of TEG curve. Reaction (R) time is the time it takes for initiation of clot formation and is reflective of coagulation factor activity. Increased R-time suggests low level of coagulation factors, therefore fresh frozen plasma (FFP) is indicated. Activated clotting time (ACT, only available in rapid TEG) also represents coagulation factor activity. Alpha angle reflects the rate of crosslinking fibrins formation from cleavage of fibrinogen. A lower alpha angle indicates there is not enough fibrinogen, therefore indicating the need for cryoprecipitate. Maximum amplitude (MA) represents the maximum clot strength and is used clinically for indication of platelet transfusion. Lastly, lysis at 30 min (LY 30) measures the extent of clot degradation 30 min after MA is achieved. It provides information regarding fibrinolysis. Increased LY-30 indicates the need to give an anti-fibrinolytic, usually tranexamic acid, which inhibits plasminogen and ultimately slows down clot breakdown.

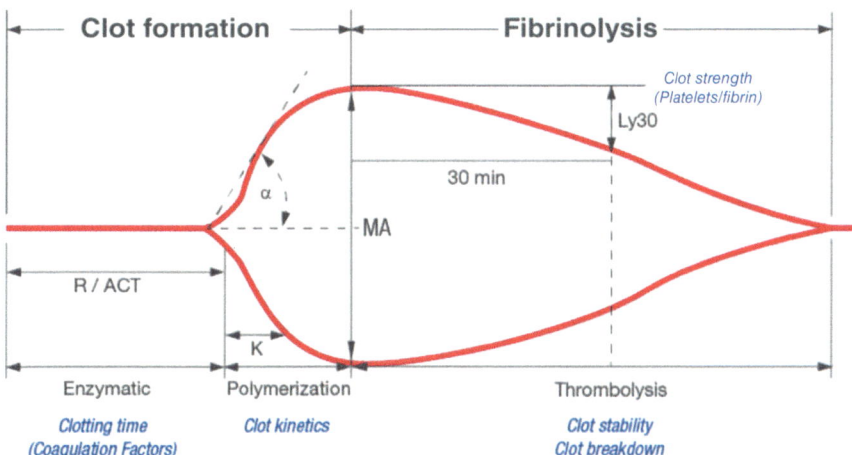

Fig. 8.1 Example of TEG tracing [7]

Available Blood Products

Low-Titer O Whole Blood (LTOWB)

Whole blood was the predominant blood product prior to component therapy becoming common. Resurging interest in the use of whole blood was brought about through the United States' involvement in the Global War on Terror. The challenges of distance from the continental United States and logistics of transportation made it challenging to make blood products available in this environment, especially platelets. A solution was found by utilizing the walking blood bank, where a unit of whole blood was donated on demand by a pool of prescreened donors and immediately transfused into a bleeding patient.

As the bleeding patient is bleeding all components that make up blood, transfusing a bleeding patient exactly what they are losing through hemorrhage makes intuitive sense. Duplicating a walking blood bank is challenging in the civilian environment, but these war time experiences motivated the consideration in using cold stored LTOWB. Just as with fresh whole blood, LTOWB contains physiologic amounts of red blood cells, coagulation factors, and platelets. It also has the advantage of containing less preservative solution than individual components.

Whole blood units are stored between 1 and 6 °C for up to 21 or 35 days, typically in the emergency department or in trauma bay for rapid accessibility.

Packed Red Blood Cells (pRBCs)

Packed red blood cells are the most transfused blood product. The pRBC is collected from donor whole blood by spinning down the donor blood and allowing dense RBCs to settle down at the bottom while liquid plasma remains on the top. To preserve red blood cells and prevent coagulation during storage, additives including citrate, dextrose, and adenine are mixed with the products [8]. Hypocalcemia is common after RBC transfusions because of the addition of citrate, which chelates calcium. Packed RBCs can be stored in refrigerated temperatures for up to 45 days. One unit of pRBC should approximately raise the hemoglobin by 1 g/dL.

RBC transfusions are indicated for acute hemorrhage and anemia to improve oxygen delivery to tissues. In normal clinical settings, restrictive transfusion strategy is recommended, i.e., transfusion threshold is hemoglobin <7 g/dL [9]. Decisions to transfuse should not be based on a single lab value, and this is particularly true in the setting of active hemorrhage in trauma or surgical patients. Hemoglobin level is not helpful in acute bleeding settings since it is a measure of concentration and the lab value may not immediately decrease even with massive hemorrhage. Active hemorrhage should be suspected based on clinical findings including tachycardia, hypotension, tachypnea, pale mucosa, mottled skin, low urine output, and change in mental status.

Platelets

Platelet infusions can be done either with apheresis platelets or pooled platelets. Pooled platelets are obtained by centrifuging a unit of whole blood, with platelets from multiple donors combined into a single unit. One apheresis unit is therapeutically equivalent to six packs of pooled donor platelet [8]. One apheresis unit is expected to raise the platelet count by $30–60 \times 10^3\ \mu L^{-1}$. Traditionally, platelets are stored at room temperature to achieve longer circulation time after infusion. Room-temperature platelets have many limitations. It has a high risk of contamination compared to other blood products, and its limited shelf-life (5 days) often leads to wastage [10].

Cold-stored (CS) platelets were recently approved by FDA to be used in actively bleeding patients when room temperature platelets are not available. It is stored at 1–6 °C for up to 14 days without agitation. Current literature has suggested that cold temperature storage significantly reduces half-life of platelet leading to shorter circulating time but appears to maintain or possibly improve platelet function (hemostasis efficacy) in the early window after transfusion [11]. With the recent FDA approval, there will be more data/study focusing on CS platelet, whether it can safely and effectively become the alternative for RT platelet.

Platelet transfusion is used for thrombocytopenia and platelet dysfunction either prophylactically or in the setting of active bleeding. The current recommendation is to transfuse one apheresis platelet prophylactically for platelet counts $<10 \times 10^3\ \mu L^{-1}$ in patients who have chronic thrombocytopenia in hospital. The threshold increases to 50×10^3 for patients who are undergoing elective major surgeries [12]. However, these recommendations are not well supported by literature and practices vary based on patient's clinical pictures and physician's experience. Viscoelastic assays can help guide the decision to transfuse as well, with platelets typically given for a maximum amplitude value of less than 55 on TEG. Platelet transfusion is also part of the massive transfusion protocol.

Fresh Frozen Plasma (FFP)

FFP is collected from whole blood centrifugation or apheresis and then stored at −18 °C for at most 24 h. It contains all the coagulation factors, fibrinolytic proteins, albumin, immunoglobulins, and many other proteins. FFP is usually given to reverse INR > 1.6 in patients who are active bleeding or anticipate major bleeding. It is part of the MTP to address coagulopathy in trauma patients. It is also a treatment option for hereditary hemangioma, to supplement Cl esterase inhibitor specifically. It should not be the first choice if the goal is only to replete fibrinogen. It has low fibrinogen concentration comparing to the next two products, i.e., will require large volume of FFP to adequately replete fibrinogen. Viscoelastic testing can be used to determine if FFP is indicated, typically by a prolonged R time.

Cryoprecipitate

This is the precipitate collected after FFP is being thawed between 1 and 6 °C. Specifically, cryoprecipitate contains a high concentration of fibrinogen and factor VIII. It also contains factor XIII, vWF, and fibronectin. Each unit should increase fibrinogen by 5–10 mg/dL. Common dosing for adult patients is 10 units at a time.

Cryoprecipitate is the product of choice for hypofibrinogenemia in the United States. Common causes for hypofibrinogenemia include massive blood loss during perioperative period (for example, cardiac surgery), hemorrhaging trauma patients, and severe liver failure. The historical targeted level for fibrinogen is 1 g/L, but some have increased the transfusion threshold to <1.5–2 g/L depending on clinical scenarios [13]. An alpha angle of less than 65° on TEG indicates the need for cryoprecipitate.

Fibrinogen Concentrates

In addition to FFP and cryoprecipitate, fibrinogen concentrate is another product that replenishes fibrinogen level. As the name suggests, it carries a higher concentration of fibrinogen. In comparison to FFP and cryoprecipitates, it has the advantage of lower viral transmission rate, faster administration time (it is a powder in room temperature that can be reconstituted just with sterile water), and lower transfusion volume [14]. However, there is no clear consensus on whether fibrinogen concentrate is preferable over cryoprecipitates in acquired hypofibrinogenemia in practice. In the United States, fibrinogen concentrate is only licensed for congenital fibrinogen disorders.

Prothrombin Complex Concentrate (PCC)

A large plasma pool is processed via ion-exchange chromatography to produce three-factor PCC (factor II, IX, X) or four-factor PCC (factor II, VII, IX, and X). The only FDA-approved indication is urgent reversal of acquired anticoagulation from vitamin K antagonists in adult patients with acute major bleeding. In addition, it is suggested that PCC is helpful to reverse other oral anticoagulants, Xa inhibitors, and direct thrombin inhibitors [15].

Hemoglobin-Based Oxygen Carrier (HBOCs)

These are semisynthetic or synthetic bioengineered surrogates of RBCs. Theorectically, they are able to carry out the therapeutic function of RBCs to provide adequate oxygenation of tissues, while avoiding many limitations encountered with RBC transfusion (limited availabilities, short shelf-life, cross-matching requirement, pathogen contamination, etc.). Currently, there is no FDA-approved product in the market, but some products have progressed to preclinical and clinical evaluations [16].

Risks

Even though transfusion can be lifesaving, it is not without risk. In the United States, it is estimated that the risk of having an adverse reaction from blood transfusion is 0.2% [10]. Transfusion-related complications can be divided into infectious and noninfectious. With development of advanced screening tools for known infectious causes, the risk of being infected by bacteria, parasites, or viruses through transfusion has decreased significantly. For example, the odds of getting HIV, hepatitis B, and hepatitis C through transfusion are 1 in 2 million, 1 in 300,000, and 1 in 1.5 million respectively [17]. Other viral agents that have been mentioned in literature include human T-lymphotropic virus 1 or 2, Creutzfeldt-Jakob disease, human herpesvirus 8, pandemic influenza, and West Nile virus [18, 19]. Bacterial contaminations of transfused product can lead to sepsis. Yersinia enterocolitica is the most common contaminant found in RBCs because of its ability to replicate in cold temperature. Other common bacteria include *Staphylococcus aureus*, coagulate-negative staphylococci, diphtheroid bacilli, streptococci, and other skin flora bacteria [10].

Noninfectious complications are much more common than infectious causes these days. There are many subtypes within this category, and we will only discuss some of them here. A full list of complications is included in Table 8.1.

Acute Hemolytic Transfusion Reaction Acute hemolytic transfusion reactions are uncommon, estimated to occur in 1 per 10,000–50,000 blood transfusions [10, 18]. In this reaction, recipients have pre-existing antibodies that are against antigens on donor RBC leading to RBC hemolysis. ABO-incompatible transfusion is a typical cause. Clinical symptoms include acute onset of fever/chills, chest/back/abdominal pain, pain at infusion site, nausea/vomiting, dyspnea, hypotension, diffuse bleeding, oliguria, or hemoglobinuria. Because the clinical presentations are nonspecific, high index of suspicion should be maintained and lead to further investigation.

Transfusion should be stopped immediately, followed adequate IV fluids administration. Other supportive measures could include oxygen for dyspnea or

Table 8.1 Non-infectious complications of blood transfusion [10, 18]

Acute phase (<24 h)	Immune mediated	Acute hemolytic transfusion reaction
		Febrile non-hemolytic transfusion reaction
		Allergic/urticarial/anaphylactic reactions
		Transfusion-related acute lung injury
	Non-immune mediated	Air embolism
		Transfusion-associated circulatory overload
		Non-immune hemolysis
Delayed phase	Immune mediated	Delayed hemolytic transfusion reaction
		Alloimmunization to: HLA antigens, platelet antigens, RBC antigens
		Transfusion-related immunomodulation
		Transfusion-associated graft versus host disease
		Posttransfusion purpura
	Non-immune mediated	Iron overload

acetaminophen for fever. Kidney function and coagulation profiles need to be closely monitored, and further reaction workup should be sent. The most common confirmatory test is a direct antiglobulin test, which detects antibodies attached to RBC.

A concern with the utilization of LTOWB has been hemolysis, though multiple experiences in the literature show this risk to be exceedingly low. Previously, the American Association of Blood Banks (AABB) required WB transfusion to be ABO group identical to recipients, which greatly limited its use in the trauma setting. Realizing this limitation, now the standard practice is to use LTOWB to mitigate the risk of hemolysis when transfusing to an unknown ABO group recipient. Knowing that Group O WB still contains anti-A and anti-B in its plasma, to decrease the risk of hemolysis from antibodies, hospitals are responsible to establish a definition for "low titer" and to determine how many units of LTOWB a patient can receive. These two parameters are currently not standardized, and each institution can determine its own practice [20].

Febrile Nonhemolytic Transfusion Reaction One of the most common transfusion reactions, with an incidence of 86 per 100,000 [18]. This reaction is caused by cytokines that are released by white blood cells in the stored blood products. As the name suggests, the defining symptom is fever, specifically a change of at least 1 °C into the febrile range during or within 4 h of transfusion. This is typically a diagnosis of exclusion. Other clinical causes and other transfusion reactions that present as fever need to be ruled out. When suspected, the first step is always to stop the transfusion and send the blood back to blood bank for investigation. Tylenol can be used for fever. Pre-storage leukoreduction significantly decreases the incidence of this reaction.

Allergic Reactions Allergic reactions to transfusions are common. They have a spectrum of presentations, from mild skin reactions (hives, pruritus, erythema, edema) to severe life-threatening anaphylaxis. Treatment therefore targets specific symptoms in addition to stopping the transfusion and can range from antihistamines and steroids to full resuscitation requiring epinephrine for anaphylaxis. Patients with IgA deficiency may experience anaphylaxis during blood transfusions.

Transfusion-Related Acute Lung Injury (TRALI) TRALI is a leading cause of transfusion-related mortality. It is defined as an acute pulmonary injury with apparent temporal association with transfusion and cannot be explained by other pathologies clinically. Clinically, patients present with respiratory distress, hypoxemia, and tachypnea. Radiographically, it mimics the finding of acute respiratory distress syndrome (ARDS) with bilateral infiltrates, except this injury usually recovers faster than ARDS once identified. The underlying mechanism is not fully understood, but anti-HLA and anti-HNA antibodies are thought to be the main players in this type of reaction. This reaction is usually managed by stopping transfusion immediately and aggressive respiratory support.

Transfusion-Associated Graft Versus Host Disease Unlike other reactions that are discussed here, this is a delayed reaction. It is exceedingly rare but usually deadly. It happens when donor T-lymphocytes engraft and proliferate in the host, trigger an immune response, and usually affect an immunocompromised host. The clinical presentation occurs 1–6 weeks after transfusion, including fever/chill, rash, liver failure, GI symptoms, and pancytopenia. Treatment is limited, so an emphasis is made to prevent it from happening. This is the rationale behind the frequent practice of giving irradiated blood products to certain cancer patients as irradiation removes the T-lymphocytes.

References

1. Kauvar DS, Lefering R, Wade CE. Impact of hemorrhage on trauma outcome: an overview of epidemiology, clinical presentations, and therapeutic considerations. J Trauma. 2006;60(6 Suppl):S3–11.
2. Holcomb JB, et al. The prospective, observational, multicenter, major trauma transfusion (PROMMTT) study: comparative effectiveness of a time-varying treatment with competing risks. JAMA Surg. 2013;148(2):127–36.
3. Holcomb JB, et al. Transfusion of plasma, platelets, and red blood cells in a 1:1:1 vs a 1:1:2 ratio and mortality in patients with severe trauma: the PROPPR randomized clinical trial. JAMA. 2015;313(5):471–82.
4. Cotton BA, et al. A randomized controlled pilot trial of modified whole blood versus component therapy in severely injured patients requiring large volume transfusions. Ann Surg. 2013;258(4):527–32; discussion 532–3.
5. Guyette FX, et al. Prehospital low titer group O whole blood is feasible and safe: results of a prospective randomized pilot trial. J Trauma Acute Care Surg. 2022;92(5):839–47.

6. Dhara S, et al. Modern management of bleeding, clotting, and coagulopathy in trauma patients: what is the role of viscoelastic assays? Curr Trauma Rep. 2020;6(1):69–81.

7. Dias JD, et al. New-generation thromboelastography: comprehensive evaluation of citrated and heparinized blood sample storage effect on clot-forming variables. Arch Pathol Lab Med. 2017;141(4):569–77.

8. AABB. Circular of information for the use of human blood and blood components (circular). 2022.

9. Carless PA, et al. Transfusion thresholds and other strategies for guiding allogeneic red blood cell transfusion. Cochrane Database Syst Rev. 2010;10:CD002042.

10. Khan AI, Gupta G. Non-infectious complications of blood transfusion. In: StatPearls. Treasure Island: StatPearls Publishing LLC.; 2022.

11. Mack JP, Miles J, Stolla M. Cold-stored platelets: review of studies in humans. Transfus Med Rev. 2020;34(4):221–6.

12. Kaufman RM, et al. Platelet transfusion: a clinical practice guideline from the AABB. Ann Intern Med. 2015;162(3):205–13.

13. Levy JH, Goodnough LT. How I use fibrinogen replacement therapy in acquired bleeding. Blood. 2015;125(9):1387–93.

14. Sørensen B, Bevan D. A critical evaluation of cryoprecipitate for replacement of fibrinogen. Br J Haematol. 2010;149(6):834–43.

15. Tomaselli GF, et al. 2017 ACC expert consensus decision pathway on management of bleeding in patients on oral anticoagulants: a report of the American College of Cardiology Task Force on expert consensus decision pathways. J Am Coll Cardiol. 2017;70(24):3042–67.

16. Sen Gupta A. Hemoglobin-based oxygen carriers: current state-of-the-art and novel molecules. Shock. 2019;52(1S Suppl 1):70–83.

17. American National Red Cross. Risks and complications. Available from: https://www.redcrossblood.org/donate-blood/blood-donation-process/what-happens-to-donated-blood/blood-transfusions/risks-complications.html#:~:text=Acute%20Immune%20Hemolytic%20Reaction&text=The%20attack%20triggers%20a%20release,back%20pain%2C%20and%20dark%20urine.

18. Hendrickson JE, Hillyer CD. Noninfectious serious hazards of transfusion. Anesth Analg. 2009;108(3):759–69.

19. Vamvakas EC, Blajchman MA. Transfusion-related mortality: the ongoing risks of allogeneic blood transfusion and the available strategies for their prevention. Blood. 2009;113(15):3406–17.

20. Yazer MH, et al. Rebirth of the cool: the modern renaissance of low titer group O whole blood for treating massively bleeding civilian patients. Ann Blood. 2022;7:17.

Chapter 9
The Primary Survey

Christopher D. Graham and Rajika Jindani

Introduction

The primary survey consists of the "ABCDEs" of trauma care which can be assessed in a quick sequence:

- Airway maintenance and cervical spine protection
- Breathing and ventilation
- Circulation with hemorrhage control
- Disability (assessment of neurologic status)
- Exposure/environmental control

There are nuanced arguments to replace "the ABCs" with "the CABs" in penetrating trauma by certain trauma centers and the military, acknowledging the need for prompt hemorrhage control in venues with higher proportions of penetrating trauma. Additionally, in tertiary trauma centers with multiple providers, multiple evaluations can occur concurrently (i.e., exposure being obtained at the same time as airway and breathing evaluation). At this time, the Advanced Trauma Life Support® (ATLS) course taught by the American College of Surgeons (ACS) still teaches "ABC" order resuscitation, presuming practice in an austere environment, as we will, in this chapter.

C. D. Graham (✉)
Rutgers New Jersey Medical School/University Hospital,
Newark, NJ, USA

Rutgers New Jersey Medical School/University Hospital, Newark, NJ, USA

R. Jindani
Department of General Surgery, Albert Einstein College of Medicine/Montefiore Medical Center, Bronx, NY, USA
e-mail: rjindani@montefiore.org

© The Author(s), under exclusive license to Springer Nature Switzerland AG 2025
T. S. Brahmbhatt, D. R. Scantling (eds.), *Trauma Surgery Clerkship*, Contemporary Surgical Clerkships,
https://doi.org/10.1007/978-3-032-01412-2_9

Adjuncts to the primary survey include chest X-ray, pelvis X-ray, and the focused assessment with sonography in trauma (FAST) exam, which can be done prior to starting the secondary survey.

Airway Maintenance and Cervical Spine Protection

- The first step in the primary survey is evaluating the patency of the patient's airway. This can be done by asking patients to state their name or asking what occurred during the event.
- If the patient is unable to respond, interventions such as suctioning the oropharynx, identifying and removing any foreign bodies, and assessing for facial and/or neck trauma or burn injury must be undertaken. This includes briefly removing a cervical collar, if present, while maintaining cervical stabilization in order to evaluate for neck trauma.

Emergencies That Need a Definitive Airway
- Patients with a depressed mental status, unable to protect their airway.
- Those with severe hemodynamic instability (importantly, this should be done following resuscitation as intubation of a hypotensive trauma patient will worsen the hypotension and may cause cardiac arrest if hypovolemia is present).
- Those with high risk for airway obstruction including facial and neck trauma.

Types of Airways
- Typically, patients that require a definite airway undergo endotracheal intubation.
- Other types of airways that can be used are laryngeal mask airway, nasotracheal intubation, a supraglottic airway device (which may be used as a temporary method to secure an open airway), and surgical airways.
- Surgical airways are established in emergency situations when the upper airway is obstructed due to massive facial trauma, obstructing foreign body, or in response to failed intubation.
- The most common emergent airway is a cricothyrotomy, which is established by inserting a tube through an incision in the cricothyroid membrane.

Breathing and Ventilation

The next step is to confirm the airway and ensure the patient is ventilating and oxygenating properly.

- On physical exam, symmetrical chest rise, tracheal position, jugular venous distention, deformities to the chest wall, such as flail chest, penetrating injuries, or significant chest wounds, and appearance of the chest wall should be evaluated.

- Both lungs should be auscultated to identify audible breath sounds and note if there are decreased or asymmetric breath sounds at any point.

Injuries That Must Be Identified and Treated Rapidly
- Tension pneumothorax
- Massive pneumothorax
- Hemothorax
- Open pneumothorax ("sucking" chest wound)
- These can be identified on physical exam, with findings of absent breath sounds, tracheal deviation, and hemodynamic instability.
- These diagnoses are confirmed with chest radiograph, and prompt action should be taken, though in extremis, definitive management should not be delayed awaiting radiographic confirmation.

Circulation with Hemorrhage Control

- Assessing a patient's circulation includes acquiring basic hemodynamic vital signs, rapidly identifying sources of hemorrhage (and intervening if possible), obtaining vascular access, and beginning resuscitation.
- Obtain the patient's vital signs. Prior to placement on a monitor, one should palpate a truncal (femoral or carotid) pulse and obtain a manual blood pressure.
- Tachycardia could be indicative of pain or stress but is a sign of hemorrhage in a trauma patient until ruled out.
- Other indicators of hemorrhage include changes in blood pressure, such as a decreased systolic blood pressure or narrowed pulse pressure.
- Hypotension in adults is a systolic blood pressure less than 90 mmHg.
- Hemodynamic instability = hypotension and tachycardia.
- Intravenous access must be established, ideally on both upper extremities in the antecubital fossa with large bore IVs, in order to ensure patient can be resuscitated adequately. In a patient with difficult IV access, intraosseous (IO) lines may be placed as a bridge to IV cannulation, and central venous lines may be placed, usually with short, wide catheters, such as Cordis catheters (and not a triple-lumen catheter).

Hemorrhagic Shock
- All traumatically injured patients in shock are assumed to be in hemorrhagic (hypovolemic) shock initially. Hemorrhagic shock must be ruled out prior to investigating other potential sources of shock.
- Hemorrhagic shock can be classified by amount of blood loss and expected physiologic responses.
- Other clinical factors should be incorporated in assessment, such as medications a patient is taking and baseline vitals.
- Classically, there are five compartments that are large enough to contain blood volumes that could cause hemorrhagic shock and death:

- Thoracic cavity
- Peritoneal cavity
- Retroperitoneum/pelvis
- Long bones, such as the femur
- The environment ("bleeding out")

- In terms of management, hemorrhagic shock can occur in three zones of the body: extremity, junctional (inguinal, axillary, neck), or truncal.

  - *Extremity bleeding* can usually be controlled with direct pressure, packing, or tourniquet application.
  - *Junctional hemorrhage* is classically more difficult to control but attempts to control can be made with direct pressure and packing, as well as junctional tourniquets.
  - *Truncal hemorrhage* usually requires surgical or interventional radiographic control.

- Patients in hemorrhagic shock should be resuscitated with immediate transfusion of blood products. Depending on the capabilities of the hospital, this should be with either whole blood (WB), or component blood (packed red blood cells (PRBC), fresh frozen plasma (FFP), and platelets) in a 1:1:1 ratio.
- Early evaluation for initiation of massive transfusion protocol (MTP) should be considered. The ABC (assessment of blood consumption) score assigns one point for each of: penetrating mechanism, positive FAST, arrival HR >120 bpm, arrival SBP <90 mmHg. Two or more points is 75% sensitive and 82% specific for predicting the need for an MTP.
- In patients undergoing MTP, rapid administration of tranexamic acid (TXA) and calcium should be considered, as these patients often present hypocalcemia and with increased fibrinolysis.

Disability

- The patient's neurologic status should be assessed by assessing gross neurologic function, pupillary size and reaction, level of consciousness, and Glasgow Coma Scale (GCS).
- The GCS (Fig. 9.1) is a tool that is used to calculate a patient's level of consciousness and can be categorized into three groups:

  - 13+: mild traumatic brain injury (TBI)
  - 9–12: moderate TBI
  - 3–8: severe TBI

- A depressed neurologic exam could be due to many factors, such as alcohol intoxication, drug or medication effects, shock state. These should be "diagnoses

Fig. 9.1 Glasgow Coma
Scale

Eye opening	
Spontaneous	4
Open to verbal command	3
Open to pain	2
No eye opening	1
Verbal response	
Oriented	5
Confused	4
Inappropriate words	3
Incomprehensible sounds	2
No verbal response	1
Motor response	
Follows commands	6
Localizes to pain	5
Withdraws to pain	4
Flexes to pain	3
Extends to pain	2
No movement	1
Total score	**3–15**

of exclusion," i.e., TBI must be ruled out prior to presuming intoxication as a cause of altered mental status.

Exposure and Environmental Control

- Expose the patient completely to assess for any missed injury.
- All clothing must be removed from the patient and patient must be log-rolled to assess for spinal tenderness, evaluate for perineal or rectal injury, and examine axilla.
- All penetrating injuries should be identified and marked with radio-opaque markers to allow for trajectory to be noted on imaging. It is our practice to use paperclips for this purpose as open paperclips on posterior injuries (vs. closed paperclips anteriorly) allow for three-dimensional trajectory interpretation.
- Patient should be covered with warm blankets to prevent hypothermia after full exposure and evaluation.

Adjuncts
- *Chest X-ray*: Obtain as part of the primary trauma survey, analyzing it methodically in an "ABCDE" pattern: ensure midline and unobstructed airway, check for hemothorax or pneumothorax, evaluate cardiac border and possible great vessel injury, assess diaphragm borders and presence of fluid or herniation, and examine for fractures, subcutaneous emphysema, and foreign bodies.
- *Pelvic X-ray*: Obtain for patients with pelvic tenderness, unstable pelvis, unexplained hemodynamic instability, unreliable exam, or significant mechanism of injury. This is used for evaluating for pelvic ring disruption, acetabular fractures, sacral fractures, and retained foreign bodies.
- Additional X-rays may be obtained based on the trauma team leader's discretion, including for missile trajectory assessment (cavitary triage) and suspected long-bone fractures, but in hemodynamically unstable patients, obtaining these images should not delay definitive care unless they provide crucial information for the patient's resuscitation.
- *FAST exam*: A rapid method to identify free fluid in the peritoneal or pericardial spaces, consisting of four views (right upper quadrant, left upper quadrant, suprapubic, and subxiphoid cardiac), with an extended version including pleural cavity views for hemo- or pneumothorax detection.

The primary survey checklist	
A	☐ Confirm airway is protected ☐ Evaluate for need for intubation ☐ If endotracheally intubated, note ET tube size and depth ☐ If intubated, confirm via $ETCO_2$ ☐ Confirm C-spine is immobilized and evaluate neck for injuries with cervical collar opened
B	☐ Check O_2 saturation ☐ Expose chest and note any signs of injury (penetrating wound, laceration, bruising, etc.) ☐ Listen for breath sounds, note chest movement ☐ If supplemental oxygen is needed, place nasal cannula or non-rebreather ☐ Based on hemodynamics and physical exam, determine if any urgent intervention indicated, such as tube thoracostomy
C	☐ Obtain manual blood pressure measurement ☐ Check for presence of truncal pulse ☐ Identify sites of external hemorrhage and control with direct pressure or tourniquet, as indicated ☐ Establish vascular access (preferably two large bore IV if accessible) ☐ Draw full set of labs with type and cross ☐ Determine whether blood products are needed
D	☐ Determine GCS ☐ State pupil size and response ☐ Note extremity movement and any lateralizing signs (i.e., hemiparesis)

The primary survey checklist	
E	☐ Expose patient by removing clothing ☐ Log roll patient, holding C-spine if necessary, checking if patient has spinal tenderness ☐ Complete a perineal/rectal exam and axillary exam bilaterally ☐ Cover with warm blanket
Repeat	☐ For any acute change in clinical course (vital signs, patient responsiveness), repeat primary survey
Adjuncts	☐ Chest X-ray ☐ Pelvic X-ray ☐ FAST exam
Monitor	☐ Confirm monitors hooked up for continuous oxygen saturation, end tidal CO_2, blood pressure, heart rate, respiratory rate ☐ Confirm waveforms on monitors
Vitals	Evaluate whether within normal limits: ☐ Heart rate ☐ Oxygen saturation ☐ Blood pressure ☐ Respiratory rate ☐ Temperature

Bibliography

1. Cannon JW. Hemorrhagic shock. N Engl J Med. 2018;378:370–9. https://doi.org/10.1056/NEJMra1705649.
2. Gondek S, Schroeder ME, Sarani B. Assessment and resuscitation in trauma management. Surg Clin North Am. 2017;97(5):985–98. https://doi.org/10.1016/j.suc.2017.06.001.
3. Kostiuk M, Burns B. Trauma assessment. [Updated 2022 May 29]. In: StatPearls [Internet]. Treasure Island: StatPearls Publishing; 2022. [Figure, Glasgow Coma Scale (GCS). Created by Michael Kostiuk, DO] Available from: https://www.ncbi.nlm.nih.gov/books/NBK555913/figure/article-30531.image.f1/.
4. McKenna P, Desai NM, Tariq A, et al. Cricothyrotomy. [Updated 2022 Dec 1]. In: StatPearls [Internet]. Treasure Island: StatPearls Publishing; 2022. Available from: https://www.ncbi.nlm.nih.gov/books/NBK537350/.
5. Mehta R, Chinthapalli K. Glasgow coma scale explained. BMJ. 2019;365:l1296. https://doi.org/10.1136/bmj.l1296. PMID: 31048343.
6. Planas JH, Waseem M, Sigmon DF. Trauma primary survey. [Updated 2022 Aug 7]. In: StatPearls [Internet]. Treasure Island: StatPearls Publishing; 2022. Available from: https://www.ncbi.nlm.nih.gov/books/NBK430800/.
7. Stead T, Lee J, Huang D, et al. Massive spontaneous pneumothorax. Cureus. 2022;14(1):e20992. https://doi.org/10.7759/cureus.20992.
8. American College of Surgeons. Trauma I – ABCs of trauma. ACS/ASE Medical Student Core Curriculum, American College of Surgeons Division of Education, Blended Surgical Education and Training for Life. https://www.facs.org/quality-programs/trauma/.
9. Nunez TC, Voskresensky IV, Dossett LA, Shinall R, Dutton WD, Cotton BA. Early prediction of massive transfusion in trauma: simple as ABC (assessment of blood consumption)? J Trauma. 2009;66(2):346–52. https://doi.org/10.1097/TA.0b013e3181961c35.

Chapter 10
The Tertiary Survey

Noelle N. Saillant and Jeffrey Melvin

Introduction

The tertiary survey is a complete head to toe physical exam performed around 24 h after traumatic injury or before discharge (if discharge is sooner than 24 h) with the purpose of detecting injuries that were not identified during the primary or secondary survey. The tertiary survey provides the opportunity to reassess identified injuries and confirm or exclude suspected injuries. It should ideally be performed in an awake, coherent and non-obtunded patient. It also serves as an opportunity to review labs, evaluate final radiology reads, and address any incidental findings on imaging.

Background

- The tertiary survey was first proposed as an adjunct to the primary and secondary survey by Dr. Blaine Enderson at the University of Tennessee Medical Center in a landmark study in 1990 after noticing that life-threatening injuries, emergent operation, or unconsciousness upon presentation interfered with a comprehensive exam and led to missed injuries [1].

N. N. Saillant
Division of Acute Care and Trauma Surgery, Boston Medical Center, Boston University
Chobanian and Avedisian School of Medicine, Boston, MA, USA
e-mail: Noelle.saillant@bmc.org

J. Melvin (✉)
Department of Surgery, Boston Medical Center, Boston University Chobanian and Avedisian
School of Medicine, Boston, MA, USA
e-mail: Jeffrey.Melvin@bmc.org

© The Author(s), under exclusive license to Springer Nature
Switzerland AG 2025
T. S. Brahmbhatt, D. R. Scantling (eds.), *Trauma Surgery Clerkship*,
Contemporary Surgical Clerkships,
https://doi.org/10.1007/978-3-032-01412-2_10

Table 3 Frequency of Various Body Region Injuries before (PRE) and after (POST) Implementation of a Formal Tertiary Trauma Survey

	PRE (1997–1998)	POST (2000–2001)
Extremity fracture	31	27
Spine fracture	16	8
Abdominal injury	16	9
Cervical spine injury	12	4
Brain injury	10	3
Pelvic fracture	5	0
Vascular injury	3	1
Diaphragm rupture	3	0
Total Injuries	96	59

- A missed injury can lead to prolonged hospital stays, readmissions, increased morbidity, and even death [2, 3].
- Since its implementation at trauma centers nationwide, it has significantly reduced the incidence of missed injury in the acutely traumatized patient, decreasing missed injuries by up to 36% (Fig. 10.1) [4, 5].

The Trauma Workup

- Trauma workup begins at the initial time of evaluation. It begins with a primary and secondary survey as discussed in the previous chapters.
- The primary survey serves to assess and treat any life-threatening injuries promptly. The secondary survey is then performed to diagnose all injuries before formulating a definitive management plan.
- The role of the tertiary survey is to reevaluate the patient to assess for more subtle injuries that may have been missed during the initial triage as the rate of missed injury has been reported to be as high as 9% [1, 2, 6].

Initial Approach to the Tertiary Survey

- The tertiary survey is a structured head to toe physical examination following major trauma and can be repeated as needed.
- It should include a comprehensive review of all imaging and laboratory work obtained during the admission.
- Many trauma centers have their own standard form and/or structure to completing the tertiary survey (Figs. 10.2 and 10.3).

SURGERY TERTIARY EXAM

GCS
GCS (Eye Opening, Motor Response, Verbal Response)

SCALP
Inspect and palpate Scalp for:
Laceration/Abrasions, Ecchymosis

FACE
Inspect and palpate Face for:
Lac/Abrasion, Swelling, Ecchymosis, Fractures

EYES
Examine Eyes / Record:
Eye movement, Pupil size/Reaction, and Visual Acuity

MOUTH
Inspect Mouth / Ears for:
Malocclusion, Teeth problem, CSF leak, Hemotympanum

NECK
Inspect Neck for:
Laceration/Abrasion, Hematoma, Swelling, Subcutaneous air, Tenderness
C-Spine cleared radiographically? and C-Spine cleared clinically?

CHEST
Inspect Chest for:
Laceration / Abrasion, Swelling, Ecchymosis and Subcutaneous air
Palpate for tenderness or deformity:
Ribs, Sternum, Clavicle, Flail and Paradoxical movement

CXR
Evaluate for hemothorax / pneumothorax and mediastinal abnormalities

ABDOMEN
Inspect Abdomen for:
Laceration/Abrasion, Swelling, and Ecchymosis
Palpate for:
Tenderness/Guarding and Masses

PELVIS
Assess stability and review pelvic X-ray

BACK
Inspect back of head/entire back for:
Laceration/Abrasion, Swelling and Ecchymosis
Inspect for tenderness and deformity
Vertebrae (T-L-S Spine) and Ribs

EXTREMITIES
Inspect upper and lower extremities for:
Laceration / Abrasion, Swelling, Ecchymosis
Palpate for tenderness or deformity and assess:
Ribs, Sternum, Clavicle, Flail chest, and Paradoxical movement

PULSES
Palpate Radial: Left, Right
Palpate Dorsal pedal: Left, Right
Palpate Posterior tibial: Left, Right

PERIPHERAL NERVES
Assess Motor: Ulnar, Median Distal, Median, Anterior Interosseus, Musculocutaneous, Radial, Axillary, Femoral, Obturator, Posterior Tibial, Superficial Peroneal, Deep Peroneal, Sciatic Nerve, Superior Gluteal and Inferior Gluteal and
Assess Sensation: Ulnar, Median Distal, Median, Anterior Interosseus, Musculocutaneous, Radial, Axillary, Femoral, Obturator, Posterior Tibial, Superficial Peroneal, Deep Peroneal, Sciatic Nerve, Superior Gluteal and Inferior Gluteal

IMAGING STUDIES
Review Final Report

Fig. 10.2   Boston Medical Center tertiary survey

The Exam

- The physical exam should be completed in a systematic and standardized way to ensure it can be done by any provider.
- It begins with determination of the patient's Glasgow Coma Score (GCS)

  - If a patient's score is anything less than 15 it is important to consider if the patient will be able to provide a reliable exam.

- The patient should not be intoxicated.
- The physical exam then continues from the head down with inspection and palpation of the scalp (where lacerations are commonly missed). It then moves to the face looking for lacerations, abrasions, and ecchymosis. Pupil response, eye movement, and visual acuity should be assessed at this time.
- The patient should be asked to open and close their mouth to assess for broken teeth and malocclusion.
- During physical exam of the neck, special attention should be paid to the cervical spine as cervical collar (C-collar) clearance can be assessed at this time.

Fig. 10.3 Primarily visual, the caption is that it is the tertiary form for university of florida. Does not need further description. From Shands Hospital at the University of Florida: Trauma and Emergency Surgery Tertiary Survey Form

Trauma and Emergency Surgery Tertiary Survey Form (page 1 of 2)

Date:
Admission Date: Admission Time:
HPI Recap (MOI, Interventions, Hospital Course):

Past Med / Surg Hist:

Social Hist:

Physical Examination	Lacerations / Abrasions / Burns (Document Location / Size)
VS:	
T: P: BP: R:	
GCS:	
Eyes: Verbal: Motor:	
HEENT:	
Neck:	
CV:	
Resp / Chest:	
Abd / Rectal:	
GU:	
Extremities:	
Neuro /CN. Extremities):	

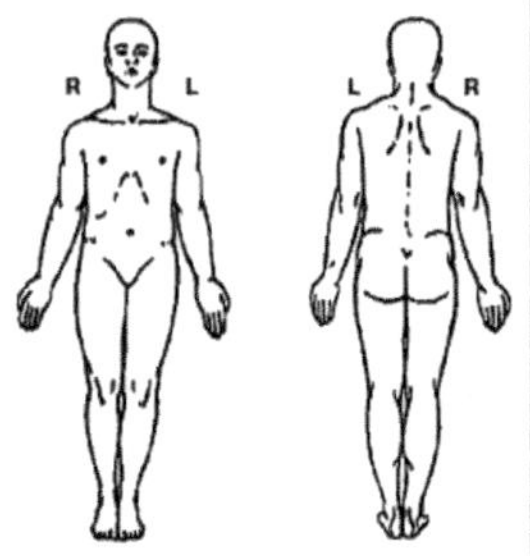

Trauma and Emergency Surgery Tertiary Survey Form (page 2 of 2)

Consults / Interventions (include dates):
Neurosurgery:

Orthopaedics:

Plastics / ENT / OMFS:

Urology:

Others:

Radiologic Findings (Please provide FINAL READS):
Plain Films
CXR:

Pelvis:

T/L/S Spine:

Extremities:

CT / MR
Chest:

Abdomen / Pelvis:

Other:

Laboratory Trends:

Plan:

MD Signature _____ MD# _____ Date / Time _____

MD Signature _____ MD# _____ Date / Time _____

Patient Name: Patient Identification #:

- Physical exam of the chest and abdomen is then performed to evaluate for any lacerations, tenderness, swelling, ecchymosis, or deformity.
    - Palpate the ribs, sternum, and clavicles
- The exam then moves to the back to assess for any spinal tenderness or deformities in the thoracic, lumbar, or sacral spine.
- Extremities can then be evaluated to look for deformities, tenderness, swelling, or lacerations
    - Do not forget the digits
- Strength and range of motion of extremities must be assessed at this stage.
- This is also a good time to assess peripheral pulses and nerves.

Timing of the Tertiary Survey

- The tertiary survey is typically completed within 24 h of a patient's initial presentation or before a discharge sooner than 24 h [4, 5].
- However, it may need to be repeated during admission as many patients may have an altered mental status that will make the exam unreliable

What to Do with New Physical Exam Findings

- If the head to toe physical exam reveals any abnormalities or concerns, there should be a low threshold to obtain further imaging studies
- Lacerations that are found and have not been repaired must be washed out to prevent infection. They should be repaired on a case-by-case basis.

C-Collar Clearance

- Many patients following major blunt trauma are placed in a C-collar in the field or upon presentation to the trauma bay.
- To clear a C-collar, one must review imaging of the cervical spine if performed (CT scan or X-ray), determine if the patient is reliable, and then perform a physical exam.
- In patients who did receive imaging for their C-spine after blunt trauma, a CT scan was effective for ruling out clinically significant injury with a sensitivity of 98.5% [7].

– In the *reliable patient*, perform a physical exam. If there is pain in the neck during any part of the physical exam, the C-collar cannot be cleared.

  • Gross inspection
  • Palpation of midline
  • Passive motion
  • Active motion

– In the *unreliable patient* (confused, intoxicated, sedated, or obtunded), physical exam will not be accurate.

  • If the patient's age is less than 65 and clinical exam cannot be performed but has negative CT imaging and is observed moving all extremities equally against gravity, then the cervical spine can be cleared.

Missed Radiologic Injuries

• Life-threatening injuries may be immediately apparent on imaging and physical exam, but occult injuries may not be seen on preliminary reports.
• All radiologic imaging obtained must be thoroughly reviewed as part of the tertiary survey.

Incidental Radiologic Findings

• Incidental findings on imaging are common with the acutely traumatized patient.
• Appropriate documentation and follow-up are important for these findings.

Classification and Examples of Incidental Radiologic Findings

• Classification [8, 9]

  – Category I: potentially severe condition requiring further diagnostic workup or intervention.
  – Category II: diagnostic workup dependent on patients' symptoms. Requires follow-up.
  – Category III: findings of minor concern requiring no diagnostic workup or follow-up.

• Incidence

  – 44.5% of patients receiving a "total body" CT (head, neck, chest, abdomen, pelvis) scan had at least one incidental finding [8].

- – Category III findings were 68.8% of the incidental findings.
- Common Incidental Findings
  - – Category I: pulmonary masses, adrenal masses, aortic aneurysms >5 cm.
  - – Category II: cardiomegaly, fatty liver disease, mediastinal lymphadenopathy, hernias, enlarged common bile duct.
  - – Category III: thyroid nodules, liver cysts, renal cysts, diverticulosis, pulmonary nodules.
- After discovery of these findings, it is important to update the patient or healthcare proxy, document the finding in the medical record, and have a plan for appropriate follow-up.

Substance Use

- Many acutely traumatized patients may have comorbid substance use disorders and their time in the hospital can serve as a jumping point for counseling and getting help.
- It is important to ask patients about their substance use and offer to refer them to counseling service.

Referrals

- Domestic violence and abuse should be appropriately referred to support and protections services where appropriate.
- Trauma patients often represent a vulnerable patient population. Using a trauma admission or observation to help patients engage with a primary care provider before discharge can be invaluable to their health.
- Incidental findings on imaging may need outpatient follow-up with the appropriate provider.

Pitfalls of the Tertiary Survey

- The Critically Ill Patient
  - – Patients in the intensive care unit (ICU), patients with traumatic brain injuries, and patients undergoing emergent surgical procedures are at highest risk of having a missed injury so it is important to have a high index of suspicion in these patients [4, 10].

- It is good practice to examine these patients at 24 h after initial presentation and again when the patient is able to participate in the exam.
- The Intoxicated Patient
  - Some patients may be under the influence of substances or pain medication during the tertiary survey, so it is important to ensure the patient is reliable before performing the tertiary survey.
  - It may be necessary to repeat the tertiary exam later on during the hospital course to ensure injuries are not missed.

References

1. Enderson BL, Reath DB, Meadors J, Dallas W, DeBoo JM, Maull KI. The tertiary trauma survey: a prospective study of missed injury. J Trauma. 1990;30(6):666–9; discussion 669–670.
2. Houshian S, Larsen MS, Holm C. Missed injuries in a level I trauma center. J Trauma. 2002;52(4):715–9.
3. Robertson R, Mattox R, Collins T, Parks-Miller C, Eidt J, Cone J. Missed injuries in a rural area trauma center. Am J Surg. 1996;172(5):564–7; discussion 567–568.
4. Biffl WL, Harrington DT, Cioffi WG. Implementation of a tertiary trauma survey decreases missed injuries. J Trauma. 2003;54(1):38–43; discussion 43–34.
5. Janjua KJ, Sugrue M, Deane SA. Prospective evaluation of early missed injuries and the role of tertiary trauma survey. J Trauma. 1998;44(6):1000–6; discussion 1006–1007.
6. Giannakopoulos GF, Saltzherr TP, Beenen LF, et al. Missed injuries during the initial assessment in a cohort of 1124 level-1 trauma patients. Injury. 2012;43(9):1517–21.
7. Inaba K, Byerly S, Bush LD, et al. Cervical spinal clearance: a prospective Western Trauma Association Multi-institutional Trial. J Trauma Acute Care Surg. 2016;81(6):1122–30.
8. Sierink JC, Saltzherr TP, Russchen MJ, et al. Incidental findings on total-body CT scans in trauma patients. Injury. 2014;45(5):840–4.
9. Paluska TR, Sise MJ, Sack DI, Sise CB, Egan MC, Biondi M. Incidental CT findings in trauma patients: incidence and implications for care of the injured. J Trauma. 2007;62(1):157–61.
10. Buduhan G, McRitchie DI. Missed injuries in patients with multiple trauma. J Trauma. 2000;49(4):600–5.

Chapter 11
Initial Imaging of the Trauma Patient

Miriam Y. Neufeld and Sabrina E. Sanchez

Introduction

For the trauma patient, it is essential to identify the presence and location of life-threatening injury quickly. Imaging in the trauma bay can provide rapid, noninvasive, and relatively accurate assessment of the location of traumatic injuries and can help inform decisions about next steps in management [1]. The use of ultrasonography and plain radiography allows for the trauma team to perform rapid cavitary triage: initial triage of all major body cavities including the chest, abdomen, and pelvis. Additionally, it can identify injury to the heart that may be contributory to shock. The ultimate goal is to identify hemodynamically significant sites of injury [2].

Imaging Assistance in Cavitary Triage

Chest

In the chest, hemodynamic instability can result from injury to the lungs, thoracic and mediastinal vasculature, or the heart. Initial imaging in the trauma bay may not be able to identify exact locations or types of injury but can show evidence of

M. Y. Neufeld
Indiana University School of Medicine, Indianapolis, IN, USA
e-mail: mneufeld1@iuhealth.org

S. E. Sanchez (✉)
Boston University Chobanian and Avedisian School of Medicine, Boston, MA, USA
e-mail: Sabrina.Sanchez@bmc.org

© The Author(s), under exclusive license to Springer Nature   91
Switzerland AG 2025
T. S. Brahmbhatt, D. R. Scantling (eds.), *Trauma Surgery Clerkship*,
Contemporary Surgical Clerkships,
https://doi.org/10.1007/978-3-032-01412-2_11

pneumothorax, hemothorax, mediastinal widening, and pericardial effusion. The rapid assessment of this body cavity facilitates prompt management of these injuries, which can often start in the trauma bay. Assessment of this cavity can be achieved with plain film radiography and ultrasound. In the absence of imaging, cavitary triage of the thorax can be achieved with placement of chest tubes and looking for physiologic signs of tamponade.

Chest Radiography

- Initial screening tool for chest injuries [3].
- Can help to identify moderate to large pneumothoraces [4] (see Fig. 11.1).
- Can identify hemothorax with greater than 250 ml of blood [5] (see Fig. 11.2).

  - Hemothorax may be visualized as blunting of costophrenic angles and haziness [5].
  - Chest radiograph done in the supine position, as is customary in the trauma bay, are more limited and may need as much as 1 L of blood before significant changes are seen [2].

- Mediastinal widening (6–8 cm) can indicate traumatic rupture of the aorta [6].

Ultrasonography of the Chest

- There is growing evidence that point-of-care ultrasound (POCUS) is useful in diagnosing hemothorax and pneumothorax, and has greater sensitivity and specificity compared to chest radiography [3].
- The extended Focused Assessment with Sonography for Trauma (eFAST) includes oblique views of the hemidiaphragms (anterior axillary line between the sixth and ninth ribs) to evaluate for dependent fluid and anterior views (left and right midclavicular line between second and third rib spaces) to evaluate for pneumothorax [7]. More details can be found in the FAST chapter of this book.

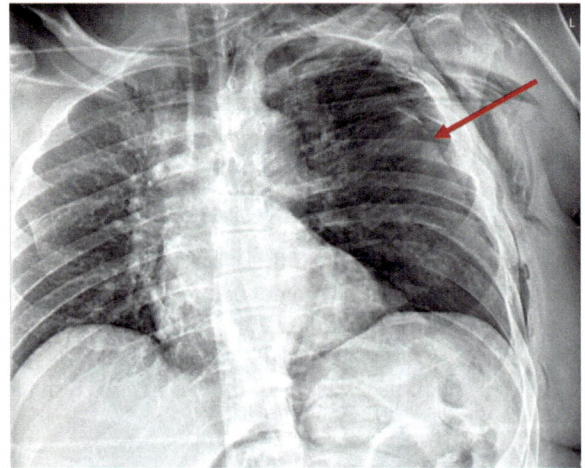

Fig. 11.1 Left-sided pneumothorax with evidence of lucency in the lateral chest, a visible visceral pleural edge, absence of lung markings beyond the line, and lucency around the pectoralis muscle indicating subcutaneous emphysema (arrow indicates edge of the pleura)

Fig. 11.2 Left-sided
hemothorax with evidence
of a fluid meniscus and
blunting of the
costophrenic angle

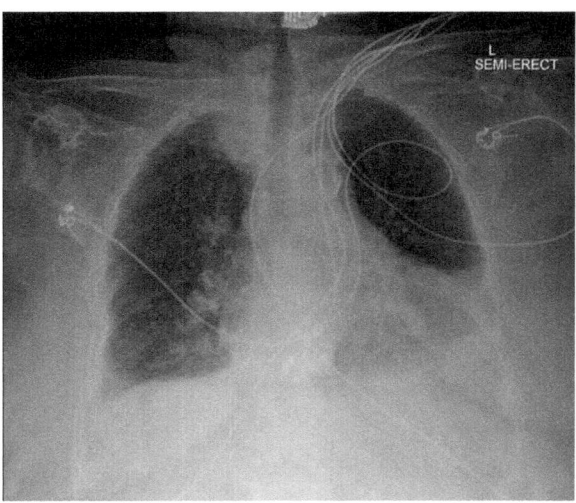

Cardiac Ultrasonography

- The pericardial view is a key component and one of the four conventional views of the FAST [1] and evaluates for hemopericardium.

- Accumulation of fluid in the pericardium prevents cardiac compliance, resulting in shock. Findings include right ventricular collapse during diastole and inferior vena cava (IVC) plethora (failure of the IVC to collapse during inspiration) [1]. More details can be found in the FAST chapter of this book.

Abdomen

Early recognition of intraabdominal hemorrhage is challenging based on physical exam alone. Differentiating the abdomen from other cavities as the source of hemodynamic instability is critical as it has significant implications on management. Ultrasonography has become ubiquitous in trauma resuscitations in evaluating for the presence of free fluid in the abdomen. Historically, direct peritoneal lavage was used to determine the presence of blood or enteral contents in the peritoneum. The FAST exam, however, is a noninvasive test that rapidly and accurately detects hemoperitoneum in the injured patient [1]. The use of ultrasonography saves time and resources in those patients who have hemodynamic instability and multiple injuries for whom accurate and rapid cavitary triage is essential. More details on the use of FAST for cavitary triage of the abdomen can be found in the FAST chapter of this book.

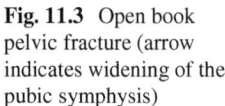

Fig. 11.3 Open book pelvic fracture (arrow indicates widening of the pubic symphysis)

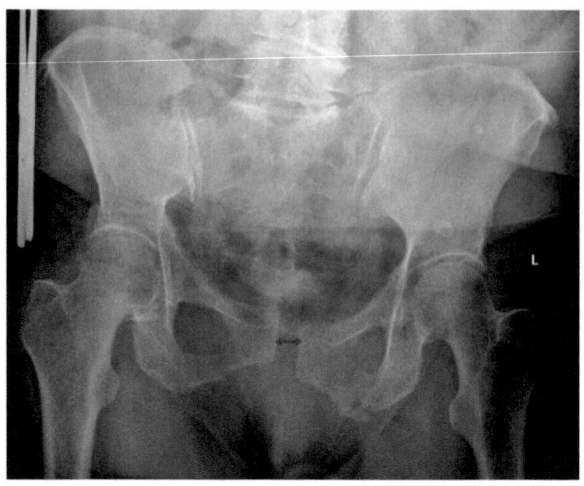

Pelvis

Pelvic trauma can lead to hemodynamically significant hemorrhage. The pelvic ring is anatomically connected to a large number of blood vessels. Hemorrhage remains a significant cause of death in those presenting with pelvic fractures [8]. While a view of the pelvis is included in the FAST exam (suprapubic view), retroperitoneal hemorrhage in this area may not be visible with ultrasonography. In addition to physical exam, plain film radiography can help to assess for pelvic fracture that may be contributing to hemodynamic instability.

Pelvic Radiography

- Best screening test for pelvic fracture and will reveal 90% of pelvic bony injuries [9].
- Anteroposterior pelvic radiograph is a rapid diagnostic tool for hemodynamically unstable patients allowing for early intervention [9] (Fig. 11.3).
- Allows for assessment of pelvic symmetry [10].

Cross-Sectional Imaging

After the initial evaluation of a trauma patient, further evaluation can be pursued with cross-sectional imaging depending on the patient's history and physical examination, clinical status, and mechanism of injury. Computed tomography (CT) is the imaging of choice to further evaluate hemodynamically stable patients after the secondary survey is completed [11].

Brain

- Adult patients with trauma to the head, altered mental status, loss of consciousness, or amnesia should get a CT scan [11].
- Pediatric patients with trauma to the head should be evaluated based on the Pediatric Emergency Care Applied Research Network (PECARN) guidelines. In specific, children with non-frontal soft tissue hematoma, brief loss of consciousness, or severe mechanism of injury but without other symptoms may undergo CT or observation, with observation being reasonable to be performed in the emergency department and discharge home possible as long as the patient has adequate follow-up [13].

Cervical Spine

- The National Emergency X-Radiograph Utilization Study (NEXUS) criteria or the Canadian Cervical Rules (CCR) are both appropriate to determine whether an awake, stable, adult patient requires CT of the cervical spine after traumatic injury [11].

  - NEXUS criteria: Patients with focal neurological deficits, midline spinal tenderness, altered level of consciousness, intoxication, or a distracting injury should have imaging of the cervical spine [14].
  - CCR: If age 65 or greater, dangerous mechanism, or extremity paresthesia, patient should have cervical spine imaging. If none of those are present and the patient has a Glasgow Coma Scale of 15 and only low-risk factors, including a simple rear-end MVC, sitting position in the emergency department, ability to ambulate at any time, delayed onset of neck pain, and absence of midline cervical spine tenderness, you can ask the patient to rotate their neck, and if they are able to, no imaging is needed. However, if you are unable to safely assess range of motion, you should proceed with cervical spine imaging [15].

- Patients with possible spinal cord injury based on imaging or physical exam concerns should undergo magnetic resonance imaging (MRI) of the cervical spine.
- Older adults have a higher rate of asymptomatic cervical spine injuries [16], so strong consideration should be given to image older patients more liberally.

Chest

- An intravenous (IV) contrast-enhanced chest CT should be obtained in all adult patients with high-energy torso trauma, traumatic findings on chest radiograph, or positive findings on physical exam [11].
- CT scan of the chest can also be considered for patients with altered mental status, distracting injuries, or clinically suspected thoracic injuries even in the absence of the criteria above, although its yield may be questionable.

Abdomen/Pelvis

- An IV contrast-enhanced CT of the abdomen and pelvis with both an arterial and a portal venous phase should be obtained in all adult patients with high-energy torso trauma or positive findings on physical exam [11].
- CT scan of the abdomen/pelvis can also be considered for patients with altered mental status, distracting injuries, or clinically suspected abdominal injuries even in the absence of the criteria above, although its yield may be questionable.
- A negative FAST does not rule out intraabdominal injury [11].
- A patient with a positive FAST that is hemodynamically normal may proceed to CT imaging for further evaluation. However, if there is a clear indication for laparotomy, imaging of the abdomen should not be obtained [11].
- In the absence of other injuries, it is safe to discharge patients home after blunt injury to the abdomen with a negative CT scan of the abdomen and pelvis as long as they do not have peritonitis [17].

Spine

- Patients with known cervical spine injuries, pain or tenderness of the thoracolumbar spine, neurologic abnormalities, distracting injuries, and high energy mechanisms should have imaging of the thoracolumbar spine [11].
- A normal CT of the spine obviates the need for an MRI unless a patient has signs or symptoms of spinal cord injury, conus medullaris, or nerve root injury [12].

Whole-Body CT

- Whole-body CT (WBCT, also called "panscan") involves non-contrast imaging of the head and neck (cervical spine) and contrast imaging of the chest, abdomen, and pelvis [12].

- WBCT is appropriate for the initial evaluation of hemodynamically stable high energy trauma patients or trauma patients with findings suggestive of multisystem injury after the primary and secondary surveys are completed [18].
- A negative WBCT in a high-energy trauma patient may allow for earlier discharge from the ED [17].

References

1. Bloom BA, Gibbons RC. Focused Assessment with Sonography for Trauma. [Updated 2022 Jul 25]. In: StatPearls [Internet]. Treasure Island: StatPearls Publishing; 2022. Available from: https://www-ncbi-nlm-nih-gov.ezproxy.bu.edu/books/NBK470479/.
2. Gondek S, Schroeder ME, Sarani B. Assessment and resuscitation in trauma management. Surg Clin N Am. 2017;97:985–98. Available from https://cbc.org.br/wp-content/uploads/2017/11/112017SCiii.pdf
3. Pumarejo Gomez L, Tran VH. Hemothorax. [Updated 2022 Aug 8]. In: StatPearls [Internet]. Treasure Island: StatPearls Publishing; 2022. Available from: https://www.ncbi.nlm.nih.gov/books/NBK538219/.
4. McKnight CL, Burns B. Pneumothorax. [Updated 2022 Aug 8]. In: StatPearls [Internet]. Treasure Island: StatPearls Publishing; 2022. Available from: https://www.ncbi.nlm.nih.gov/books/NBK441885/.
5. Weerakkody Y, Yap J, Feger J, et al. Hemothorax: Reference Article. Accessed on Nov 30 2022. Available from: https://radiopaedia.org/articles/24341
6. Wackerman L, Gnugnoli DM. Widened Mediastinum. [Updated 2022 Jul 25]. In: StatPearls [Internet]. Treasure Island: StatPearls Publishing; 2022. Available from: https://www.ncbi.nlm.nih.gov/books/NBK539890/.
7. American College of Emergency Physicians. ACEP Now. EFAST- Extended Focused Assessment With Sonography for Trauma. Accessed on 30 Nov 2022. Available from: https://www.acep-now.com/article/efast-extended-focused-assessment-sonography-trauma/4/?singlepage=1
8. Geeraerts T, Chhor V, Cheisson G, et al. Clinical review: initial management of blunt pelvic trauma patients with haemodynamic instability. Crit Care. 2007;11:204. Available from: https://ccforum.biomedcentral.com/articles/10.1186/cc5157
9. Davis DD, Foris LA, Kane SM, et al. Pelvic Fracture. [Updated 2022 Aug 7]. In: StatPearls [Internet]. Treasure Island: StatPearls Publishing; 2022. Available from: https://www.ncbi.nlm.nih.gov/books/NBK430734/.
10. Mirza A, Ellis T. Initial management of pelvic and femoral fractures in the multiple injured patient. Crit Care Clin. 2004;20:159–70. Available from: https://ubccriticalcaremedicine.ca/academic/jc_article/Pelvic%20and%20Femoral%20Fractures%20in%20Multitrauma%20Management%20Review%20(Feb-14-08).pdf
11. ACS TQIP Best practice guidelines in imaging. 2018. Available from: https://www.facs.org/media/oxdjw5zj/imaging_guidelines.pdf.
12. Kupperman N, Holmes JF, Dayan PS, et al. Pediatric emergency care applied research network (PECARN). Identification of children at very low risk of clinically-important brain injuries after head trauma: a prospective cohort study. Lancet. 2009;374(9696):1160–70.
13. Hoffman JR, Mower WR, Wolfson AB, et al. Validity of a set of clinical criteria to rule out injury to the cervical spine in patients with blunt trauma. National Emergency X-radiography utilization study group. N Engl J Med. 2000;343(2):94–9.
14. Stiell IG, Wells GA, Vandemheen KL, et al. The Canadian C-spine rule for radiography in alert and stable trauma patients. JAMA. 2001;286(15):1841–8.
15. Healye CD, Spillman SK, King BD, et al. Asymptomatic cervical spine fractures: current guidelines can fail older patients. J Trauma Acute Care Surg. 2017;83(1):119–25.

16. Livingston DH, Lavery RF, Passannante MR, et al. Admission or observation is not necessary after a negative abdominal computed tomographic scan in patients with suspected blunt abdominal trauma: results of a prospective multi-institutional trial. J Trauma. 1998;44(2):273–80. discussion 280–2

17. Treskes K, Saltzherr TP, Luitse JSK, et al. Indications for total-body computed tomography in blunt trauma patients: a systematic review. Eur J Trauma Emerg Surg. 2017;43:35–42.

18. Salim A, Sangthong B, Martin M, et al. Whole body imaging in blunt multisystem trauma patients without obvious signs of injury: results of a prospective study. Arch Surg. 2006;141(5):468–75.

Chapter 12
Post-trauma Bay Considerations: OR, CT, IR?

Abdimajid Mohamed and Crisanto M. Torres

Introduction

Following a rapid initial patient assessment in the trauma bay, a decision must be made to either proceed with additional diagnostic workup or to pursue immediate limb or lifesaving intervention. Standard options in the pathway include direct operating room (OR) transit, interventional radiologic (IR) management, or computed tomography (CT) scanning to supplement the secondary evaluation. All modalities have risks and benefits.

Post-trauma bay disposition relies on rapidly identifying patients who require emergent intervention; this is the first and most critical step in the decision-making pathway. Findings from the primary survey can indicate which patient will likely decompensate in the trauma bay or shortly after transport from the bay. Therefore, a rapid yet careful decision to proceed to the OR, IR, or CT is strongly influenced by findings from the primary trauma survey.

Computed tomography (CT) scan is a valuable adjunct to the secondary survey in identifying a wide range of injuries that may be difficult to identify on physical exam, X-ray, or extended focused assessment for the sonography of trauma (eFAST) exam.

A. Mohamed
Department of General Surgery, Boston University School of Medicine, Boston, MA, USA
e-mail: abdimajid.mohamed@bmc.org

C. M. Torres (✉)
Department of General Surgery, Boston University School of Medicine, Boston, MA, USA

Division of Trauma and Acute Care Surgery, Boston Medical Center, Boston, MA, USA
e-mail: crtorres@bu.edu; Crisanto.torres@bmc.org

T. S. Brahmbhatt, D. R. Scantling (eds.), *Trauma Surgery Clerkship*, Contemporary Surgical Clerkships,
https://doi.org/10.1007/978-3-032-01412-2_12

It is important to note that the initial evaluation of the patient is a dynamic process that requires ongoing assessment and adjustment of treatment plans based on individual patient characteristics and clinical judgment. In some cases, a patient may initially appear to be in a stable and satisfactory condition. However, it is important to recognize that their apparent well-being can rapidly deteriorate due to undetected examination findings that do not accurately represent the true extent of their injuries. Additionally, there are instances where patients may exhibit unexpected transient responses to resuscitation, further complicating the assessment of their condition.

In the context of fluid resuscitation in the trauma bay, responders are patients who exhibit a positive physiological response to the administration of fluids. These individuals show improvements in vital signs, such as blood pressure, heart rate, and urine output, indicating that their circulatory system is effectively responding to fluid therapy.

Transient responders, on the other hand, are patients who initially demonstrate positive physiological changes following fluid resuscitation but subsequently revert to a compromised state. These individuals may experience a temporary improvement in their vital signs but fail to maintain a sustained response, suggesting that their underlying condition requires further intervention or a different approach to management.

Non-responders are patients who do not exhibit any meaningful improvement in their physiological parameters despite receiving fluid resuscitation. These individuals fail to show the expected response to fluid therapy, indicating a more severe or refractory condition that may necessitate alternative treatment strategies beyond fluid administration alone.

Differentiating transient responders from sustained responders and non-responders is vital in the trauma bay. It facilitates timely interventions, prevents clinical deterioration, optimizes resource allocation, and ultimately improves patient care and outcomes.

In scenarios involving unstable trauma patients, immediate surgical or angiographic management should be prioritized over additional diagnostic assessments to ensure timely and essential intervention. Surgery is the imperative and definitive intervention for the rapidly bleeding hemodynamically unstable patient. When necessary, angiographic management should also be promptly considered as a potential intervention for these patients. However, in emergent situations, surgical intervention can be initiated promptly, as it does not require additional time for diagnostic imaging or the setup of angiographic equipment. This time-saving factor is crucial for unstable patients who require immediate lifesaving measures.

Computed Tomography Evaluation

The Role of CT Scan

Physical examination of the injured patient can often be misleading, which may lead to missed or delayed diagnosis of injuries. Distracting injuries, mental obtundation, and drug or alcohol intoxication are commonly known factors that may mask the identification of other injuries.

CT imaging can provide a rapid and detailed assessment of intra-abdominal, retroperitoneal, thoracic, musculoskeletal, and central nervous system injuries that may not be clinically evident on physical exam or extended focus assessment for the sonography of trauma (eFAST) exam.

Multidetector CT scans have improved diagnostic accuracy and the detection of clinically unsuspecting or occult injuries (Fig. 12.1) [1].

The use of whole-body CT in patients with major trauma after blunt injury is associated with increased survival probability, likely due to earlier identification and subsequent definitive management of critical injuries [2].

Hemodynamically stable patients with positive clinical findings concerning underlying injury, those with high-risk injury mechanisms, or those with unreliable exams should proceed from the trauma bay to the CT scanner for additional secondary evaluation.

Drawbacks of CT Scan

Patients must be transported from the readily accessible, resuscitation-equipped trauma bay to the resource- and staff-limited CT suite, and no provider can be in the room during sometimes lengthy imaging.

Figure 12.1 CT imaging of a hemodynamically stable patient with a penetrating wound

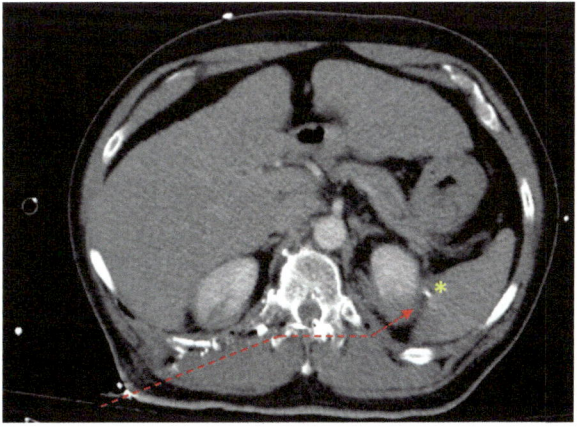

Unsuspected transient responders to resuscitation may manifest with acute and rapid deterioration while in the scanner.

Patient transfer from the stretcher to the scanner table may lead to dislodged tubes, catheters, and intravenous lines that are critical for access.

Uncooperative patients can make CT scanning difficult. This may lead to providers administering pharmacologic sedation, further eliciting clinical decompensation or the need for a definitive airway.

Diaphragmatic, mesenteric, pancreatic, and hollow viscus injuries are commonly missed on initial CT imaging.

Overutilization of CT scanning for injuries that have definitively been ruled in or out can delay surgical or radiologic intervention.

Immediate OR Transit

The goal of proceeding directly to the operating room from the trauma bay is to provide definitive surgical intervention for time-sensitive, limb, or life-threatening injuries.

For hemodynamically unstable patients, the primary assessment is usually sufficient in identifying those who warrant emergent operative intervention; additional diagnostic tests such as CT scans may be unnecessary and thus delay definitive treatment or expose the patient to fatal delays in hemorrhage control.

For patients requiring operative intervention, decreasing the time to definitive surgical care is known to improve patient outcomes. Hemodynamically unstable patients should be taken expeditiously to the operating suite, as the success of surgical management appears to be time-dependent [3].

Common indications for immediate operative intervention include refractory hemodynamic instability, peritonitis, evisceration, and uncontrolled bleeding. Overt signs indicative for uncontrolled or life-threatening bleeding include pulsatile bleeding or a rapidly expanding hematoma (Table 12.1).

OR Preparation

Expedient coordination and clear communication with the OR staff are critical to patient outcome. Every minute delay portends a poorer prognosis for critically injured patients.

A brief description of the type of surgical procedure should be provided to the OR team to assist with selecting the most appropriate surgical set-up for the type of procedure expected. For example, a laparotomy tray would contain surgical instruments most compatible with an exploratory laparotomy procedure.

Table 12.1 Common indications for immediate operative intervention

Abdominal
Hemodynamic instability
Evisceration
Peritonitis
Gross rectal bleeding
Gross hematemesis
Extremity
Mangled extremity
Compartment syndrome
Pulsatile bleeding
Expanding hematoma
Absent pulse in the involved limb
Pale and cold limb
Chest
Bloody chest tube drainage >1200–1500mL or thoracic injury with hemodynamic instability
Pericardial effusion on eFAST with hemodynamic instability
Neck
Expanding hematoma
Pulsatile bleeding
Neurologic deficit
Airway compromise

Often patients with severe injuries that necessitate immediate OR management have multiple injuries that warrant operative repair. Therefore, the surgeon must understand the role and timing of requesting additional assistance that may involve emergent consultation with other surgical subspecialties.

Interventional Radiology

With the increasing role and utilization of selective non-operative management of various injuries, IR has become a critical component for the management and disposition of trauma patients.

Often massive hemorrhage can obscure the operative field, creating a substantial challenge for the surgeon to obtain rapid hemorrhage control. Typically performed after initial damage control surgery and, if necessary, IR management can provide temporizing or definitive intervention that can complement surgical control of bleeding.

Minimally invasive techniques such as angioembolization provide the benefit of definitive hemorrhage control while increasing the ability to salvage solid organs.

Injury-Specific Considerations for IR

Pelvis

Complex pelvic fractures with hemodynamic instability without an indication for laparotomy should be considered for immediate transport to the IR suite from the trauma bay for emergent angioembolization.

Often patients will have a negative eFAST, unremarkable abdominal exam, presence of a complex pelvic fracture on X-ray, and with labile hemodynamics.

Spleen

Non-operative management has emerged as the gold standard treatment in patients with hemodynamically stable splenic trauma or in those who durably respond to transfusion.

The American Association for the Surgery of Trauma (AAST) developed a splenic injury scale to assign grades based on the severity of injury [4].

Splenic artery embolization should be considered in hemodynamically stable patients with grade IV/V splenic injury or with imaging or evidence of active splenic hemorrhage.

Liver

Approximately 80% of blunt liver injuries are managed non-operatively [5].

Angiographic evaluation with embolization is the mainstay treatment for hemodynamically stable patients with evidence on imaging of active extravasation, pseudoaneurysm, or arteriovenous/arterioportal fistula.

At times, initial OR temporizing measures such as peri-hepatic packing are performed for hemodynamically unstable patients, followed by definitive hemorrhage control through IR embolization.

Kidney

There is limited use for IR embolization for renal trauma; however, it may be valuable when performed.

Active extravasation on CT or an expanding retroperitoneal hematoma that is not surgically explored should be considered for IR management.

Renal artery thrombosis is an uncommon finding after blunt trauma. Patients are at risk for renal failure and subsequent renal loss. IR endovascular management is ideal to increase the odds of organ salvageability, especially if within 6 hours of injury [6].

Logistical Challenges and Considerations

IR management relies on several technical and logistical issues for which prudent decision-making is critical for success. An experienced and savvy proceduralist serves no purpose without the assistance of a readily accessible team, resources, and appropriate timing.

Twenty-four-hour IR availability is imperative when deciding to proceed with IR management. Conversely, the absence or unreliable service accessibility should direct the decision to move immediately to the OR to manage hemodynamically unstable traumatic bleeding.

Time to intervention is a critical factor associated with overall patient outcomes. Therefore, rapid mobilization of the IR team, resources, and IR-capable suites are important to improve patient morbidity and survival.

For American College of Surgeons-verified level 1 and 2 trauma centers, radiologists are to be available for interventions within 60 min of request [7].

Once the decision has been made to proceed with IR intervention, the next step is deciding whether the patient would be more appropriate for a hybrid angiographic-OR room or the IR angiographic suite.

Complications of Angiography

Pseudoaneurysms at the access site are not uncommon and may need to be embolized or repaired.

Arterial embolization may cause unintended end-organ ischemia and necrosis.

Biloma, hepatic ischemia/necrosis, liver abscess, and gallbladder necrosis can be seen with hepatic embolization.

Splenic infarct, abscess, and sepsis can develop with splenic embolization.

Dashed red arrow indicates bullet trajectory and track. Yellow asterisk illustrates hyper-attenuated bullet fragment.

References

1. Mirvis SE, Shanmuganathan K. Abdominal computed tomography in blunt trauma. Semin Roentgenol. 1992;27(3):150–83. https://doi.org/10.1016/0037-198X(92)90027-Y.
2. Huber-Wagner S, Lefering R, Qvick L, et al. Effect of whole-body CT during trauma resuscitation on survival: a retrospective, multicentre study. Lancet (British edition). 2009;373(9673):1455–61. https://www.clinicalkey.es/playcontent/1-s2.0-S0140673609602324. https://doi.org/10.1016/S0140-6736(09)60232-4.
3. Hoyt DB, Shackford SR, McGill T, Mackersie R, Davis J, Hansbrough J. The impact of in-house surgeons and operating room resuscitation on outcome of traumatic injuries. Arch Surg (Chicago. 1960). 1989;124(8):906–10. https://doi.org/10.1001/archsurg.1989.01410080036005.
4. Kozar RA, Crandall M, Shanmuganathan K, et al. Organ injury scaling 2018 update: Spleen, liver, and kidney. J Trauma Acute Care Surg. 2018;85(6):1119–22. https://www.ncbi.nlm.nih.gov/pubmed/30462622. https://doi.org/10.1097/TA.0000000000002058.

5. Velmahos GC, Toutouzas K, Radin R, et al. High success with nonoperative management of blunt hepatic trauma: the liver is a sturdy organ. Arch Surg (Chicago. 1960). 2003;138(5):475–81. https://doi.org/10.1001/archsurg.138.5.475.
6. Bittenbinder EN, Reed AB. Advances in renal intervention for trauma. Semin Vasc Surg. 2014;26(4):165–9.   https://www.clinicalkey.es/playcontent/1-s2.0-S0895796714000301. https://doi.org/10.1053/j.semvascsurg.2014.06.012.
7. American college of surgeons. resources for optimal care of the injured patient. 2022. 2022.

Chapter 13
Cricothyroidotomy

Julia Lerner, Thomas J. Martin, and Tareq Kheirbek

Introduction

The primary survey in the assessment of trauma patients starts with evaluating and securing a patent and protected airway. In most cases, patients can protect the airway and are breathing spontaneously. However, in some cases the trauma team needs to establish a secure airway, commonly via endotracheal intubation. Approaches to endotracheal intubation and rescue methods for difficult airway management are not discussed in this chapter. In very rare occasions, the provider will be faced with a *"cannot ventilate, cannot intubate"* scenario. This occurs when there is a significant disruption or swelling of the upper airway that it prohibits the provider from safely performing endotracheal intubation despite all available rescue methods. In these occasions, it becomes important to perform a "surgical airway" via cricothyroidotomy [1]. It is vital that all providers who participate in the assessment and care of trauma patients be familiar with the indications for and the surgical techniques needed to secure airway access via the cricothyroid membrane without delay. While the majority of cricothyroidotomies are performed in the emergency department, it is possible that an emergent surgical airway becomes indicated in other settings, such as the operating room or the hospital wards. The hospital should establish protocols and surgical airway teams staffed with providers who are familiar with and skilled in performing emergent cricothyroidotomy. Simulation modules

J. Lerner · T. Kheirbek (✉)
Warren Alpert Medical School, Brown University, Providence, RI, USA
e-mail: tareq_kheirbek@brown.edu

T. J. Martin
Department of Surgery, Brigham and Women's Hospital, Boston, MA, USA
e-mail: tmartin28@bwh.harvard.edu

© The Author(s), under exclusive license to Springer Nature Switzerland AG 2025
T. S. Brahmbhatt, D. R. Scantling (eds.), *Trauma Surgery Clerkship*, Contemporary Surgical Clerkships,
https://doi.org/10.1007/978-3-032-01412-2_13

should be developed and implemented frequently to improve provider's comfort in performing surgical airway [2].

Indications

- Cricothyroidotomy is indicated when there is a "cannot ventilate, cannot intubate" situation. In trauma, this can occur secondary to direct airway injury, significant facial fractures, large or expanding neck hematoma, significant swelling, or airway contamination due to emesis or bleeding in the oropharynx.
- Communication among the trauma team members regarding the state of the airway and the ease of intubation or ventilation should be clear.
- Advanced rescue methods and interventions should be attempted to maintain adequate ventilation and oxygenation.
- When there is concern for impending loss of airway patency, a separate team member should begin preparing for a surgical airway immediately—even as further nonsurgical attempts continue.
- The neck should be immediately evaluated in preparation for a possible cricothyroidotomy, and appropriate instruments, lighting, and personal protective equipment (i.e., mask, safety goggles, or visor) should be immediately worn.

Anatomy Considerations

- The provider should be familiar with the anatomy of the airway and be able to easily and quickly identify the cricothyroid membrane (Fig. 13.1) [3].
- Ideally, the neck would be extended to facilitate palpation of the anterior airway structures. However, the neck is likely to be immobilized during the initial assessment of a trauma patient.
- A cervical collar may be removed to facilitate access to the neck and manual stabilization instead performed.
- The most prominent structure in the neck is the thyroid cartilage. Below that, the cricothyroid membrane is located between the thyroid cartilage and the cricoid cartilage.
- The first step to correctly identify the membrane is to palpate the thyroid cartilage in the midline with the index finger.
- The provider then rolls the index finger inferiorly until they feel a "drop," which would be the location of the cricothyroid membrane. The membrane should be relatively superficial with no major structure anterior to it.
- Continuing to roll the index finger inferiorly will help identify the tracheal rings, which begin to feel deeper in the neck due to direction of the trachea and the presence of the thyroid gland and strap muscles anteriorly. Attempting to access

Fig. 13.1 Palpation of
the cricothyroid
membrane between the
thyroid cartilage and the
cricoid cartilage

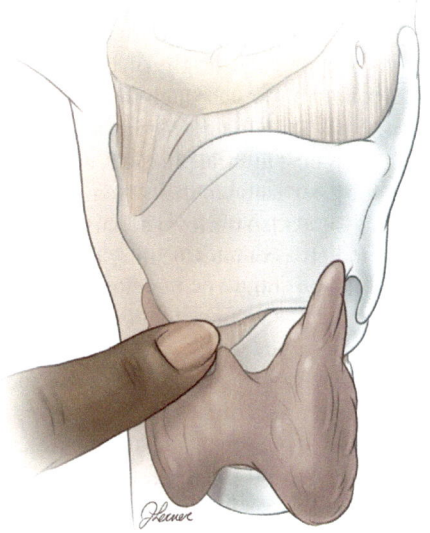

the airway emergently at this level can be difficult and result in unnecessary
blood loss which would compromise the procedure and delay securing a protected airway.

- A common pitfall is to mistakenly identify the thyrohyoid membrane as the cricothyroid membrane. The thyrohyoid membrane is superior to thyroid cartilage.
Performing the surgical airway through the thyrohyoid membrane could result in
a significant injury to the vocal cords.
- Providers who are expected to perform cricothyroidotomy are encouraged to palpate their own neck to be familiar with the structures and develop fingertip memory for when it becomes necessary.

Procedure

There are two main approaches to place a cricothyroidotomy tube—open and percutaneous using a Seldinger technique [4, 5]. Needle cricothyroidotomy using only
an angiocatheter or needle-style device can be used when instruments are not readily available. It is, however, considered a temporary option only. It allows for oxygenation, but it is not sufficient to effectively ventilate the patient. It can be also
used in a young pediatric patient as a bridge to a more definitive airway. Due to the

funnel shape of the airway in young children, a cricothyroidotomy can result in a significant subglottic stenosis and, therefore, should be avoided if possible [6].

Open Cricothyroidotomy

- The provider should anticipate the need for an emergent surgical airway based on assessment of patient's injuries and oropharynx.
- The provider should ensure that instruments are readily accessible, and the patient is appropriately positioned.
- Neck extension provide a better visualization of the anterior neck but may not be feasible if there is concern for cervical spine injury. In this case, manual neck immobilization should be maintained during the procedure.
- Neck prep can be achieved with any available antiseptic solution but should not delay the procedure.
- The provider should use sterile gloves and don personal protective equipment, including eye protection.
- The provider should then palpate the neck to identify the cricothyroid membrane between the thyroid cartilage and the cricoid cartilage. Other landmarks should also be identified such as the sternal notch and the thyrohyoid membrane.
- The nondominant hand should stabilize the airway by holding the thyroid cartilage. This also helps orienting the provider to the midline of the neck.
- A vertical midline incision is made over the cricothyroid membrane to avoid injury to the lateral vascular structures. This can be performed using size 15 blade scalpels, but any available blade should be used in emergency (Fig. 13.2).
- A gentle spread of the subcutaneous tissue exposes the cricothyroid membrane. The membrane can then be incised horizontally using the scalpel. Alternatively, the provider can use the back of the scalpel handle, a hemostat, or a Kelly clamp to enter the airway through the membrane bluntly. This should be done with caution if using the scalpel handle given the risk of injury to the proceduralist (Fig. 13.3).
- The cricothyroidotomy should be dilated by spreading a hemostat or through digital dilation (Fig. 13.4).
- Although often unnecessary, a tracheal hook can be used to maintain the opening in the cricothyroid membrane until a tube is inserted.
- An endotracheal tube or a tracheostomy tube can then be inserted into the airway either directly or placed over the bougie (preferred) using the Seldinger technique (Fig. 13.5).
- If an endotracheal tube is used, it should only be advanced for a few centimeters (2–3 cm) into the airway to avoid main-stem bronchial intubation and a small tube, such as a size 6, should be used.
- The tube is secured around the neck and ventilation is initiated. Tracheal placement is confirmed using end-tidal CO_2 waveform or colorimetric capnography (Fig. 13.4).

Fig. 13.2 Vertical
incision over the
cricothyroid membrane

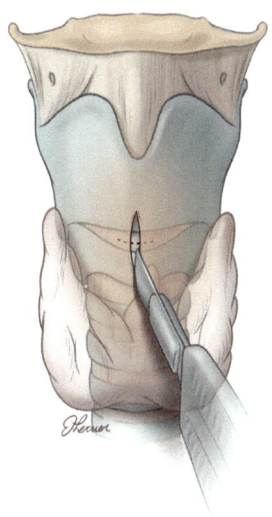

Fig. 13.3 Dilatation of
the cricothyroidotomy

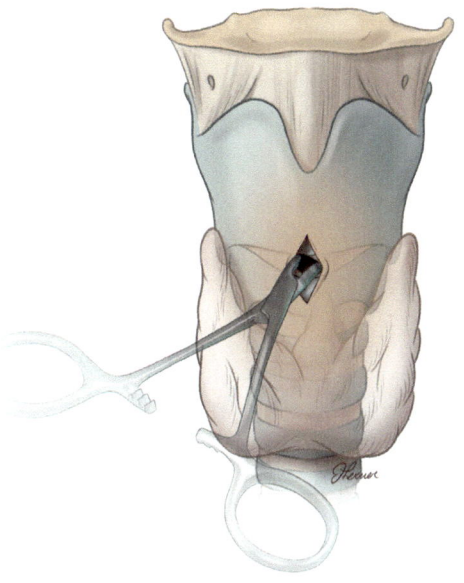

Fig. 13.4 Bougie is inserted into the cricothyroidotomy to guide placement of tube

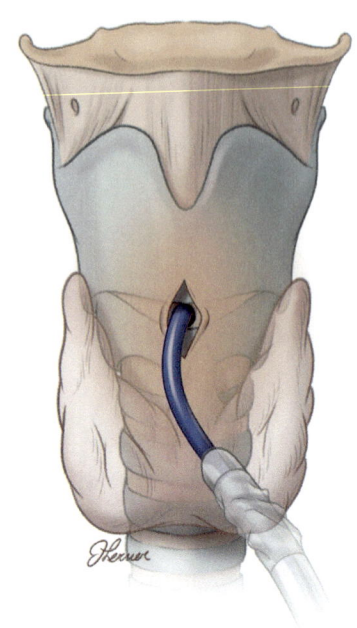

Fig. 13.5 Cricothyroidotomy tube is inserted and secured

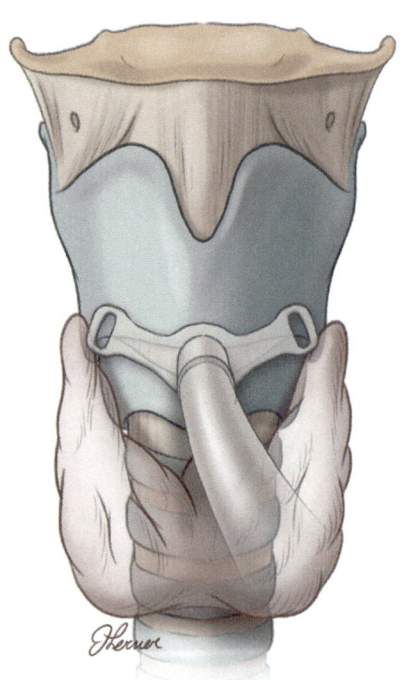

Percutaneous Cricothyroidotomy

- As an alternative to the open approach, one can establish an airway using a percutaneous Seldinger-based approach.
- This technique may be preferable in patients with significant subcutaneous tissue where open exposure under nonideal (e.g., bedside) exposure can hamper access to the deep structures.
- There are variations of this technique depending on the several commercial kits that are available. Providers should familiarize themselves with the kits that are in use at each institution [7].
- The common approach involves making a midline vertical incision over the cricothyroid membrane while the nondominant hand stabilized the airway similar to the open approach.
- A needle attached to a fluid-filled syringe is then inserted into the airway through the membrane while aspirating.
- The syringe is then removed, and guidewire is passed into the airway.
- The needle is removed, and a cricothyroidotomy tube inserted over the wire into the airway.
- The wire is removed, and ventilation is initiated.

Post-cricothyroidotomy Care

A cricothyroidotomy tube is considered a stable and secure airway. Routine conversion to a tracheostomy tube is not supported [8]. The tube should be removed when ventilatory support is not further required and the oropharynx or the airway injuries are fixed.

Complications

- Rates of procedure-specific complications after cricothyroidotomy vary depending on comfort and expertise of the provider, location of the procedure, available support, and injury and patient characteristics.
- The common complications are bleeding, misplacement, and injury to the posterior wall of the trachea.
- Bleeding is often venous and stops spontaneously. Direct pressure should be sufficient to assist in bleeding control. Rarely, suture control of the bleeding site would be required.
- Misplacement can be avoided by accurate identification of the anatomical landmarks and the use of bougie to guide entrance into the airway.

- Posterior tracheal wall injury can occur if forceful blunt entry is performed. This may be associated with an esophageal injury. Prompt identification of these complications and correction are critical.
- Other rare complications include laryngeal fracture, vocal cords injury, recurrent laryngeal nerve injury, infection, and airway stenosis.

References

1. Bair AE, Filbin MR, Kulkarni RG, Walls RM. The failed intubation attempt in the emergency department: analysis of prevalence, rescue techniques, and personnel. J Emerg Med. 2002;23(2):131–40. https://doi.org/10.1016/s0736-4679(02)00501-2.
2. McMurray H, Kraemer LS, Jaffe E, Raiciulescu S, Switzer JM, Dosal GC, et al. Development of a simulation surgical Cricothyroidotomy curriculum for novice providers: a learning curve study. Mil Med. 2021;188:e1028–35. https://doi.org/10.1093/milmed/usab520.
3. Dover K, Howdieshell TR, Colborn GL. The dimensions and vascular anatomy of the cricothyroid membrane: relevance to emergent surgical airway access. Clin Anat. 1996;9(5):291–5. https://doi.org/10.1002/(SICI)1098-2353(1996)9:5<291::AID-CA1>3.0.CO;2-G.
4. Kempema JM, Brown CVR. Airway management. In: Moore EE, Feliciano DV, Mattox KL, editors. Trauma, 8e. New York, NY: McGraw-Hill Education; 2017.
5. Bribriesco A, Patterson GA. Cricothyroid approach for emergency access to the airway. Thorac Surg Clin. 2018;28(3):435–40. https://doi.org/10.1016/j.thorsurg.2018.04.009.
6. Black AE, Flynn PE, Smith HL, Thomas ML, Wilkinson KA, Association of Pediatric Anaesthetists of Great B, et al. Development of a guideline for the management of the unanticipated difficult airway in pediatric practice. Paediatr Anaesth. 2015;25(4):346–62. https://doi.org/10.1111/pan.12615.
7. Vadodaria BS, Gandhi SD, McIndoe AK. Comparison of four different emergency airway access equipment sets on a human patient simulator. Anaesthesia. 2004;59(1):73–9. https://doi.org/10.1111/j.1365-2044.2004.03456.x.
8. Choi J, Anderson TN, Sheira D, Sousa J, Borghi JA, Spain DA, et al. The need to routinely convert emergency Cricothyroidotomy to tracheostomy: a systematic review and meta-analysis. J Am Coll Surg. 2022;234(5):947–52. https://doi.org/10.1097/XCS.0000000000000114.

Chapter 14
Chest Tubes

Heba Elassar and Aaron Richman

Overview

- Chest tubes are used to drain air or fluid from the pleural cavity.
- Chest tubes are available in a variety of sizes for different uses.
- Careful consideration of anatomy and indication is imperative when placing a chest tube.
- Once a chest tube is inserted, it is attached to a sealed drainage system.
- Chest tube management is not universal and must be tailored to the patient.
- Proper chest tube removal technique is critical to avoid recurrent pneumothorax.

Background

Air or fluid can accumulate in the pleural space after traumatic injury, thoracic surgery, or due to other thoracic pathology. If sufficient volume of air or fluid accumulates, it can compress the lung and mediastinum compromising cardiopulmonary function. Chest tubes, also known as thoracostomy tubes, are inserted into the pleural space to drain air or fluid thereby restoring normal pulmonary function and hemodynamics. Management of the tube after placement varies depending on the patient's pathology.

H. Elassar · A. Richman (✉)
Boston Medical Center/Boston University Chobanian and Avedisian School of Medicine, Boston, MA, USA
e-mail: Heba.Elassar@bmc.org; Aaron.Richman@bmc.org

© The Author(s), under exclusive license to Springer Nature Switzerland AG 2025
T. S. Brahmbhatt, D. R. Scantling (eds.), *Trauma Surgery Clerkship*, Contemporary Surgical Clerkships,
https://doi.org/10.1007/978-3-032-01412-2_14

Chest tubes are available in a variety of sizes, shapes, and materials tailored to the indication for placement. Tubes are typically made of PVC or silicone and constructed with fenestrations at the distal end that is inserted into the chest. Smaller tubes are used to manage pneumothoraces or thin fluid pleural effusions, while larger chest tubes are used in cases of thicker fluid collections like blood or empyema. A common variety of small-bore chest tube is a pigtail catheter, so named because the tip coils like a pig's tail to prevent dislodgement.

Once the chest tube is inserted, it is connected to a closed drainage system and typically placed on suction. The drainage system consists of three chambers: the suction chamber, the water seal chamber, and the collection chamber. When the system is on water seal, it allows the chest tube to drain to gravity but does not allow air to re-enter the chest. Using these devices, suction pressure can be controlled, and drainage can be characterized and measured [1, 2].

Current Practice

- Indications for chest tube placement include pneumothorax, hemothorax, pleural effusion, empyema, pleurodesis, and post-operative care.
- Chest tubes are commonly available in sizes ranging from 6 French to 40 French.
- Tubes are available in a variety of configurations including straight, angled, or pigtail.
- The proper tube size and shape should be selected to properly drain the pleural space.
- Coagulopathy, prior thoracic surgery, and ipsilateral diaphragmatic hernia are relative contraindications to bedside tube thoracostomy.

Chest Tube Placement

- Chest tubes can be placed at the bedside or in the operating room.
- Standard chest tube placement is at the mid-axillary line of the fourth or fifth intercostal space.
- The "triangle of safety" for tube insertion is defined anteromedially by the lateral border of pectoralis major, posteriorly by the anterior border of latissimus dorsi, and inferiorly by a horizontal line at the level of the nipple or inframammary fold.[3].
- Open dissection, Seldinger/wire-guided, and trocar techniques can be used for placement.
- Open dissection is typically used for large bore tubes (≥20 French) (Fig. 14.1).
- Seldinger/wire-guidance is typically used for small bore tubes (<20 French).
- Tube placement can be guided with CT or ultrasound to target the pathology.

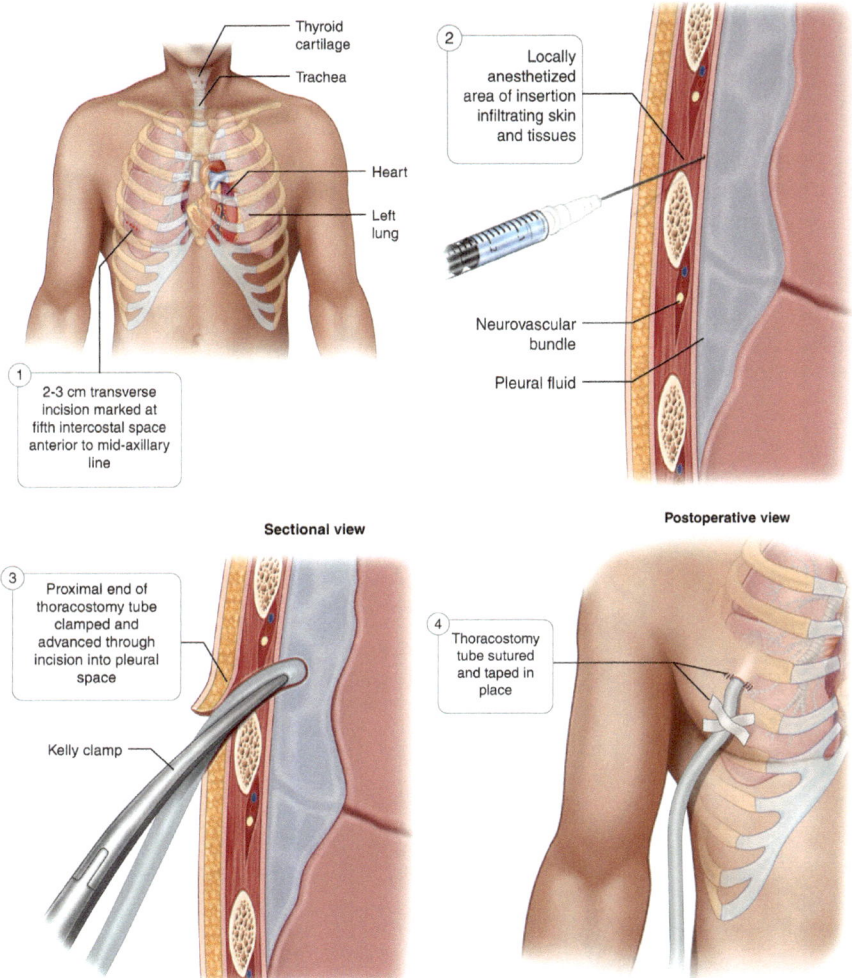

Fig. 14.1 Open chest tube placement procedural steps [3]

- Placement should be along the superior edge of the rib to avoid injuring the inter-costal artery, vein, and nerve within the intercostal bundle.[3].
- For pneumothoraces, the chest tube is oriented with the tip toward the apex of the chest.
- For hemothorax or pleural effusion, the chest tube is guided posterior and basilar where the fluid typically settles.
- Complications include bleeding, surgical site infection, injury to the lung, dia-phragm, spleen, or liver.

Chest Tube Management

- Tube management is tailored to the patient and their pathophysiology.
- The tube is connected to a closed drainage system (Fig. 14.2), sometimes called pleural drainage unit (PDU).
- Chest tubes can be placed to suction, water seal, or much more rarely clamped based on the stage of management.

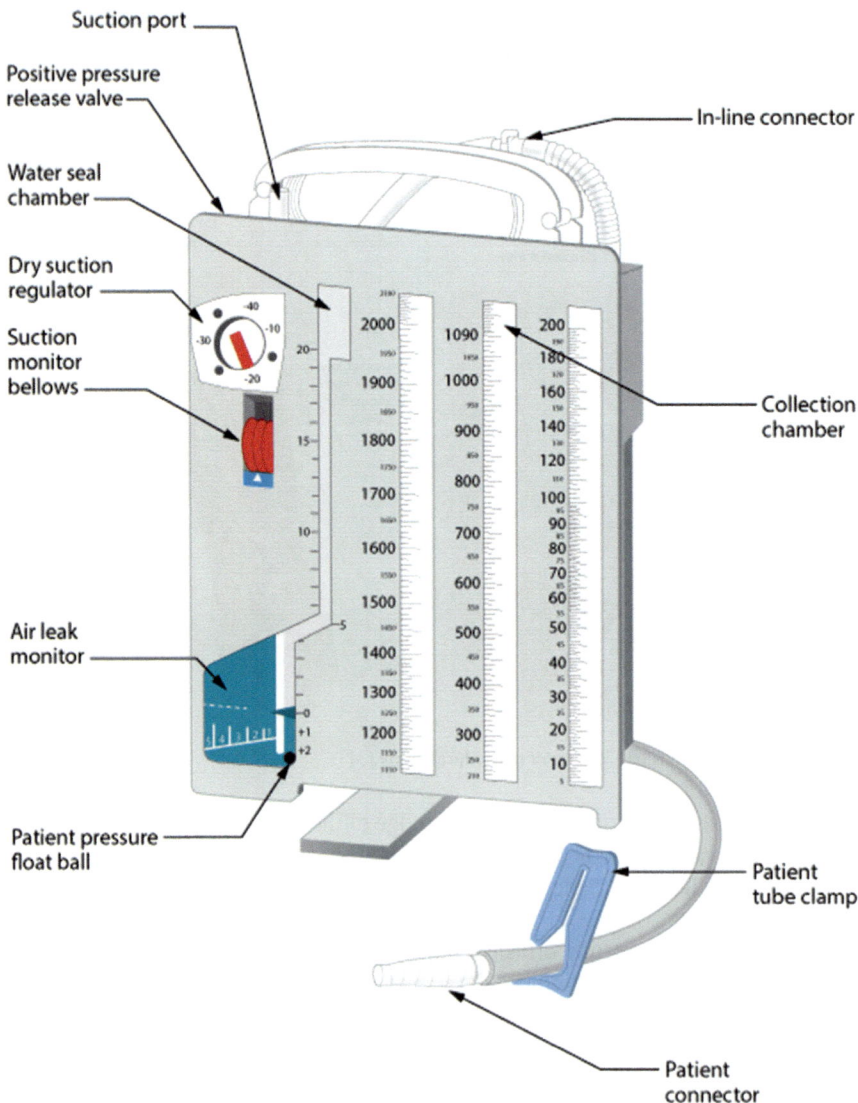

Fig. 14.2 Closed suction pleural drainage unit [4]

- Suction pressure is controlled by the "dry suction regulator" valve on the PDU, not by the source of suction. Of note, this valve will read the set suction pressure even if disconnected from suction. The suction monitor bellow, or "accordion" shows whether the suction is actually active. [2, 4].
- Output from the tube is measured and examined regularly.
- Traumatic hemothorax with output >1.5 L immediately or 200 cc for 4 h should prompt surgical evaluation, but it should always be considered that hemodynamically unstable patients may still need operative intervention regardless of chest tube output and that blood may clot (in the pleural space or the pericardium) and not exit the chest to be measured. Repeat chest XR may help evaluate for retained blood. [5].
- Bubbling in the PDU indicates an air leak, this can be from the lung, the chest wound, or a break in the drainage system, such as a disconnection between the tube and drainage system.
- Bubbling with a cough typically indicates a leak from the lung parenchyma.
- An air leak lasting more than a few days may need surgical exploration.
- Daily chest X-rays are typically obtained to follow the progression of the disease process and to ensure the tube remains in good position.
- The tube fenestrations should remain within the pleural space until the tube is removed.

Chest Tube Removal

- No universal guidelines exist for chest tube removal.
- A tube can generally be considered for removal if the following conditions are true:
  - Resolution of any air leaks, and resolution of or minimal residual pneumothorax.
  - Daily fluid output <150–400 cc.
  - Fluid output thin and serosanguinous (e.g., not a substance that requires further drainage regardless of output).
- Tube removal should be synchronized with the patient's breath to avoid removing it upon inspiration.
- Removal during inspiration creates a pressure gradient that can draw air along the tract leaving a residual pneumothorax.
- The tube site is covered with an occlusive dressing.
- Sometimes a U-stitch is placed to ensure wound closure.
- A chest X-ray is often obtained after chest tube removal to ensure no reaccumulation of pneumothorax or effusion.

Key Points for Patient Care

- Chest tubes are used to drain air or fluid from the pleural space and re-expand the lung.
- Chest tubes are common, and it is important for all providers to be familiar with their use.
- In most cases of chest tube placement, patients generally have a good outcome, but chest tube placement does come with its own risks.

References

1. Anderson D, Chen SA, Godoy LA, Brown LM, Cooke DT. Comprehensive review of chest tube management: a review. JAMA Surg. 2022;157:269–74.
2. Cooke DT, David EA. Large-bore and small-bore chest tubes: types, function, and placement. Thorac Surg Clin. 2013;23:17–24, v.
3. Wegerif G, Savage EB. Chest tube thoracostomy. In: Rosenthal RJ, Rosales A, Lo Menzo E, Dip FD, editors. Mental conditioning to perform common operations in general surgery training. Cham: Springer; 2020. p. 47–50.
4. Doyle GR, McCutcheon JA. Clinical procedures for safer patient care. BCcampus; 2015.
5. Chest Tube – StatPearls – NCBI Bookshelf. https://www.ncbi.nlm.nih.gov/books/NBK459199/. Accessed 9 Mar 2023

Chapter 15
Emergency Department Thoracotomy

Carl A. Beyer and Mark J. Seamon

Overview

The initial treatment of the trauma patient in extremis presents a clinical, logistical, and sometimes ethical challenge. The patient's physiology and clinical presentation should guide the immediate work-up and treatment. While emergency cardiothoracic surgery is ideally conducted in the operating room, traumatic cardiac arrest may mandate an immediate emergency department thoracotomy (EDT). The decision to perform EDT must balance the chance of meaningful survival, the risk of poor neurologic outcome, the hazard due to occupational exposure, and the consideration for human dignity at the end of life. EDT enables rapid thoracic hemorrhage control, release of pericardial tamponade, aortic cross clamping, and the ability to perform open cardiac massage to increase perfusion. To maximize survival, EDT must be performed in conjunction with balanced blood product transfusion and rapid transport to the operating room for definitive surgery.

C. A. Beyer (✉)
Division of Acute Care Surgery, Morsani School of Medicine, University of South Florida, Tampa, FL, USA

M. J. Seamon
Division of Traumatology, Surgical Critical Care and Emergency Surgery, University of Pennsylvania, Philadelphia, PA, USA
e-mail: mark.seamon@pennmedicine.upenn.edu

© The Author(s), under exclusive license to Springer Nature Switzerland AG 2025
T. S. Brahmbhatt, D. R. Scantling (eds.), *Trauma Surgery Clerkship*, Contemporary Surgical Clerkships, https://doi.org/10.1007/978-3-032-01412-2_15

Background

History

Trauma remains the leading cause of mortality for the population aged 1–44, and roughly one-third of trauma deaths occur prior to hospital arrival [1, 2]. With dismal survival rates after traumatic cardiac arrest, EDT has emerged as an extension of cardiopulmonary resuscitation (CPR) in an attempt to improve survival in the most critically injured patients [1, 3]. The first thoracotomy for trauma was described in 1896 in a patient with a cardiac stab wound, and Beall provided the initial formal report of immediate thoracotomy for the moribund trauma patient in 1967 [4, 5]. In 1976, indications for EDT were expanded by Ledgerwood's description of pre-laparotomy thoracotomy with aortic cross clamping for control of abdominal hemorrhage [6]. Despite this long history, EDT remains controversial. Significant research has been devoted to understanding the predictors for survival and futility to enable the targeting of this procedure to patients that can potentially benefit.

Predictors of Survival

The important known predictors of EDT survival include the injury mechanism, anatomic location of injury, the duration of cardiac arrest, and the presence of signs of life [7]. Patients are more likely to survive EDT following penetrating injury compared to blunt mechanisms of injury. Despite an aggressive resuscitation protocol using EDT and epinephrine infusion, Moriwaki reported only 3% survival to hospital discharge after blunt traumatic cardiac arrest with most survivors in a persistent coma [8]. The uniformly poor outcomes in the medical literature following EDT for blunt trauma mandate very selective use in this patient population. When penetrating injuries are further subdivided, survival is also higher for stab wounds compared to firearm injuries [9].

The anatomic location of major injury also influences the chances for survival after EDT. A large meta-analysis showed that isolated cardiac injuries had the best survival (19.4%), followed by other thoracic injuries (10.7%) and abdominal injuries (4.5%) [9]. This survival pattern reflects the immediate improvement after release of pericardial tamponade and the possibility for direct control of hemorrhage in the thoracic cavity during thoracotomy.

Perhaps the primary predictor of survival after EDT is patient physiology at the time of the procedure. A shorter duration of cardiac arrest and the presence of signs of life are surrogate markers for salvageable physiology which have repeatedly been associated with EDT survival. A large multicenter prospective observational study showed no survivors with prehospital CPR duration greater than 15 min [10]. The American College of Surgeons' Committee on Trauma has defined a sign of life as "pupillary response, spontaneous ventilation, the presence of a carotid pulse, measurable or palpable blood pressure, extremity movement, or any cardiac electrical activity." [11].

Decision-Making Algorithms

The decision to undertake EDT for the resuscitation of a trauma patient in extremis relies on the rapid evaluation and synthesis of survival predictors and the possible benefit in each individual clinical scenario. In recognition of the challenge presented by this decision point, national trauma surgery societies have created guidelines to evaluate the available evidence. The Western Trauma Association algorithm stratifies patients first by signs of life, recommending thoracotomies for all patients with signs of life regardless of injury mechanism. For patients without signs of life, this algorithm recommends a 10-min cutoff for blunt injury and a 15-min cutoff for penetrating injury [12]. The Eastern Association for the Surgery of Trauma guideline similarly recommends resuscitative thoracotomies for all patients with signs of life. However, this guideline recommends termination of resuscitation for bluntly injured patients who present to the ED without signs of life regardless of CPR duration [13].

Current Practice

Initial Evaluation and Decision-Making

- When time allows, the team leader should prepare the trauma team for the arrival of a patient in extremis—ensure there are well-defined roles for which team member will perform the primary survey and possible procedures.
- A concise hand-off from the transport team should relay the mechanism of injury, duration of CPR, and any signs of life in the field.
- Initial evaluation should follow the principles of the Advanced Trauma Life Support primary survey and quickly determine the presence of any signs of life.
- Rolling the patient early in the evaluation for penetrating trauma allows the identification of all wounds and the assessment of possible anatomic trajectories of injury.

  - If bilateral thoracic wounds are identified, consider immediate clamshell thoracotomy.
  - If a transcranial trajectory is identified, consider immediate termination of the resuscitation.

Fig. 15.1 Pericardial effusion (*white asterisk*) identified during the Focused Assessment with Sonography in Trauma (FAST)

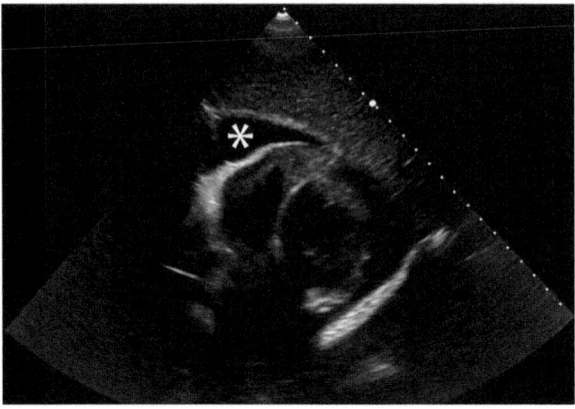

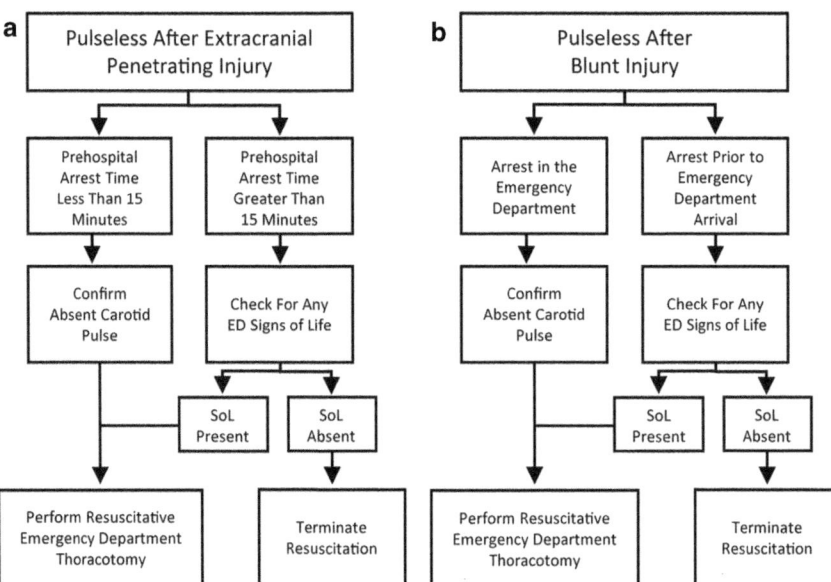

Fig. 15.2 (**a**) Example emergency department thoracotomy decision algorithm for penetrating injury. (**b**) Example emergency department thoracotomy decision algorithm for blunt injury. Signs of life (SoL) include motion or effusion on cardiac ultrasound, cardiac electrical activity, spontaneous breathing or movement, measurable blood pressure, and pupillary reactivity

- Focused Assessment with Sonography in Trauma (FAST) can be performed with attention to the cardiac window to evaluate for tamponade and cardiac motion, which can indicate a rapidly reversible cause of cardiac arrest (Fig. 15.1).
- An institutional algorithm can help the trauma team leader rapidly synthesize data and decide between proceeding with EDT or terminating the resuscitation efforts (Fig. 15.2).

Emergency Department Thoracotomy Procedural Steps

- Limit the number of individuals around the bed to the minimum required and ensure maximal personal protective equipment use by all team members to reduce the risk of inadvertent injury and bodily fluid exposure.
- Confirm patient location on the stretcher is adequate for the simultaneous performance of endotracheal intubation, vascular access, and right tube thoracostomy by other available team members during the EDT.
- Position the patient supine with the left arm above the patient's head.
- Make the thoracotomy incision sharply in the fourth intercostal space just above the fifth rib. The level of the nipple in males and the inframammary crease in females usually corresponds to the correct rib space.
- The incision should follow the curve of the rib and extend from the right sternal border to the left posterior axillary line (Fig. 15.3).
- Once in the thoracic cavity, use the Finochietto retractor to spread the ribs for maximal exposure. Place the handle of the retractor toward the axilla in case the incision needs to be extended to the right chest for additional exposure.
- Open the pericardium longitudinally to release any tamponade, taking care to stay anterior to the phrenic nerve and to avoid laceration to the underlying heart. The pericardium should be opened fully to allow delivery of the heart for complete inspection and open cardiac massage (Fig. 15.4).
- Retract the lung anteriorly to expose the descending thoracic aorta. The left inferior pulmonary ligament may need to be divided.
- Develop anterior and posterior windows in the parietal pleura overlying the descending thoracic aorta and place a non-crushing vascular clamp (Fig. 15.5).

Fig. 15.3 Thoracotomy incision (*black dashed line*) follows the curve of the rib and extends from the right sternal border to the left posterior axillary line

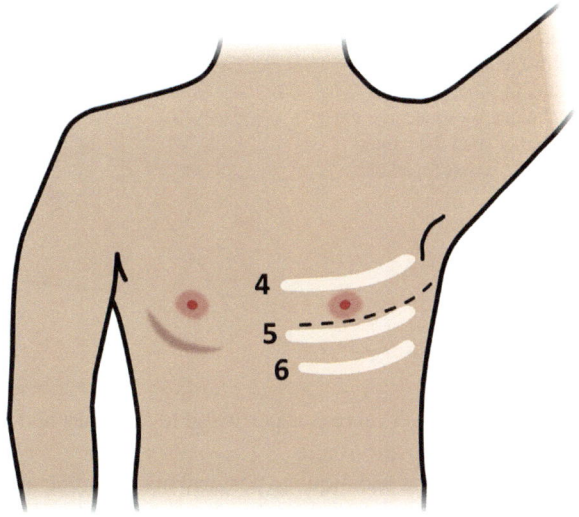

Fig. 15.4 Pericardial incision (*black dashed line*) opens the pericardium longitudinally anterior to the phrenic nerve (*yellow line*)

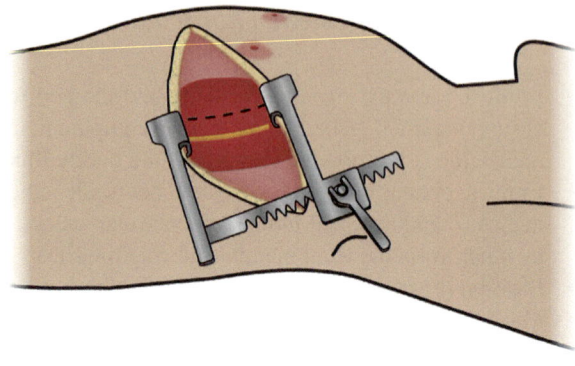

Fig. 15.5 Surgeon's left hand retracts the lung anteriorly to expose the descending thoracic aorta. The non-crushing clamp is placed on the aorta to limit subdiaphragmatic hemorrhage and augment perfusion to the heart and brain

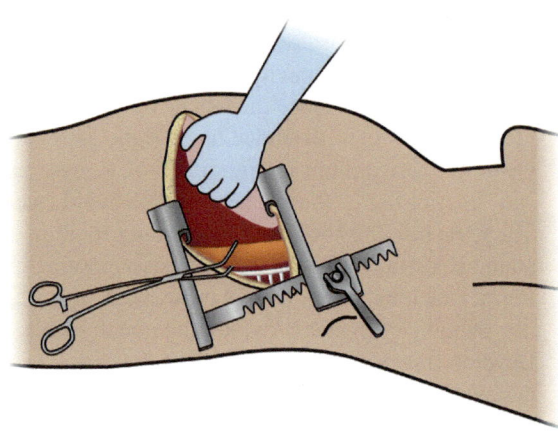

Fig. 15.6 Open cardiac massage is performed using the "bellows" technique by squeezing the heart between the palms with the wrists together

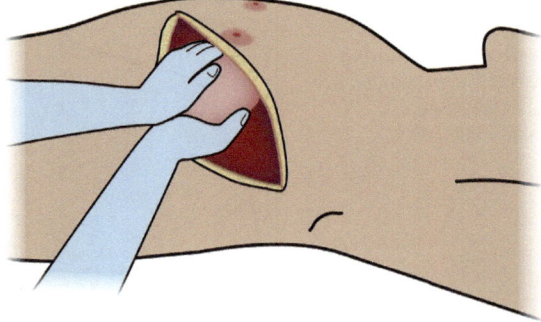

This maneuver increases perfusion to the heart and brain while reducing subdiaphragmatic hemorrhage.

- Use a bellows technique to perform open cardiac massage by squeezing the heart between the palms of both hands while keeping the wrists together (Fig. 15.6).

- If hemothorax is encountered during right tube thoracostomy, the thoracotomy incision should be extended and mirrored onto the right chest to facilitate hemorrhage control.
- Treatment of ventricular tachycardia or fibrillation can be performed by specifically designed open defibrillation paddles applied directly across the heart.

Temporizing Techniques for Specific Injuries

- Cardiac Injury.
  - Direct manual pressure with one or two fingers will control many cardiac injuries.
  - Consider temporarily closing ventricular wounds with skin staples.
  - Consider Satinsky clamp closure for thin-walled atrial lacerations.
  - When appropriate, definitively repair cardiac wounds with non-absorbable monofilament suture using pledgets. Be sure to avoid coronary vasculature while repairing cardiac injuries.
  - Inspect coronary arteries for presence of bubbles which indicates air embolism.

- Lung Injury.
  - Many lung injuries can be controlled by packing or by clamping the injured lung parenchyma with a Duval clamp.
  - If more localized control cannot be obtained, a large vascular clamp can be applied directly to the pulmonary hilum.
  - Alternatively, a maneuver termed the "hilar twist" can be used. The inferior pulmonary ligament is fully mobilized, and the lung is spun around the hilum to fully occlude the vascular structures and bronchus.

- Abdominal Injury.
  - Consider aortic cross clamping as the first maneuver to limit subdiaphragmatic hemorrhage.

Emergency Department Thoracotomy Completion

- If return of spontaneous circulation is achieved, priority must be to continue a balanced damage control resuscitation with expedient transfer to the operating room for definitive hemorrhage control.
- The clinical decision to terminate resuscitation efforts after EDT relies on the experience of the team leader and must consider the ongoing resource use, burden of injury, and likelihood of survival.

- If resuscitation efforts are terminated, there should be a moment of reflection to recognize the efforts of the team and acknowledge the human dignity of the life lost.

Outcomes

- The reported survival after EDT is between 5% and 25% in most studies depending on methodology and patient population. [9, 7, 14].
- Favorable neurologic outcome is reported in many EDT survivors; however, long-term functional outcomes after this procedure remain less well characterized. Survivors would likely benefit from long-term follow-up with multidisciplinary therapy and rehabilitation. [14, 15].
- A survey of 1360 healthcare workers following 305 EDTs showed an occupational exposure to potentially infectious fluids at a rate of 1.6% per worker per event. [16].

Take-Home Points for Patient Care

- EDT presents a challenging decision point for the trauma surgeon, balancing the heroic attempt at patient salvage with the competing interests of neurological outcome, risk of exposure to the trauma team, and human dignity.
- In appropriately selected patients, there is a reasonable chance for success— institutional algorithms and professional society guidelines can help with decision-making.
- A systematic approach to the procedure enables high performance in a chaotic and stressful environment.

References

1. Heron M. Deaths: leading causes for 2019. National Vital Statistics Reports; vol 70 no 9. Hyattsville: National Center for Health Statistics. p. 2021.
2. Sauaia A, Moore FA, Moore EE, Moser KS, Brennan R, Read RA, Pons PT. Epidemiology of trauma deaths: a reassessment. J Trauma. 1995;38:185–93.
3. Zwingmann J, Mehlhorn AT, Hammer T, Bayer J, Sudkamp NP, Strohm PC. Survival and neurologic outcome after traumatic out-of-hospital cardiopulmonary arrest in a pediatric and adult population: a systematic review. Crit Care. 2012;16(4):R117.
4. Rehn L. Ueber penetrirende herzwunden und herznaht. Archiv fur Klinische Chirurgie. 1897;55:315–29.
5. Beall AC, Diethrich EB, Cooley DA, DeBakey ME. Surgical management of penetrating cardiovascular trauma. Southern Med J. 1967;60:698–704.

6. Ledgerwood AM, Kazmers M, Lucas CE. The role of thoracic aortic occlusion for massive hemoperitoneum. J Trauma. 1976;16:610.
7. Seamon MJ, Chovanes J, Fox N, Green R, Manis G, Tsiotsias G, Warta M, Ross SE. The use of emergency department thoracotomy for traumatic cardiopulmonary arrest. Injury. 2012;43(9):1355–61.
8. Moriwaki Y, Sugiyama M, Yamamoto T, Tahara Y, Toyoda H, Kosuge T, Harunari N, Iwashita M, Arata S, Suzuki N. Outcomes from prehospital cardiac arrrest in blunt trauma patients. World J Surg. 2011;35(1):34–42.
9. Rhee PM, Acosta J, Bridgeman A, Wang D, Jordan M, Rich N. Survival after emergency department thoracotomy: review of published data from the past 25 years. J Am Coll Surg. 2000;190:288–98.
10. Moore EE, Knudson MM, Burlew CC, Inaba K, Dicker RA, Biffl WL, Malhotra AK, Schreiber MA, Browder TD, Coimbra R, Gonzalez EA, Meredith JW, Livingston DH, Kaups KL, WTA Study Group. Defining the limits of resuscitative emergency department thoracotomy: a contemporary Western Trauma Association perspective. J Trauma. 2011;70:334–9.
11. Working group. Ad Hoc Subcommittee on Outcomes. American College of Surgeons' Committee On Trauma. Practice management guidelines for emergency department thoracotomy. J Am Coll Surg. 2001;193:303–9.
12. Burlew CC, Moore EE, Moore FA, Coimbra R, McIntyre RC, Davis JW, Sperry J, Biffl WL. Western Trauma Association critical decisions in trauma: resuscitative thoracotomy. J Trauma Acute Care Surg. 2012;73(6):1359–63.
13. Seamon MJ, Haut ER, Arendonk KV, Barbosa RR, Chiu WC, Dente CJ, Fox N, Jawa RS, Khwaja K, Lee JK, Magnotti LJ, Mayglothling JA, McDonald AA, Rowell S, To KB, Falck-Ytter Y, Rhee P. An evidence-based approach to patient selection for emergency department thoracotomy: a practice management guideline from the Eastern Association for the Surgery of Trauma. J Trauma Acute Care Surg. 2015;79(1):159–73.
14. Shi D, McLaren C, Evans C. Neurological outcomes after traumatic cardiopulmonary arrest: a systematic review. Trauma Surg Acute Care Open. 2021;6(1):e817.
15. Keller D, Kulp H, Maher Z, Santora TA, Goldberg AJ, Seamon MJ. Life after near death: long-term outcomes of emergency department thoracotomy survivors. Trauma Acute Care Surg. 2013;74(5):1315–20.
16. Nunn A, Prakash P, Inaba K, Escalante A, Maher Z, Yamaguchi S, Kim DY, Maciel J, Chiu WC, Drumheller B, Hazelton JP, Mukherjee K, Luo-Owen X, Nygaard RM, Marek AP, Morse BC, Fitzgerald CA, Bosarge PL, Jawa RS, Rowell SE, Magnotti LJ, Ong AW, Brahmbhatt TS, Grossman MD, Seamon MJ. Occupational exposure during emergency department thoracotomy: a prospective, multi-institution study. J Trauma Acute Care Surg. 2018;85(1):78–84.

Chapter 16
E-FAST Exam Book Chapter

Ryan M. Brzycki and Allyson M. Hynes

Overview

- Focused assessment with sonography for trauma (FAST) examination serves as a screening tool to identify intrapleural hemorrhage, intrapericardial hemorrhage, or intraperitoneal hemorrhage. It has been incorporated into advanced trauma life support (ATLS) for the past several decades.
- The FAST exam has a vital role in the unstable patient aiding in multicavity triage.
- The windows (views obtained) include the pericardial space, the hepatorenal space, the perisplenic space, the paracolic gutters, and the pouch of Douglas.
- The extended FAST (E-FAST) adds bilateral thoracic windows to detect underlying hemo/pneumothoraces.

R. M. Brzycki (✉)
Department of Emergency Medicine, University of Arizona Medical Center,
Tucson, AZ, USA

A. M. Hynes
Department of Emergency Medicine, University of New Mexico School of Medicine,
Albuquerque, NM, USA

Department of Surgery, University of New Mexico School of Medicine,
Albuquerque, NM, USA
e-mail: ahynes@salud.unm.edu

131

T. S. Brahmbhatt, D. R. Scantling (eds.), *Trauma Surgery Clerkship*,
Contemporary Surgical Clerkships,
https://doi.org/10.1007/978-3-032-01412-2_16

Background

- Ultrasound (US) has several advantages as a rapid, reliable, noninvasive, easily repeatable, inexpensive, and portable method of cavitary triage without associated radiation.
- FAST examination has essentially replaced diagnostic peritoneal lavage in most centers and the presence of free fluid typically mandates surgical intervention in the unstable patient.
- The FAST examination can expedite the decision to place a thoracostomy tube.
- The E-FAST exam does have several drawbacks: [1] it cannot locate the source of hemorrhage; [2] it cannot evaluate hollow viscous injuries, mesenteric injuries, retroperitoneal injuries (including pancreatic injuries), and solid abdominal viscera; [3] it is dependent on operator expertise and interpretation; [4] inherent limitations in certain patient populations (obese, extensive subcutaneous emphysema, pneumoperitoneum, pneumomediastinum, bowel gas) and limitations in its ability to distinguish type of fluid; [5] ongoing bleeding may not be initially obvious in the rapidly transported patients.
- The sensitivity and specificity of the FAST examination are similar in women who are pregnant compared to those who are not pregnant [1]..

Current Practice: Clinical Indications

- In the blunt trauma victim, the decisional tree will depend on both the results of the FAST and the hemodynamics of the patient.
- In the penetrating trauma victim, the FAST exam should be utilized when a provider is uncertain if immediate surgery is warranted.
- In an unstable abdominal gunshot wound, the pericardial window has a role in multicavity triage and may guide surgical exposure decisions (sternotomy versus thoracotomy).
- A FAST examination is static, and the treating clinician should have a low threshold to repeat the negative examination as the sensitivity of the exam increases with worsening pathology (i.e., increase in hemoperitoneum).

Detection of Free Intraperitoneal Fluid, Intrapericardial Hemorrhage, Intrapleural Hemorrhage, and Pneumothoraces

- When performed in multiple quadrants, FAST examination has a sensitivity of 87%, specificity of 100%, and accuracy of 98% for detecting intraperitoneal free fluid [2].

- As little as 100 mL of fluid can be detected on US depending on the proficiency of the US operator [3]. A small anechoic (black) stripe in Morison's pouch represents approximately 250 mL of fluid and a 0.5 cm anechoic stripe corresponds to more than 500 mL of free intraperitoneal fluid [4].
- Pericardial tamponade physical exam findings are present in less than 40% of patients. POCUS has been shown to expedite this surgical decision through rapid diagnosis. A positive pericardial view in an unstable patient typically requires that the patient to be taken directly to the operating theatre.
- Upright CXR requires 50–100 mL of blood to be detected; a supine CXR (as is typical in the trauma bay) requires 175 mL [5]; meanwhile, US requires as little as 20 mL.
- E-FAST and CXR have equal sensitivity (96%), specificity (100%), and accuracy (100%) for detecting pleural fluid [6] and the E-FAST has similar or superior sensitivity in detecting pneumothoraces (PTX) [7].
- US can delineate pleural fluid, pleural thickening, and pulmonary contusions.

Anatomical Considerations of the Abdomen and Thorax

- The location of fluid accumulation depends on patient position and source of bleeding as fluid accumulates in the dependent regions.
- The peritoneal compartment is further divided into the supramesocolic and inframesocolic compartments; connected by the paracolic gutters. The right paracolic gutter connects Morison's pouch (potential space between the liver and the right kidney) with the pelvis.
- In the supine patient, free fluid accumulates in Morison's pouch before overflowing into the pelvis as the left paracolic gutter's connection to the splenorenal recess is blocked by the phrenicocolic ligament.
- Free blood in the left upper quadrant (LUQ) accumulates in the left subphrenic space first, not the splenorenal recess before overflowing into the pelvis [8].
- Free fluid in the pelvis accumulates in the retrovesical pouch in supine males and retrouterine pouch in supine females.
- Repositioning to Trendelenburg or decubitus may redistribute the free fluid, although clotted blood may not redistribute.
- Normally, visceral and parietal pleural oppose one another with a scant amount of lubricating fluid between them; allowing for lung sliding during respirations. When air is present, the layers will separate, and sliding will be lost. When lung sliding is present, this almost eliminates the possibility of PTX. Subcutaneous emphysema may give the appearance of normal lung sliding (false positive); thus, it is imperative to clinically correlate.

How to Scan

- A 3.5 MHz phased array transducer or curvilinear probe are commonly utilized. The phased array is smaller, allowing for better scanning between the ribs; however, it has limited utility in obese patients where a curvilinear probe is often preferred.
- Using a sweeping motion, obtain both a longitudinal (sagittal) and a transverse view for each view.
- The order of view selection will vary based on clinical status and operator dependence. During periods of hemodynamic instability, starting with the sub-xiphoid four-chamber view of the heart quickly excludes the presence of pericardial tamponade. Otherwise, one may start with the pericardium or the hepatorenal recess, which statistically has the highest probability of finding free fluid. Then moving to the splenorenal recess and the pelvis. Finally, one can utilize the transthoracic views of the left and right thorax for lung sliding. The inexperienced provider may start with views that have a statistically lower chance of containing free fluid to have a baseline comparison view.

Technique Pericardial

- Subxiphoid four-chamber view (Fig. 16.1): lay the probe flat in the subxiphoid space angling toward the heart with the probe indicator (a dot or ridge on one side of the probe) toward the patient's left shoulder.
- Briefly assesses global cardiac function, chamber size, and presence of fluid in the pericardial space.
- Normal pericardium should be hyperechoic (a white line).

Fig. 16.1 Subxiphoid view: A normal view demonstrating the heart, four cardiac chambers (*RA* right atrium, *RV* right ventricle, *LV* left ventricle, *LA* left atrium) with the surrounding pericardium (hyperechoic line)

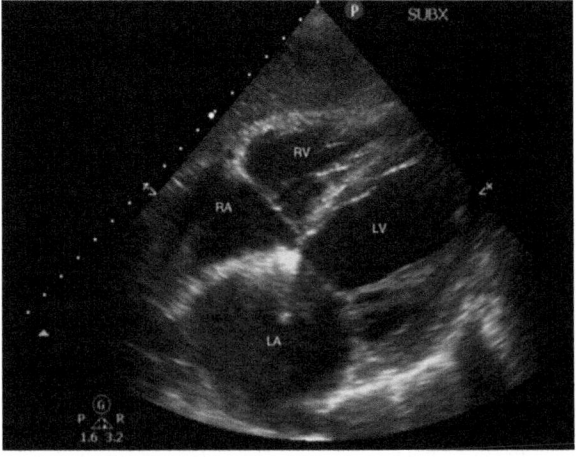

- A pericardial fat pad may be mistaken for a pericardial effusion. Pericardial fat pads are hypoechoic, and they are almost always anterior to the right ventricle.
- Pericardial fluid or hemorrhage will be in both the anterior and posterior pericardial spaces. Clotted blood will move independently of cardiac motion.
- A small amount of physiological fluid may be visualized in the pericardium during systole.
- The sensitivity of the FAST examination decreases with an adjacent hemothorax as blood may decompress from the injured pericardial sac into the thoracic cavity.

Abdominal

- RUQ (Fig. 16.2a): Visualize the right diaphragm, right lobe of the liver, and right kidney by placing the probe in the right midaxillary line between the eighth and 11th ribs with the probe marker cephalad and on an oblique scanning plane. If the rib shadows are blocking the underline structures, then rotate the probe counterclockwise to obtain optimal views. Angle the probe cephalad to assess for pleural fluid superior to the diaphragm. The diaphragm will be a hyperechoic line; pleural fluid will be an anechoic stripe superior to the diaphragm and the spine can be visualized (spine sign).
- Next, assess the LUQ (Fig. 16.2b) for left pleural effusion and free fluid in the splenorenal recess by repeating the RUQ technique. If the left kidney is identified first, then point the probe more cephalad to locate the spleen.
- The left kidney is often more difficult to visualize than the right kidney as it is higher in the abdomen, and it has a higher likelihood of being obscured by bowel gas. Additionally, the spleen is smaller than the liver, limiting its ability to serve as an acoustic window. Visualization of the kidneys can be improved by having the patient hold a deep breath.

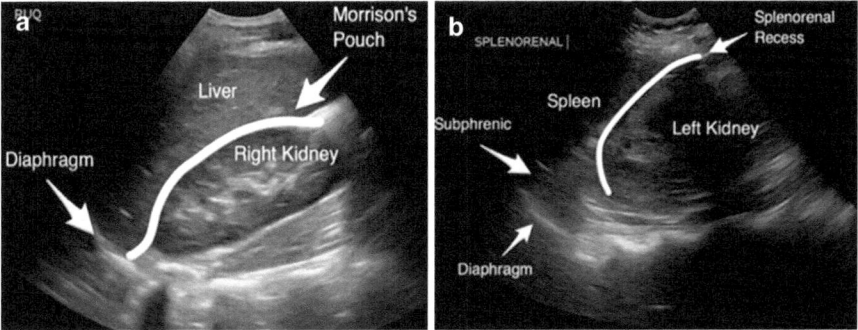

Fig. 16.2 (**a**): Right upper quadrant view: A normal view demonstrating the liver, diaphragm, right kidney, and Morrison's pouch (hepatorenal/subhepatic recess). (**b**): Left upper quadrant view: A normal view demonstrating the spleen, the diaphragm, left kidney, subphrenic space, and splenorenal recess

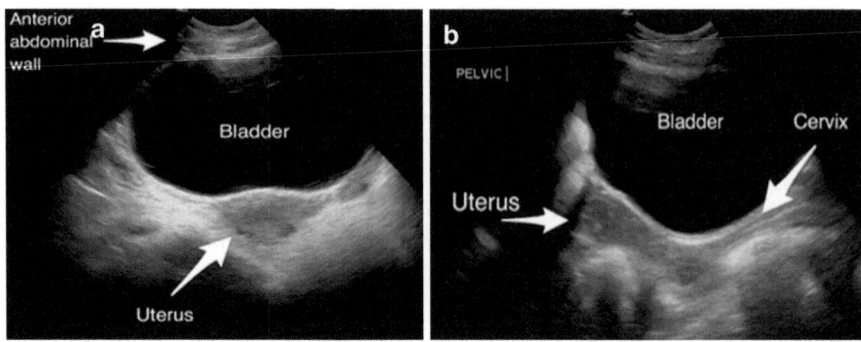

Fig. 16.3 (**a**) Pelvic view: A normal longitudinal view demonstrating the bladder, uterus, and anterior abdominal wall (**b**): A normal transverse view demonstrating the bladder, uterus, and cervix

- On the left, fluid most often accumulates in the paracolic gutters and subphrenic space. It is rare to find it only in the splenorenal space. Thus, it is paramount to obtain multiple views including the left diaphragm and left subphrenic space [8].
- Next, assess the pelvis (Fig. 16.3a, b) by inspecting the bladder, prostate or uterus, and lateral walls of the pelvis.
- Place the probe midline 2 cm superior to the pubic symphysis with the marker facing the patients right (longitudinal view). Rotate the probe 90 degrees with the marker facing the patient's head (sagittal view).
- Fluid in a filled bladder appears well circumscribed and anechoic.
- Free intraperitoneal fluid is often irregular, anechoic, and external to the visualized bladder. Hemoperitoneum is usually more echogenic with visible clots, thereby making it distinguishable from simple fluid. Clotted blood is often located in the cul-de-sac, and it can distort the contour of the bladder whereas liquid blood and ascites are often adjacent to the bladder and anterior peritoneum. US is unable to differentiate free fluid from urine. Other sources of fluid may result in a false positive examination.

Thoracic

- Place the linear high frequency or curvilinear probe between two ribs with the marker cephalad at the midclavicular line, creating a perpendicular image. The ribs will be separated by a pleural line ("Bat wing" sign). Examine it for sliding.
- Motion mode (M-mode) can facilitate detection of pneumothorax by tracking motion and velocity over time. Either the absence of lung sliding (stratosphere sign) or normal lung sliding (seashore sign) will be depicted (Fig. 16.4).
- The most specific sign for pneumothorax is the presence of a "lung point," a transition point between normal sliding pleura and the pneumothorax (i.e.,

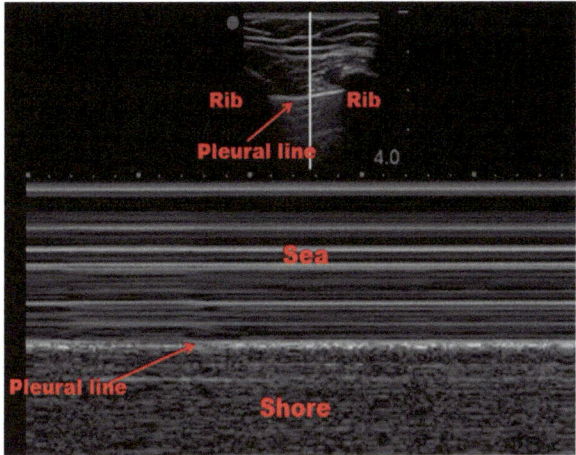

Fig. 16.4 Top picture depicts "bat sign": Two ribs with posterior shadowing which represents the wings of a bat with the hyperechoic pleural line as the body. Meanwhile, the bottom pictorial is in M-mode illustrating the "seashore sign," which is a normal finding. The hyperechoic pleural line divides the image with the motionless top ½ portion creating the horizontal "waves," while the sliding below the pleural line creates a granular pattern called the "sand"

generating an alternating pattern of the stratosphere and seashore signs) with a sensitivity of 79% and specificity of 100% [9].
- Adhesions (e.g., COPD or interstitial lung disease) and periods of apnea inhibit lung sliding. In large pneumothoraces, the lung will never contact the parietal pleura, thus no lung point will be detected.
- "B lines" are artifact arising from the pleural lining when the US beam encounters the physiological fluid that separates the pleural layers. They can only be seen when the pleural are in contact with each other. When a PTX is present, air separates the pleural layers and B lines disappear. If both lung sliding and B lines are present, the clinician can reliably exclude PTX at the examined location.

Take-Home Points for Patient Care

- E-FAST examination consist of six different US views that assess the thorax to the pelvis (pericardium, Morison's pouch, perisplenic space, pouch of Douglas, and bilateral thoracic windows).
- This technique aids in cavitary triage and guides decision-making, including choice of incision and post-trauma bay destination.
- Begin with the sub-xiphoid four-chamber view of the heart, moving next to the hepatorenal recess, then the splenorenal recess, then finally moving to the pelvis. Then assess the transthoracic views of the left and right thorax for lung sliding.

- While intraperitoneal hemorrhage manifests as free fluid, other sources of fluid exist (ruptured cyst, ascites, ruptured bladder).
- Intra-abdominal injury may exist even in the setting of a negative fast exam, as solid organ, enteric, and diaphragmic injuries are often undetectable on ultrasound. It is paramount to visualize the left diaphragm and left subphrenic space.
- A thoracic ultrasound can only detect a pneumothorax directly under the ultrasound probe. Thus, scanning multiple sites is necessary to detect an underlying pneumothorax.

References

1. Goodwin H, Holmes JF, Wisner DH. Abdominal ultrasound examination in pregnant blunt trauma patients. J Trauma [Internet]. 2001;50(4):689–93. discussion 694. Available from: http://www.ncbi.nlm.nih.gov/pubmed/11303166
2. Ma OJ, Kefer MP, Mateer JR, Thoma B. Evaluation of hemoperitoneum using a single- vs multiple-view ultrasonographic examination. Acad Emerg Med [Internet]. 1995;2(7):581–6. Available from: http://www.ncbi.nlm.nih.gov/pubmed/8521202
3. Goldberg BB, Goodman GA, Clearfield HR. Evaluation of ascites by ultrasound. Radiology [Internet]. 1970;96(1):15–22. Available from: http://www.ncbi.nlm.nih.gov/pubmed/5420399
4. Tilling T, Bouillon B, Schmid A. Ultrasound in blunt abdomino-thoracic trauma. In: Border JR, Allgöwer M, Hansen Jr ST, Rüedi TP, editors. Blunt multiple Trauma: comprehensive pathophysiology and care. 1st ed. New York: M. Dekker; 1990. p. 415–33.
5. Juhl J. Disease of the pleura, mediastinum, and diaphragm. In: Juhl J, Crummy A, editors. Essentials of radiologic imaging. 6th ed. Philadelphia: Lippincott Compnay; 1993. p. 1026.
6. Ma OJ, Mateer JR. Trauma ultrasound examination versus chest radiography in the detection of hemothorax. Ann Emerg Med [Internet]. 1997;29(3):312–5. discussion 315–6. Available from: http://www.ncbi.nlm.nih.gov/pubmed/9055768
7. Alrajab S, Youssef AM, Akkus NI, Caldito G. Pleural ultrasonography versus chest radiography for the diagnosis of pneumothorax: review of the literature and meta-analysis. Crit Care [Internet]. 2013;17(5):R208. Available from: http://www.ncbi.nlm.nih.gov/pubmed/24060427
8. O'Brien KM, Stolz LA, Amini R, Gross A, Stolz U, Adhikari S. Focused assessment with sonography for Trauma examination: reexamining the importance of the left upper quadrant view. J Ultrasound Med [Internet]. 2015;34(8):1429–34. Available from: http://www.ncbi.nlm.nih.gov/pubmed/26206829
9. Lichtenstein DA, Mezière G, Lascols N, Biderman P, Courret J-P, Gepner A, et al. Ultrasound diagnosis of occult pneumothorax. Crit Care Med [Internet]. 2005;33(6):1231–8. Available from: http://www.ncbi.nlm.nih.gov/pubmed/15942336

Chapter 17
Resuscitative Endovascular Balloon Occlusion of the Aorta

Randoll T. Christopher, Shyam Murali, and Jeremy W. Cannon

Overview

- Non-compressible torso hemorrhage represents the leading cause of potentially preventable death following trauma [1].
- Significant number of patients will exsanguinate prior to definitive control of bleeding.
- Aortic occlusion has historically been part of the armamentarium of resuscitation for patients with significant torso hemorrhage: [2]

  - Direct clamping (thoracotomy vs laparotomy).
  - Endovascular approach.

- Aortic occlusion can serve as an adjunct in other clinical scenarios:

  - Pelvic bleeding—invasive placental conditions, postpartum hemorrhage.
  - Elective orthopedic procedures.
  - Ruptured abdominal aortic aneurysm (AAA).

R. T. Christopher
Department of General Surgery, Mercy Catholic Medical Center, Philadelphia, PA, USA
e-mail: Randoll.Christopher@mercyhealth.org

S. Murali · J. W. Cannon (✉)
Division of Traumatology, Surgical Critical Care & Emergency Surgery, Perelman School of Medicine at the University of Pennsylvania, Philadelphia, PA, USA
e-mail: Shyam.Murali@Pennmedicine.upenn.edu; Jeremy.Cannon@pennmedicine.upenn.edu

© The Author(s), under exclusive license to Springer Nature Switzerland AG 2025
T. S. Brahmbhatt, D. R. Scantling (eds.), *Trauma Surgery Clerkship*, Contemporary Surgical Clerkships, https://doi.org/10.1007/978-3-032-01412-2_17

Physiology

- Hypovolemia → Cross clamping→ Increased SVR → Increased Afterload.
  - Increases brain and myocardial perfusion.
  - Lowers effective circulating volume.

History of REBOA

- First endovascular balloon was used by the military in the 1950s during the Korean War. However, the lack of endovascular technology and infrastructure limited its further evolution, and it remained as a lesser used technique in damage control resuscitation, taking a back seat to emergency thoracotomy and Military Anti-Shock Trousers (MAST) [3].
- The past two decades saw an explosion of advances in endovascular technology and balloon occlusion became an established technique for nontraumatic hemorrhage control (e.g., in ruptured AAAs).
- Initial animal studies suggested a benefit to REBOA for the treatment of massive non-compressible hemorrhage.
- Translational studies confirmed similar findings in early clinical studies.
- Continued research and development led to the creation of several commercially available REBOA devices, including the following:
  - ER-REBOA (Prytime Medical, Boerne, TX).
  - CODA balloon catheter (Cook Medical, Bloomington, IN).
  - Rescue Balloon Occlusion Catheter (Tokai Medical Products, Kasugai, Japan).
  - ResQ™ Occlusion Balloon Catheter (Qx Médical, Roseville, MN).
  - pREBOA-PRO (Prytime Medical, Boerne, TX) allows for partial occlusion of the aorta to maintain some perfusion to the lower body and limit ischemia-reperfusion injury (Fig. 17.1).

Fig 17.1 pREBOA-PRO catheter can perform partial occlusion of the aorta to allow for continued perfusion beyond the balloon. Note the balloon is filled with blue dye for improved visualization. (Image courtesy Shyam Murali, MD)

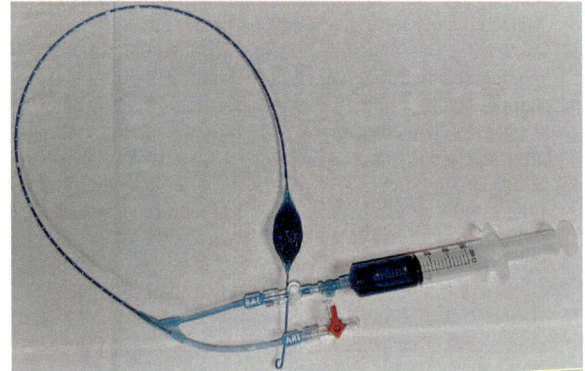

Relevant Anatomy

Zones of Occlusion (Fig. 17.2):

- Zone 1—Between takeoff of left subclavian and celiac axis

  - Occludes abdominal viscera, pelvis, lower extremities
  - Limit: Total balloon occlusion time < 30 min*

- Zone 2—Between celiac trunk and lower renal artery

  - Known as "Zone of NO occlusion".
  - Theoretical risk of intimal flaps at ostial opening

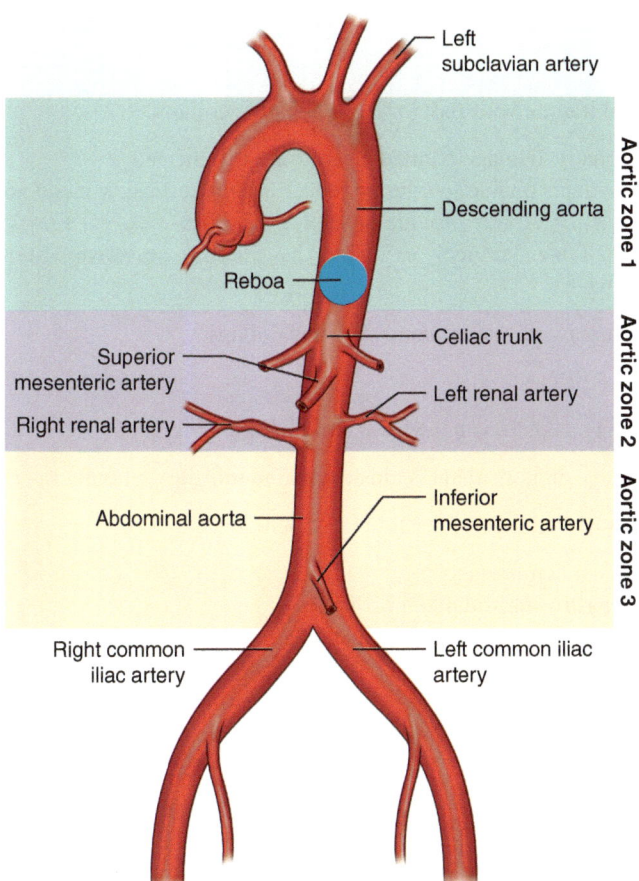

Fig. 17.2 Zones of the aorta. Occlusion is limited to Zones 1 and 3. (Image courtesy Rafael H. Cuello)

- Zone 3—Infra-renal aorta

  - Controls pelvic and lower extremity hemorrhage
  - Limit: Total Balloon occlusion time < 90 min*

  - *Maximal occlusion time may be extended with partial occlusion

Current Anatomic Limits

- Use for bleeding source in the thorax, currently limited.
- No studies evaluating REBOA in neck or axillary junctional hemorrhage.

Indications

- Abdominal trauma with risk for hemodynamic collapse

  - Traditionally, damage control laparotomy is indicated
  - Some patients unable to tolerate reduction in afterload (general anesthesia)
  - Zone 1 REBOA may provide physiologic bridge
  - Can facilitate surgical exposure by limiting massive intra-abdominal hemorrhage

- Pelvic Trauma with risk of hemodynamic collapse

  - Zone 3 REBOA

    - as long as there is no evidence of abdominal injury

  - Advantage of more distal occlusion, maintaining abdominal visceral perfusion

- Other causes of non-compressible torso hemorrhage

  - Obstetrical hemorrhage
  - Severe gastro-intestinal hemorrhage
  - Surgical procedures with anticipated large-volume blood loss

- Hemodynamic Threshold:

  - Patients with initial SBP < 90 with no response to resuscitation

Contraindications

- Significant thoracic hemorrhage
- Pericardial tamponade

- Inability to gain femoral arterial access (relative contraindications)

  - Patients with prior femoral vascular procedures
  - Stigmata of peripheral vascular disease (calcified vessels)

Technique

The technique described here will be specific to the Prytime Medical ER-REBOA device [4].

Insertion

1. Establish common femoral artery access with a 7Fr sheath.

   (a) Most commonly obtained under ultrasound guidance.
   (b) This can be the rate-limiting step.

      (i) In patients who have potential indications for REBOA, early femoral arterial access for blood pressure monitoring can be a useful first step
      (ii) If the patient already has a femoral arterial line, this can be up-sized to a 7Fr sheath

2. Determine the depth of insertion of the REBOA device by holding it over the patient. For Zone 1 insertion, the tip should be positioned at the sternal notch, and at the xiphoid process for Zone 3 insertion.
3. Test the balloon with saline to ensure there are no leaks. When deflating the balloon ensure that all the air is removed by holding the catheter upside down.
4. Straighten out the P-tip with the orange peel-away sheath and insert the sheath into the main port of the 7Fr arterial access sheath. You should get back-bleeding from the top of the orange peel-away sheath.
5. Stabilizing the top of the peel-away sheath, begin to slowly insert the REBOA device into the arterial access sheath. Once the 20-cm mark disappears behind the peel-away sheath, you can pull back the peel-away sheath to the back of the REBOA device.
6. Continue to insert the REBOA device slowly into the arterial access sheath until you reach the pre-determined depth of insertion.
7. Secure it by holding it manually or by using a rubber central line securing device. Suture between the bifurcation of the two access ports if needed (Fig. 17.3).
8. Slowly inflate the balloon with the appropriate amount of saline

   (a) Maximum of approximately 8 mL for Zone 1 and 2 mL for Zone 3
   (b) pREBOA-PRO has a safety valve that prevents over-inflation

9. Proceed with definitive hemostasis

Fig. 17.3 Securing the REBOA device to prevent it from backing out under pulsatile aortic pressure. Arrows denote suture locations. (Image courtesy Shyam Murali, MD)

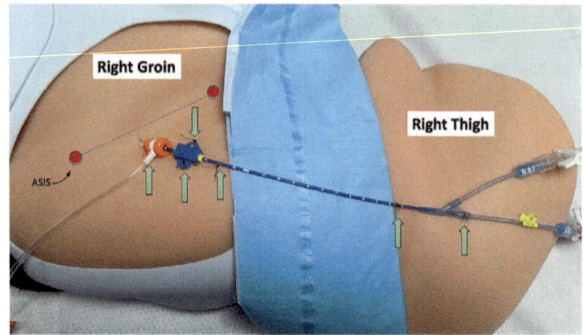

(a) Operative control
(b) Angio-embolization

Removal

1. After definitive hemostasis, alert anesthesia and other staff about the plan to deflate the REBOA balloon and remove the device. Check an arterial blood gas to ensure that the patient is well-resuscitated.
2. Slowly (i.e., one milliliter every 10 s or slower) deflate the REBOA balloon. Pay close attention to hemodynamics and active bleeding within the abdomen.
3. Once the balloon is fully deflated, remove the REBOA device from the arterial access sheath. When the balloon is near the arterial access sheath, use a corkscrew maneuver to safely remove the device without shearing the balloon.
4. Check coagulation studies (TEG, PT/INR, PTT, ACT) prior to removing the 7Fr arterial access sheath. Hold pressure. In certain situations, primary repair of the artery may be necessary.

Patient Management During Occlusion

- During balloon occlusion, arterial blood pressure above and below the balloon should be monitored.
- Resuscitation goals should target a proximal systolic blood pressure goal 90–100 mm Hg or a mean arterial pressure of 65 mm Hg.
- Continue damage control resuscitation to correct any underlying coagulopathy and maintain euvolemia with blood product administration.

  - Remain attentive to Ca++ levels throughout the resuscitation.

- Balloon deflation results in a much larger volume of distribution (lower half of the body now perfused), can wash out a large volume of ischemic by-products (e.g., K+ and metabolic acids), and can result in reperfusion injury.

Complications

- Ischemia to abdominal organs and lower extremities from aortic occlusion: aortic occlusion time should be kept as short as possible (ideally less than 30 min in Zone 1 and 90 min in Zone 3) to minimize ischemic complications [5, 6].

  - pREBOA-PRO device allows for partial balloon inflation and titration of blood flow past the balloon.

- Ischemia to lower extremities from arterial sheath: if malpositioned or placed in a small vessel, the arterial sheath can limit blood flow to the lower extremity. Frequent monitoring of neurovascular status is imperative to prevent long-term damage.

  - Target vessel for insertion is the common femoral artery.

- Ischemia-reperfusion injury: sudden physiologic derangements can occur as a result of reperfusion injury during balloon deflation. This is thought to be due to a rapid release of ischemic metabolites causing vasodilation and refractory hypotension. This can be mitigated by slow deflation, good communication with anesthesia, and rapid correction of electrolyte and acid-base abnormalities.
- Vessel dissection, rupture, perforation: these complications are rare but devastating. Misplacement of the balloon within the arterial system (e.g., migration into a renal artery) can result in vessel rupture and rapid hemorrhage.
- Embolization of thrombus: this can cause occlusion of distal vessels and further ischemia.
- Balloon rupture from overinflation.

References

1. King DR. Initial care of the severely injured patient. N Engl J Med. 2019;380(8):763–70. https://doi.org/10.1056/NEJMra1609326.
2. Weare S, Gnugnoli DM. Emergency room thoracotomy. [Updated 2022 Jul 25]. In: StatPearls [Internet]. Treasure Island: StatPearls Publishing; 2022. Available from: https://www.ncbi.nlm.nih.gov/books/NBK560863/.
3. Hughes CW. Use of an intra-aortic balloon catheter tamponade for controlling intra-abdominal hemorrhage in man. Surgery. 1954;36(1):65–8.
4. Morrison JJ, Galgon RE, Jansen JO, Cannon JW, Rasmussen TE, Eliason JL. A systematic review of the use of resuscitative endovascular balloon occlusion of the aorta in the man-

agement of hemorrhagic shock. J Trauma Acute Care Surg. 2016;80(3):554. https://doi. org/10.1097/TA.0000000000000913.

5. Ribeiro Junior MAF, Feng CYD, Nguyen ATM, et al. The complications associated with Resuscitative Endovascular Balloon Occlusion of the Aorta (REBOA). World J Emerg Surg. 2018;13:20. Published 2018 May 11. https://doi.org/10.1186/s13017-018-0181-6.

6. Osborn LA, Brenner ML, Prater SJ, Moore LJ. Resuscitative endovascular balloon occlusion of the aorta: current evidence. Open Access Emerg Med. 2019;11:29–38. Published 2019 Jan 14. https://doi.org/10.2147/OAEM.S166087.

Chapter 18
Interventional Radiology

Jessica Shi, Emily Ball, and Mikhail C. S. S. Higgins

Overview

- Introduction
- Tools for endovascular hemorrhage control
- IR interventions for:

  - Splenic injuries
  - Hepatic injuries
  - Renal injuries
  - Pelvic injuries

- Role of IR in a multidisciplinary trauma team

J. Shi
Interventional Radiology Integrated Resident, Beth Israel Deaconess Medical Center, Boston, MA, USA
e-mail: Jessica.Shi@bmc.org

E. Ball
Boston Medical Center, Boston, MA, USA
e-mail: Emily.Ball@bmc.org

Mikhail C. S. S. Higgins (✉)
The Bahamas Fibroid & Interventional Clinic (BFIC), Eleuthera, Bahamas
e-mail: Mikhail.Higgins@bmc.org

© The Author(s), under exclusive license to Springer Nature Switzerland AG 2025
T. S. Brahmbhatt, D. R. Scantling (eds.), *Trauma Surgery Clerkship*, Contemporary Surgical Clerkships,
https://doi.org/10.1007/978-3-032-01412-2_18

Introduction

Trauma remains the leading cause of death for those 45 and under, with hemorrhage accounting for up to 40% of all deaths from trauma in the United States [1–2]. Penetrating traumas may inflict complete or partial transection of vasculature. The coup-contrecoup impact of blunt injuries can have shearing impact on vessels, promote formation of pseudoaneurysms, and even truncate vasculature. Utilizing a predominately endovascular approach, interventional radiologists can provide expeditious and targeted control of the source of bleeding. Control of hemorrhage can be obtained via temporary or permanent modalities. Although current guidelines for the role of interventional radiology in trauma continue to evolve, injury mechanism, presentation, and imaging findings help to drive critical decision-making, particularly in the acute clinical care setting. While patients who are durably responsive to resuscitation and blood products are candidates for interventional radiology interventions, patients who are transiently responsive or unresponsive to transfusion should proceed directly to the operating room for open intervention and hemorrhage control.

Tools for Endovascular Hemorrhage Control

Transcatheter Arterial Embolization (TAE)

- Vascular embolization consists of administering an occlusive agent to a target vasculature.
- Along with angiography, flexible catheters and microcatheters guide precise selection of target vessel(s).
- TAE is particularly advantageous for controlling bleeds in trauma as it allows for control of the angiographically delineated source of hemorrhage while maintaining adequate perfusion to vital tissue through minimally invasive approaches.

Embolic Materials

Temporary Embolic Agent

Gelatin Sponge (gelfoam)

- Mechanism: Its high absorptive characteristic lends itself to swelling when injected and rehydrated. This causes hemostatic compression and mechanical obstruction of the vasculature, an acute full-thickness necrotizing arteritis of the arterial wall, regional edema with an associated interruption of the elastic interna of the vessel coupled with an acute inflammatory reaction, as well as delayed foreign body reaction [3]. Thrombus formation is induced which can be observed months post-treatment, although vessels embolized with gelfoam do typically recanalize.

- Typically, sheets of gelatin sponge are cut and formed into a slurry, which are injected into the vasculature of choice.
- Strengths:
  - Rapidly effective as a temporizing agent, with effects lasting up to weeks.
  - Inexpensive and widely available.
- Shortcomings:
  - Slurry has particles of varying sizes, which limits predictability of where embolic material will lodge in vasculature.
  - Gelatin sponges may retain air bubbles, which can promote aerobic infections [3].
  - Recanalization and reabsorption of the gelfoam can result in delayed hemorrhage [3].

Permanent Embolic Agents

PVA (polyvinyl alcohol) Particles

- Mechanism: PVA particles adhere to vessel walls and congregate, triggering an inflammatory angionecrosis response, leading to vessel fibrosis over time [3].
- Strengths:
  - Inexpensive and widely available.
- Shortcomings:
  - Outcome of embolization is size dependent: particles that are too large will lodge too proximally, with ineffective embolization resulting. Particles that are too small will lodge too distally, with possible distal ischemia and end-organ damage [3].
  - Due to the irregularity in size, high tendency to aggregate, with the possibility of catheter or proximal vessel occlusion [3].

Microspheres

- Mechanism: Similar to PVA, microspheres elicit an inflammatory angionecrosis response [3].
- Available in different formulations (PVA, trisacryl gelatin, polymethylmethacrylate with a coat of lyzene-F, copolymer), with different compositions lending themselves to different embolic purposes.

- Strengths:

  - Uniform smooth spherical shape.
  - Unlike PVA particles, microspheres rarely aggregate, thus reducing the risk of catheter occlusion [3].
  - Formulated in a variety of sizes, a clear advantage as microspheres have a predictable correlation between size of microsphere and diameter of vessel in which occlusion can occur [3].

- Shortcomings:

  - Risk of allergic reaction due to porcine gelatin composition.
  - Must be agitated to maintain suspension and prevent sedimentation.
  - Unintentional embolization of distal vessels may cause tissue ischemia [3].

Coils and Microcoils

- Mechanism: Bare coils effectively embolize through mechanical occlusion, by slowing or even blocking blood flow. Resultant damage to inner vessel wall endothelium triggers localized coagulation [3]. It may also be covered with thrombogenic fibers that are designed to promote thrombosis.
- Strengths:

  - Coils are deployed at the desired vessel location per the operator, offering precision.
  - Low risk of infarction due to preservation of the distal vasculature.
  - Detachable coils are retrievable, allowing for repositioning of the coil nest prior to final detachment.
  - Inexpensive, widely available.
  - Soft coils are available to prevent vessel dissection, perforation, or rupture.
  - By causing complete vessel occlusion, they are comparable to surgical ligation in outcome [3].

- Shortcomings:

  - Jailing of target vessels from re-access may occur if coil embolization is performed proximal to the site of a new or recurrent bleed.
  - Must optimize matching of the coil size to vessel diameter (20%–30% larger than target vessel diameter) [3].
  - Ineffective in setting of coagulopathy (thrombocytopenia, abnormal clotting factors, etc.) given its dependence on patients' ability to form thrombus [3].
  - Occlusion of non-target vessels can occur.
  - Coil migration can result in stroke or myocardial infarction.
  - Risk of vessel dissection, perforation, or rupture.

Choice of embolic material depends on target vasculature, intended duration of embolization, and operator preference and proficiency.

Balloon Occlusion

- Angioplasty balloons offer a temporary solution to hemorrhage.
- When inflated in a manner that allows for direct abutment of the delineated source of vascular injury, therapeutic balloon occlusion may effectively tamponade the bleeding resulting in its reduction or cessation [4].
- Temporary hemostatic stability may be used to bridge patients for definitive operative or endovascular management.

Stent Grafts

- Stent grafts allow for the reconstruction of vessels and are the cornerstone of thoracic and abdominal aortic repair in trauma. They help maintain the continuity of vasculature in cases in which the integrity of vessel walls has been compromised [4].
- Stents are deployed in vessels and may be post-dilated to desired sizes using angioplasty balloons.
- May be considered for treating ruptures, aneurysms, and dissections, allowing for exclusion of the aforementioned, with preservation of vascular flow to the distal vessel and organ.

IR Interventions for Splenic Injuries

In blunt abdominal trauma, the spleen is the most commonly injured visceral organ [5]. Given its vascular nature, splenic injuries can quickly become life-threatening. For patients who remain hemodynamically stable, non-operative, conservative management is the current standard of care. However, this approach has a failure rate of up to 34%, with even higher failure rates among patients with high-grade splenic injuries [8]. Yet, operative management via splenectomy confers a lifelong risk of infection [7]. Transcatheter splenic artery embolization is an angiographically supported splenic salvaging treatment option that allows for preservation of immunity and is appropriate for all grades of splenic injuries provided the patient is hemodynamically stable. Reports of splenic salvage rates range as high as 97% [8].

The two techniques utilized for embolization are proximal splenic artery embolization (PSAE) and super-selective distal embolization [9].

Proximal Splenic Artery Embolization

- The proximal splenic artery embolization (PSAE) is the IR equivalent of the surgical splenic artery ligation [4].
- Using a catheter, the splenic artery is selected and embolic coils are selectively deployed beyond the origin of the dorsal pancreatic artery, allowing for preserved collateral flow through the pancreatic arterial arcade.
- By occluding the main splenic artery, proximal splenic artery embolization decreases splenic arterial pressure, thus mitigating splenic hemorrhage, but while maintaining perfusion to the spleen via collateral pathways (such as short gastric arteries, pancreatic arteries, and gastroepiploic arteries) [4].
- This ultimately promotes healing and hemostasis, while preserving splenic perfusion and function.

Super-Selective Distal Embolization

- In scenarios where vascular injury can be localized angiographically to a select number of culprit vessels, distal splenic artery embolization can help focus embolization efforts.
- Similar to PSAE, a catheter (in this case, a coaxially advanced microcatheter) is advanced until the vasculature of interest is selected for embolization.
- Unlike PSAE, this technique allows for embolization distally in the splenic vasculature, as close as possible to the site of vascular injury.
- As such, hemostasis post-embolization is achieved only regional to the area of injury, while perfusion is preserved for the remaining spleen.
- This therapeutic technique is ideal for treating and excluding sites of vessel truncation, pseudoaneurysms, and focal extravasation of contrast-enhanced blood.

	Proximal splenic artery embolization	Superselective distal embolization
Duration of procedure	Shorter duration of procedure, limiting fluoroscopy time and radiation dose	Longer duration of procedure: Selection of small splenic arterial branches may be time-consuming
Strengths	Lower risk of ischemia/infarct	Preservation of vasculature and tissue not involved in the injury site
Shortcomings	Limits treatment of rebleeding that occurs distal to embolization site	More time-intensive: Not suitable for patients requiring rapid hemorrhage control Higher rate of splenic infarcts

Complications

- Possible complications include rebleeding, splenic pseudoaneurysm formation, splenic artery dissection, splenic abscess formation, delayed splenic infarction, and coil migration.
- Patients may require future splenectomy or repeat splenic angiography and intervention.

IR Interventions for Hepatic Injuries

Given its large size and rich vascularity, the liver is unsurprisingly the second most commonly injured solid organ in abdominal trauma, with a 10%–15% mortality rate. Although there is no consensus regarding timeline and patient selection for hepatic TAE, the Society of Interventional Radiology recommends consideration of embolization for hemodynamically stable patients with clinical evidence or imaging indications of ongoing hepatic bleeding or suspicion of bleeding even after surgical management.

- Hemodynamically stable grade I–III injuries can usually be treated non-operatively with medical management although active bleeding may still require angiographic intervention [6].
- Like high-grade splenic injuries, higher grade [4, 5] liver injuries can still be managed non-operatively although they often require further angiographic intervention for bleeding and additional interventions and monitoring for bile leaks.
- Unstable patients who undergo laparotomy often still require concurrent angiographic evaluation and intervention after bleeding is temporized with packing or other surgical means.
- Unlike the spleen, the liver receives the majority of its blood supply from the portal veins, with some contribution from hepatic arteries. As such, risk of infarction post-TAE is rare [4].
- However, the liver's extensive network of collateral circulation can reinforce bleeding even when injury sites are addressed with embolization [10]. Distal and proximal embolization of injury lesions can prevent this phenomenon [10]. Initial angiography may discern these collateral networks and variant vascular anatomy.
- TAE can be performed with super-selective catheterization followed by embolization. Alternatively, a less selective "scatter" embolization may be employed, which is a more regionally dispersive embolic technique that is useful when expeditious territorial control of hemorrhage is required [4].

Complications

- Notable but infrequent complications after embolization may include biloma formation, gallbladder infarction (requiring cholecystectomy), hepatic necrosis, or abscess formation, although the risk of necrosis is decreased when super-selective embolization is pursued [11].
- Most post-embolization complications can be treated conservatively.

IR Interventions for Renal Injuries

The retroperitoneal location of the kidneys confers some protective mechanism in the setting of traumatic injury. As such, the kidneys are rarely injured, and when injuries do occur, the majority are minor injuries such as low-grade lacerations or contusions [13].

- Conventionally, stable patients with grade I/II lesions are managed conservatively with observation.
- Grade III/IV/V lesions can be considered for angiography and embolization to allow for vascular injury selection to maximize renal tissue perfusion preservation while higher grade injuries (IV–V) may require nephrectomy [6].
- Delayed nephrectomy can be pursued for patients who require subsequent interventions.

IR Interventions for Pelvic Injuries

Pelvic hemorrhage carries a high mortality risk, particularly for patients who are hemodynamically unstable and have pelvic fractures [14]. Without an expeditious intervention, patients are at high risk of rapid exsanguination [4].

- TAE should be first-line therapy and standard of care for pelvic traumas over surgical management [6].
- Indications for an arterial endovascular intervention may include pelvic ring fractures and CT evidence of acute arterial vascular injury (e.g., contrast agent extravasation, expanding hematoma, pseudoaneurysm, vasospasm, vascular "cutoff" sign, arteriovenous fistula) [6].

Role of IR in a Multidisciplinary Trauma Team

The interventional radiology team provides an invaluable clinical service to patients presenting with traumatic injuries due to their unique diagnostic and therapeutic expertise. As such, their active and regular involvement in emergent trauma activations supports promotion of rapid triage and optimized multidisciplinary care.

Advantages Include the Following

- Efficient, effective, and durable hemorrhage control for anatomic regions that are difficult to access or clinically challenging to engage surgically.
- Preservation of perfusion to tissues not directly supplied by vessels impacted by the traumatic injury.
- Less physiologically taxing interventions than conventional surgical management [12].
- Beneficial in occurrences of post-operative re-bleeding as patients may not tolerate repeat laparotomy and post-operative anatomical distortion may impair successful surgical intervention.

Limitations Include the Following

- Ability to perform endovascular interventions is limited by accessibility of angiography suites with fluoroscopy capabilities.
- Endovascular interventions are not without their own set of complications; arterial access poses risk for the development of access site hematomas, arteriovenous fistulae, and arterial pseudoaneurysms. The target vessel may dissect or rupture with endovascular manipulation. When pursuing TAE, non-target embolization may result in the unintended infarction or necrosis of previously viable tissue.
- Early and routine engagement of the Interventional Radiology team is critical in abdominopelvic trauma management. Continued blood loss from the untreated injury along with hemodilution from aggressive resuscitation combined with the onset of hypothermia and acidosis may predispose patients to heightened mortality [12].

References

1. Rhee P, Joseph B, Pandit V, Aziz H, Vercruysse G, Kulvatunyou N, Friese RS. Increasing trauma deaths in the United States. Ann Surg. 2014;260(1):13–21.
2. Kauvar DS, Lefering R, Wade CE. Impact of hemorrhage on trauma outcome: an overview of epidemiology, clinical presentations, and therapeutic considerations. J Trauma. 2006;60(6):S3–S11.
3. Vaidya S, Tozer KR, Chen J. An overview of embolic agents. Semin Intervent Radiol. 2008 Sep;25(3):204–15.
4. Gould JE, Vedantham S. The role of interventional radiology in trauma. Semin Intervent Radiol. 2006 Sep;23(3):270–8.
5. Cinquantini F, Simonini E, Di Saverio S, et al. Non-surgical Management of Blunt Splenic Trauma: a comparative analysis of non-operative management and splenic artery embolization-experience from a European trauma center. Cardiovasc Intervent Radiol. 2018;41:1324–32. https://doi.org/10.1007/s00270-018-1953-9.
6. Padia SA, Ingraham CR, Moriarty JM, Wilkins LR, Bream PR, Tam AL, Patel S, McIntyre L, Wolinsky PR, Hanks SE. Society of interventional radiology position statement on endovascular intervention for trauma. J Vasc Interv Radiol. 2020;31(3):363–369.e2.
7. Demetriades D, Scalea TM, Degiannis E, et al. Blunt splenic trauma: splenectomy increases early infectious complications: a prospective multicenter study. J Trauma Acute Care Surg. 2012;72:229–34. https://doi.org/10.1097/TA.0b013e31823fe0b6.
8. Clements W, Joseph T, Koukounaras J, Goh GS, Moriarty HK, Mathew J, Phan TD. SPLEnic salvage and complications after splenic artery EmbolizatioN for blunt abdomINal trauma: the SPLEEN-IN study. CVIR Endovasc. 2020;3(1):92.
9. Quencer KB, Smith TA. Review of proximal splenic artery embolization in blunt abdominal trauma. CVIR Endovasc. 2019;2(1):11.
10. Roberts R, Sheth RA. Hepatic trauma. Ann Transl Med. 2021 Jul;9(14):1195. https://doi.org/10.21037/atm-20-4580.
11. Kozar RA, Moore JB, Niles SE, et al. Complications of nonoperative management of high-grade blunt hepatic injuries. J Trauma. 2005;59:1066–71.
12. Zealley IA, Chakraverty S. The role of interventional radiology in trauma. BMJ. 2010;340:c497.
13. Wessells H, Suh D, Porter JR, et al. Renal injury and operative management in the United States: results of a population -based study. J Trauma. 2003;54:423.
14. Papakostidis C, Kanakaris N, Dimitriou R, Giannoudis PV. The role of arterial embolization in controlling pelvic fracture haemorrhage: a systematic review of the literature. Eur J Radiol. 2012;81:897–904.

Chapter 19
Outline: Operating Room Practices

Anna E. Garcia Whitlock and Niels Martin

Introduction

- Often definitive care for the injured trauma patient can only be achieved in the operating room.
- Despite the uncertainty of acute injury, preparation and teamwork are paramount to ensuring each injury is adequately addressed.
- A standardized approach to every trauma operation ensures the best outcome for the patient including minimizing the risk of missed injuries.
- The team must decide which injuries require surgical intervention and when.
- Familiarity with the operating room equipment and procedures enables students to be helpful in an emergent situation.
- Critically ill trauma patients exhibit unique physiology that dictates which injuries can be addressed at the index operation.
- Sometimes the best operation is one that temporizes the injury and provides time for resuscitation in the intensive care unit until the patient is stable for a more definitive repair (i.e., damage control).

A. E. Garcia Whitlock
Department of Surgery, Perelman School of Medicine, University of Pennsylvania, Philadelphia, PA, USA
e-mail: Anna.Garcia@pennmedicine.upenn.edu

N. Martin (✉)
Division of Traumatology, Surgical Critical Care, and Emergency Surgery Department of Surgery, Perelman School of Medicine, University of Pennsylvania, Philadelphia, PA, USA
e-mail: Niels.Martin@pennmedicine.upenn.edu

© The Author(s), under exclusive license to Springer Nature Switzerland AG 2025
T. S. Brahmbhatt, D. R. Scantling (eds.), *Trauma Surgery Clerkship*, Contemporary Surgical Clerkships,
https://doi.org/10.1007/978-3-032-01412-2_19

To Operate or Not to Operate

- One of the biggest decisions to be made in the trauma bay is if the patient will require an operation.
- The primary and secondary surveys are critical components of identifying which injuries may require operative interventions.
- Imaging adjuncts such as plain films, ultrasound, and CT can be invaluable tools in the process of identifying, triaging, and repairing injuries, but only if the patient is stable enough to undergo them.
- Sometimes an unstable patient is not able to undergo imaging or even complete the primary or secondary survey—in these situations, it is necessary to proceed directly to the operating room.

Make a Plan

- Even though trauma surgery can be unpredictable, it still requires preoperative planning.
- The type of injuries discovered in the trauma bay combined with patient hemodynamics will largely dictate what surgeries the patient needs and when.
- Efficient planning requires a multidisciplinary approach, including at a minimum anesthesiology.
- For every case, it is important to make a plan that considers the following questions:
  - *How stable is the patient?* Operative planning must balance the patient's simultaneous needs for resuscitation and definitive repair. Stable patients might be able to undergo repair of all their injuries in one operation, while unstable patients might require a staged approach to repair known as damage control surgery.
  - *Which surgery (or surgeries) do they need?* It is important to take inventory of the patient's injuries so that you can prioritize the order in which they should be repaired. *This is often dictated by which injury is the most life-threatening*, but it might also be influenced by available equipment or timing of help from surgical consultants if needed.
  - *Should the patient go directly to the operating room?* Often the trauma patient will proceed to the operating room upon completion of the primary and secondary survey including imaging adjuncts. However, there are situations where a patient's trip to the operating room might be accelerated or delayed. For example, an unstable patient might proceed directly to the operating room without completing imaging.
  - *Where should the surgery take place?* If the patient requires vascular, neurosurgery, or interventional radiology assistance, one should consider the availability of hybrid operating rooms (rooms with special imaging to guide

interventional procedures such as angiography) where such interventions can take place alongside the surgery without the patient having to be moved from room to room.

- *What is the operative approach?* Operative approach will differ depending on the location of the injury. While most patients will receive a traditional midline laparotomy in the supine position for abdominal injuries, some situations such as subtle diaphragm injuries might benefit from starting with laparoscopy or an isolated rectal injury might need to start in lithotomy position. Similarly, the laterality and location of a thoracotomy will differ depending on the suspected location of the actual injury as will the location and type of incision in neck injury.

- *What equipment do you need?* The suspected operative approach will often dictate the equipment needed. Although there is a standard trauma laparotomy equipment set, you may need for additional retractors, instruments, or equipment depending on the injury location. This may be on a centralized cart (Fig. 19.1) or you may need to ask for the supplies. For example, a suspected rectal injury might need proctoscopy or flexible sigmoidoscopy set to evaluate the rectal mucosa from below. Similarly, bronchoscopy or esophagogastroduodenoscopy (EGD) scopes are other tools that may be necessary to evaluate the trachea and esophagus, respectively.

Fig. 19.1 Trauma cart with various supplies

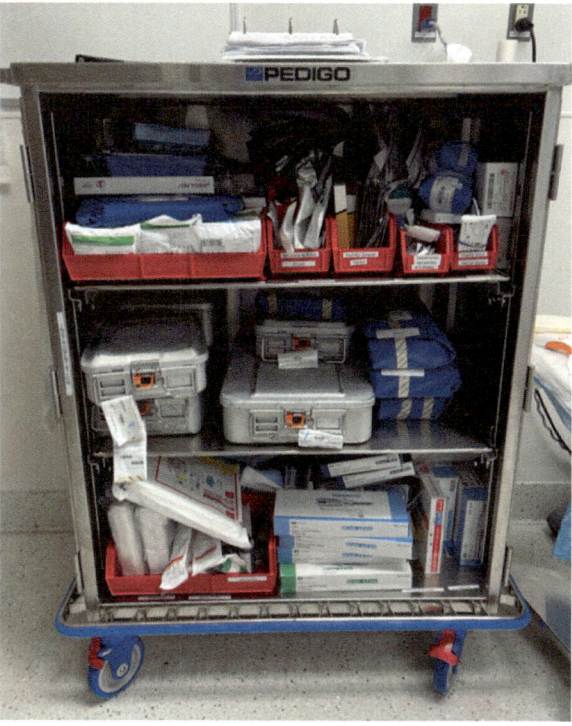

- *Do you need help from other specialties?* Although the trauma surgeon can address almost any injury, it is important to consider the availability of other specialties that might be of help. For example, vascular surgery can help with a complex vascular injury or interventional radiology can angioembolize bleeding vessels in the case of pelvic injuries or solid organ injuries.
- *Where will the patient recover?* Often patients will require additional monitoring or resuscitation in the intensive care unit (ICU). It is important to let the ICU team know early that this patient might be coming to their care so be sure that they are in the loop.

  How long do you think it will take? **The trauma bay is unpredictable. Thus, it is important to have a plan in case more patients show up. This can include leaving some members of the team in the trauma bay and having additional surgeons on back up to help if needed.**

- Things to review to make the plan include the following:

  - Clinical stability.

    - Need for intubation in the trauma bay for airway compromise.
    - Vital signs including changes from presentation and trends.
    - Need for blood pressure adjuncts including vasopressors.
    - Transfusion requirements including if they are responding to blood products.
    - Massive blood loss including need for massive transfusion protocol.

  - Primary and secondary survey.

    - Number and location of injuries including mechanism of injury.
    - History of prior surgeries including trauma (or at least location of surgical scars).
    - Relevant past medical history, medications, or allergies.

  - Laboratory and Imaging data.

    - Plain films, ultrasound, and CT imaging including if imaging suggests a trajectory in the setting of penetrating trauma.
    - Radiology interpretation of the reads including real-time discussions with the radiologist if the final reads are not back or there are lingering questions.
    - Signs of coagulopathy including the need for thromboelastography (TEG).

Assemble (and Know) the Team

- The trauma team consists of more than just the attending trauma surgeon and their trainees. There are many other providers across the trauma bay, operating room, surgical floor, and ICU who have extensive experience in trauma that you can call upon to help you execute your OR plan [2].

- Example of OR trauma team members includes the following:

  - Trauma attending surgeons, residents, and advance practice providers such as nurse practitioners and physician assistants.
  - Consultants such as orthopedics, vascular, thoracic surgery, and interventional radiology.
  - Nurses, paramedics, medical assistants, technicians, respiratory therapists, social workers and chaplains in the trauma bay.
  - Charge nurse, circulators, scrub nurses, and peri-operative assistants in OR (Fig. 19.2).
  - Anesthesia attendings, residents, nurse anesthetists, and technicians in the OR.
  - Critical care attendings, trainees, and advanced practice providers in the ICU.

- Once you have decided that the patient needs to go to the operating room, it is important to update these relevant teams with the plan:

  - *Trauma team*—Decide with the rest of the trauma team who will be going to the operating room and who will remain behind to continue to cover the trauma bay.
  - *Operating room*—A representative from the trauma team needs to call the operating room, specifically the OR charge nurse, to let them know that a patient will be coming to the operating room. It is important to relay your operative plan so that they can pull the equipment you need. It is also important to let them know when you need to be in the OR, i.e., whether this is someone who needs to be in the OR now.
  - *Anesthesia*—Similar to the OR staff, they need to know your plan including the patient's hemodynamic stability status including if the patient is already intubated or will need to be intubated in the OR. They also need to know about product administration including need for additional intravenous access or arterial blood pressure monitoring. Finally, type of injury or past medical history might influence their plan including intubation approach or type of anesthetic.

Fig. 19.2 Scrub nurse setting up the instrument table for trauma surgery

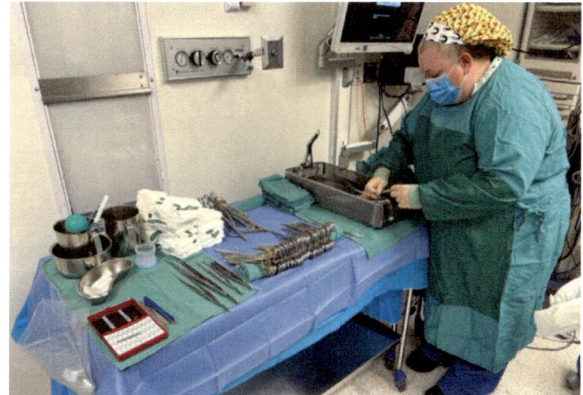

- *Blood bank*—Involving the blood bank early can help with the timely administration of blood products, especially if the patient requires massive transfusion protocol or targeted product administration based on TEG.
- *Consultants*—It is important to coordinate the prioritization and timing of intervention if multiple surgical services are required. Even if you aren't sure if you will definitively need a given consultant, it is often best to err on the side of asking them early to be on standby rather than wait until you need them imminently.

OR Physiology and Resuscitation Strategies

- Lethal Triad.

  - The lethal triad refers to a combination of hypothermia, acidosis, and coagulopathy seen in severely injured trauma patients (Fig. 19.3).
  - The lethal triad is especially common in patients who are hypotensive or have experienced hemorrhage [3].
  - Failure to prevent the lethal triad is associated with worse outcomes including death.
  - Clinical signs of the lethal triad include the following:

    - Low temperature refractory to warming measures.
    - Acidosis including large base deficit or elevated lactate.
    - Excess bleeding or abnormal labs including TEG.

- Damage Control Resuscitation.

  - This resuscitation strategy prioritizes minimizing detrimental physiologic derangements associated with injury, hemorrhage, or other major physiology insults [3].
  - Major principles include the following:

Fig. 19.3 The Lethal Triad consisting of coagulopathy, hypothermia, and acidosis

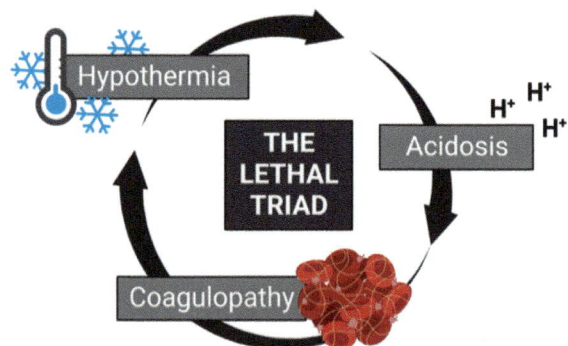

- Permissive hypotension.

  - Prioritize sufficient organ perfusion rather than normotension.
  - Goal systolic blood pressure 80–90 mm Hg—pursuing normotension may increase bleeding and coagulopathy.
  - The exception is traumatic brain injury which needs increased cerebral perfusion.

- Limit crystalloid infusion.

  - Prioritize transfusing blood products rather than crystalloid in the setting of acute blood loss.
  - Crystalloid can worsen acidosis, dilute coagulation factors, exacerbate inflammation, and lower oxygen-carrying capacity.

- Hemostatic transfusion.

  - Infuse blood product early and in a balanced ratio of platelets, plasma, and red blood cells to mimic the whole blood loss they are experience and limit coagulopathy.
  - Specifically, the Pragmatic, Randomized Optimal Platelet and Plasma Ratios (PROPPR) trial found that product administration in a balanced ratio (1:1:1 plasma to platelets to red blood cells) was associated with better outcomes [4]

- Resuscitate patients based on targeted clinical endpoints such as:

  - Vitals.
  - Urine output.
  - Lactate and/or base deficit.
  - Hemoglobin and hematocrit.
  - Conventional measures of coagulopathy such as PT and INR.
  - Viscoelastic tests including thromboelastography.
  - Ultrasound for intravascular volume.

- Damage Control Resuscitation in the OR.

  - It is important to be in constant communication with anesthesia to identify patients with the lethal triad who would benefit from damage control resuscitation strategies.
  - Damage control physiology can develop intra-operatively, potentially altering the care pathway mid procedure.
  - Minimize hypothermia by keeping the patient warm via both active and passive forms of warming including blankets," Bair Huggers," fluid warmers and rapid transfusion device.
  - Obtain blood products early including considering activating massive transfusion protocol.
  - Minimize time in the operating room including prioritizing life-threatening injuries and delayed definitive repair, i.e., damage control surgery [6].

Preparing the Trauma Operating Room

- OR Set UP.

  - The operating room should be large enough so that there is room for the trauma team including nursing and anesthesia, consulting teams, and all the necessary equipment (Fig. 19.4).
  - The operating room should be warm (70–80F) to minimize patient hypothermia and insensible losses that could lead to exacerbation of the lethal triad.

- A wide variety of instrument trays and other supplies should be immediately available to the trauma OR [5]:

  - Laparotomy tray with self-retaining multi blade retractor.
  - Sternotomy tray with sternal saw and closure wires.
  - Thoracotomy tray with Finochietto retractor.
  - Amputation tray with Gigli saw.
  - Vascular tray with shunts and catheters.
  - Resuscitative Endovascular Balloon Occlusion of the Aorta (REBOA) kits.
  - Emergency airway kit and tracheostomy.
  - Chest tubes and drains.
  - Temporary abdominal closure supplies.
  - Suction catheters and cannister.
  - Laparotomy pads with radiopaque tracer tags.
  - Adult and pediatric code carts with pacing wires.
  - Rapid infusion device and fluid warmer.
  - Auto transfuser.

Fig. 19.4 Example trauma operating room layout

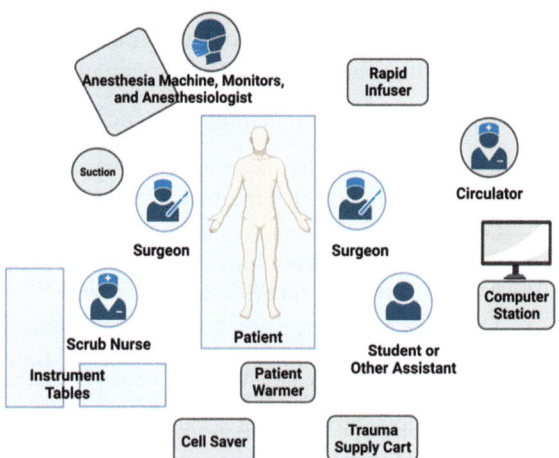

- Other more equipment might be necessary based on the injury location and mechanism, for example:

  - C-arm imaging machine for fluoroscopy.
  - Hybrid OR room if anticipate interventional radiology needs.
  - Bronchoscope or gastroscope for neck or chest injury in need of being prepared for pan-endoscopy.
  - Proctoscope or flexible sigmoidoscopy for rectal injury.

General Operating Principles

- Standard practices apply.

  - Even though the operation is emergent, it is still imperative that anesthesia administer antibiotics prior to or close to incision.
  - Same for the "time out for patient safety"—the team should still time out if time allows.
  - At a minimum keep anesthesia in the loop in terms of progress and expected physiology including a debrief upon entering the OR concerning product administration, most recent vitals and suspected operative needs as well as periodic updates throughout the operation itself.

- Preparing the patient.

  - Keep the patient warm.
  - Patient will likely need an orogastric or nasogastric tube, preferably the latter if will need decompression or enteral access postoperatively.
  - A foley is useful for both bladder decompression and hemostatic monitoring.
  - Ensure the patient has adequate vascular access including two large bore intravenous lines.

    - The patient might also benefit from a central venous line for infusion or arterial line for hemodynamic monitoring.
    - The trauma team is also able to place lines within the sterile fields.

- Positioning the patient.

  - Most of time the patient will be positioned supine with arms out.
  - Prep widely—"Chins to knees" (Fig. 19.5) [1]

    - Cover the patient with betadine soap from under the chin all the way down to the knees and down to the table laterally.
    - This is necessary in case there is a need to perform a thoracotomy, use the groin for vascular access, place a colostomy, or harvest a vein for vascular injury.
    - Can cover the groin with a sterile cloth.

Fig. 19.5 Typical trauma prep from "chin to knees" [1]

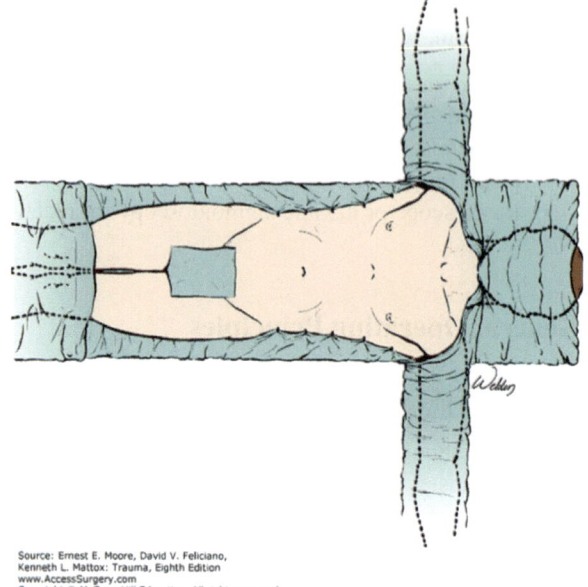

Fig. 19.6 Betadine soap prep kit used to prep widely

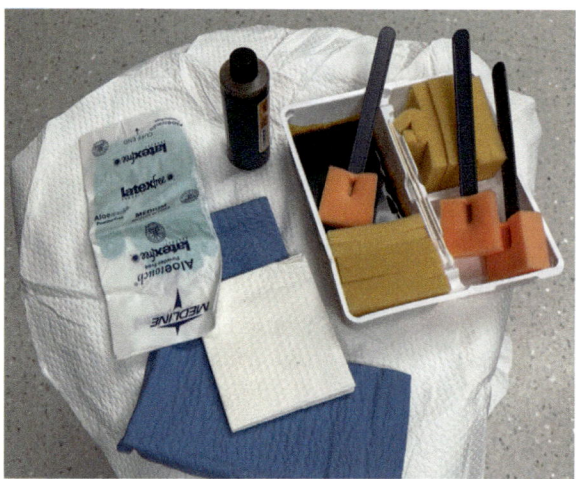

- Positioning and prepping the patient is a great opportunity to be helpful as a student and facilitate a timely operation, namely applying betadine soap (Fig. 19.6).

- Planning an incision.

  - The long midline incision from xiphoid to symphysis pubis is the most common incision in trauma as it provides extensive exposure of all organs in the abdomen.

- However, other incisions are of utility depending on the location and severity of injuries, thus the first incision or order of multiple incisions is informed by most life-threatening injury.

  - Pericardial window can help rule out tamponade.
  - Neck exploration incision can vary widely including anterior sternocleido-mastoid, collar incision, or median sternotomy.
  - Thoracotomy or median sternotomy are best to access great vessel bleeding.

    - Thoracotomy for posterior mediastinum or lung apices.
    - Median sternotomy for cardiac and hilar injuries.

After the OR

- A member of the trauma team should be sure to call the family to update them.
- ICU is the preferred location for a postop trauma patient still in shock. It is important to call the critical care team early and update them with the patient's story including how they did in the operating room.

  - A member of the trauma team along with a member of the anesthesia team should be present upon patient arrival to the ICU to provide a "warm" hand off and answer any additional questions about the patient's course.

Conclusions

- Efficient preoperative planning and teamwork is critical to operative success in trauma.
- Trauma patients exhibit unique physiology that dictates their resuscitation and operative needs.
- Because trauma is unpredictable, it is important to have a wide array of equipment available in the OR.
- In situations where there are multiple injuries, one must address the most life-threatening issues first.
- The key components of the trauma laparotomy are controlling bleeding, identify injuries, control contamination, and repair of injuries.
- Definitive repair in unstable trauma patients is delayed in favor of continued resuscitation and stabilization in the ICU.

Acknowledgments We would like to acknowledge Biorender.com regarding creation of figures and thank the overnight surgery team at Penn Presbyterian Hospital for help with the images.

References

1. Salotto J, Jurkovich GJ. Trauma laparotomy: principles and techniques. In: Moore EE, Feliciano DV, Mattox KL, editors. Trauma, 8e. New York, NY: McGraw-Hill Education; 2017.
2. Mecklenburg BSL, Inaba K. Trauma operating room. In: Demetriades D, Inaba K, Velmahos G, editors. Atlas of surgical techniques in trauma. 2nd ed. Cambridge: Cambridge University Press; 2020. p. 1–6.
3. Cannon JW. Hemorrhagic shock. N Engl J Med. 2018;378(19):1852–3.
4. Holcomb JB, Tilley BC, Baraniuk S, Fox EE, Wade CE, Podbielski JM, et al. Transfusion of plasma, platelets, and red blood cells in a 1:1:1 vs a 1:1:2 ratio and mortality in patients with severe trauma: the PROPPR randomized clinical trial. JAMA. 2015;313(5):471–82.
5. Jacobs LM, editor. Trauma laparotomy. Woodbury: Ciné-Med; 2010.
6. Martin N, Sarani B. In: Bulger EMC, Collins KA, editors. Management of the open abdomen in adults. Waltham: UpToDate; 2020.

Chapter 20
Operative Approaches to the Neck in Trauma

Loreski Collado and Frederick Thurston Drake

Introduction

The neck contains a total of nine organ systems, some of which, if injured, can lead to rapid and devastating clinical decline. Given these vital structures, neck trauma requires rapid evaluation and prompt intervention. The mechanism of injury resulting in neck trauma is broadly divided into blunt or penetrating. As with all traumas, adhering to the principals of ATLS (Advanced Trauma Life Support) is imperative; however, in neck trauma there is an emphasis on prompt assessment of the airway. Certain overt signs or symptoms suggest severe injury that should prompt immediate surgical exploration. In less acute scenarios, computed tomography (CT) angiography plays an important role in early management.

Types of Neck Trauma

- Blunt neck trauma compromises 5% of all neck traumas [1].
- The most common cause of blunt neck trauma is motor vehicle collisions. The neck is injured via acceleration and deceleration, direct contact from the dashboard or steering wheeling, or improper seat belt use. Other causes of blunt neck trauma include falls, strangulation, clothesline injuries, assault, and cervical manipulation (e.g., chiropractic manipulations).

L. Collado · F. T. Drake (✉)
Department of Surgery, Boston University Chobanian & Avedisian School of Medicine,
Boston Medical Center, Boston, MA, USA
e-mail: loreski.collado@emory.edu; frederick.drake@bmc.org

© The Author(s), under exclusive license to Springer Nature Switzerland AG 2025

T. S. Brahmbhatt, D. R. Scantling (eds.), *Trauma Surgery Clerkship*,
Contemporary Surgical Clerkships,
https://doi.org/10.1007/978-3-032-01412-2_20

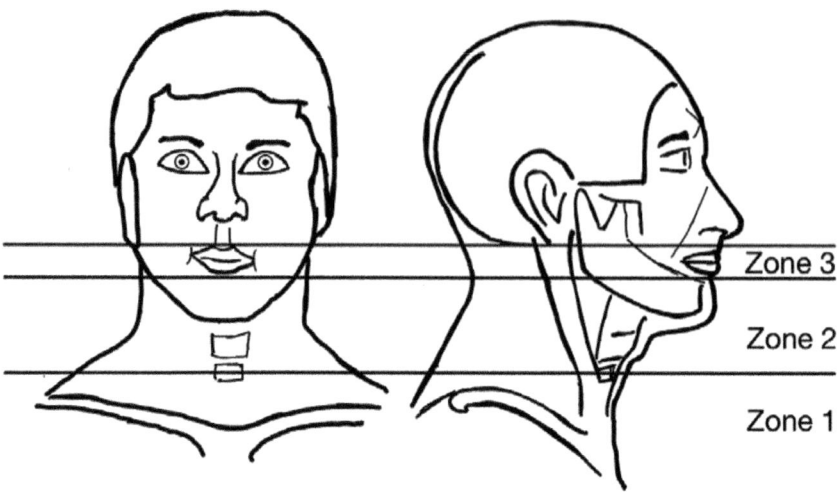

Fig. 20.1 Schematic demonstrating the zones of the neck [4]

- Penetrating trauma to the neck is typically caused by stab wounds or gunshot wounds. Knowledge of the three anatomic zones of the neck is necessary to help triage which underlying structures could be potentially damaged (Fig. 20.1), but does not dictate which wounds are operatively explored (as was previously the case).
- Historically, penetrating injury that violated the platysma mandated operative exploration. However, this resulted in non-therapeutic neck exploration rates as high as 50%–60% [2, 3].
- Now, in contemporary management of neck trauma, patients who are hemodynamically stable with injuries that penetrate the platysma can be evaluated by CT angiography. This approach has resulted in a more selective, conservative approach as to which patients can be monitored without surgical exploration and has proven to be safe among experienced surgeons [2, 3].

Presentation

- Emergency signs and symptoms in patients with neck trauma include profound shock from hemorrhage and pending airway compromise resulting in asphyxiation [5].
- Hard signs of aerodigestive injury include subcutaneous emphysema, bubbling or sucking neck wounds, large-volume hematemesis, or hemoptysis.
- Hard signs of vascular injury include bruit or thrill, expanding pulsatile hematoma or hematoma greater than 10 cm, pulsatile or severe hemorrhage, pulse deficit, or neurological deficit [3, 4].

- Other signs that neck structures have been injured include dysphonia, stridor, pneumomediastinum, and respiratory distress.
- Providers should note focal neurological deficits as these may result from cerebrovascular injury, cervical spine injury, cranial nerve injury, or brachial plexus injury [2].

Anatomy

- The platysma is a thin skeletal muscle that arises inferiorly from the deep fascia of the pectoralis major and deltoid and inserts to the lower margin of the mandible superiorly [4, 5].
  - An injury breaching the platysma can injury any number of vital structures.
- The deep cervical fascia subdivides into the investing layers, the pretracheal layer, the prevertebral layer, and the carotid sheath.
  - The fascial layers are clinically important as they can tamponade bleeding from damaged vasculature.
  - Additionally, their continuity with the thoracic fascia is important in the setting of esophageal injuries in which descending mediastinitis can develop.
- Deep to the platysma and deep cervical fascia lie the sternocleidomastoid (SCM), strap, and trapezius muscles which envelop the neck.
- Within the deep cervical fascia are eight additional organ systems (Fig. 20.2) [2, 5]:
  - Vascular system: the major components are the common, internal, and external carotid arteries, the vertebral arteries, and the internal and external jugular veins.
  - Gastrointestinal system: oropharynx, parotid/salivary glands, and cervical esophagus, which is predominantly but not entirely a left-sided structure.
  - Respiratory system: larynx and cervical trachea.
  - Nervous system: cervical spinal cord, brachial plexus, and cranial nerves (specifically, the facial [VII], glossopharyngeal [IX], vagus [X], spinal accessory [XI], and hypoglossal [XII] nerves).
  - Endocrine system: thyroid and parathyroid glands.
  - Lymphatic system: thoracic duct (left neck).
  - Skeletal system: hyoid bone, cervical vertebrae, mandible, clavicles.
  - Immune system: cervical extension of the thymus.
- The larynx extends from the epiglottis and the aryepiglottic folds to the cricoid cartilage. It communicates with the hypopharynx superiorly and with the trachea inferiorly. The larynx is made of cartilages and ligaments that are essential to its role in phonation.
- Zones of the neck (Table 20.1).

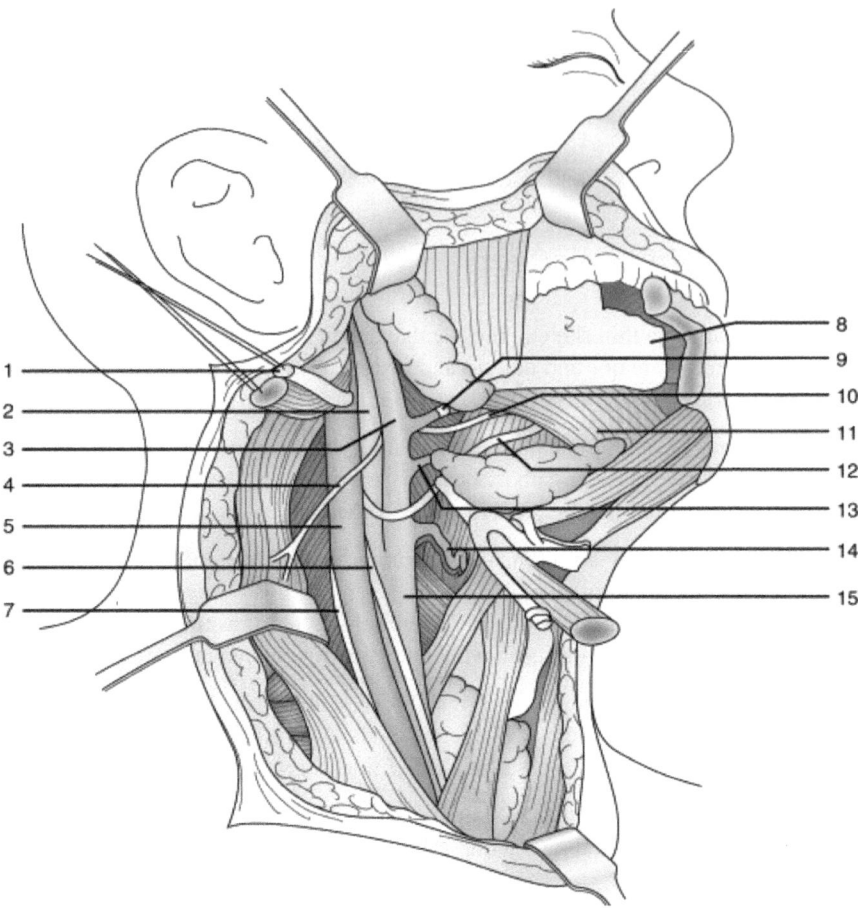

Fig. 20.2 Anatomic structures of zone II [2]. (1). Facial nerve; (2). Internal carotid artery; (3). External carotid artery; (4). Spinal accessory nerve; (5). Internal jugular vein; (6). Vagus nerve; (7). Cervical plexus; (8). Mandible; (9). Facial artery; (10). Lingual nerve; (11). Mylohyoid muscle; (12). Hypoglossal nerve; (13). Lingual artery; (14). Superior thyroid artery; (15). Common carotid artery

- Monson and colleagues developed a nomenclature widely used today dividing the neck into three zones anterior to the SCM [2, 3, 5, 6]. Note that this nomenclature is different from triangles of the neck.
- Zone I begins at the thoracic inlet and is delineated superiorly by the cricothyroid membrane.
- Zone II is between zone I and zone III, the cricothyroid membrane up to the angle of the mandible.
- Zone III is above the angle of the mandible and the base of the skull.

Table 20.1 Zones of the neck with anatomical structures and possible operative exposure [2, 4]

Zone	Anatomical boundaries	Anatomical structures	Operative exposure
I	Thoracic inlet to cricothyroid membrane	Proximal common carotid arteries Vertebral arteries Subclavian veins Jugular veins Trachea Esophagus Thoracic duct Spinal cord Cranial nerves Proximal brachial plexus	Median sternotomy with cervical extension or High anterolateral thoracotomy or Supraclavicular incision with claviculectomy
II	Cricothyroid membrane to angle of the mandible	Common carotid arteries and bifurcation Vertebral arteries Internal jugular veins Larynx Cervical tracheal Cervical esophagus Spinal cord Cranial nerves X, XI, XII	Ipsilateral oblique incision along the anterior border of SCM or High anterior collar incision with oblique extensions
III	Angle of the mandible to the base of the skull	Internal carotid arteries Vertebral arteries Internal jugular veins Pharynx Spinal cord Cranial nerves VII, IX, X, XI, XII Sympathetic chain	Subluxation of temporomandibular joint or vertical ramus mandibulotomy

Operative Approach

- A crucial step in approaching patients with neck trauma is early airway management.

  - Options to control the airway include traditional orotracheal intubation, nasotracheal intubation, awake fiberoptic intubation, awake tracheostomy and in an emergency setting, a cricothyroidotomy.
  - Tools that can be used to assist in successful intubation include video laryngoscopy, fiberoptic bronchoscopes, and a bougie with a coude tip used as a tracheal tube introducer via the Seldinger technique of inserting the endotracheal tube over the bougie and thus between the vocal cords into the airway.

- Note that while the use of a bougie has resulted in more successful first-attempt intubation in the patient with a difficulty airway, one should use caution in patients with unknown but suspected laryngeal trauma [6].
- If an emergency airway is needed and the vocal cords cannot be visualized because of blood or vomit, it is appropriate to perform a cricothyroidotomy; in the view of these authors, all healthcare providers should be familiar with the basics of emergency surgical airway (Chap. 13).

- Once the airway is secured and operative intervention is deemed necessary, an incision is chosen based on presumed zone of injury. There are several standard options (Fig. 20.3):

  - The most common approach is a vertical incision along the anterior border of the SCM extending from the angle of the mandible to the sternoclavicular joint.
  - A horizontal incision (also known as a high anterior collar incision) can be used to access multiple zones or to access bilateral neck injuries, subplatysmal flaps have to be developed for this incision, the midline raphe of the sternohyoid muscles is opened, and the sternohyoid muscles must be separated from the SCM.

- The great vessels in the thoracic inlet can be palpated and occasionally visualized by identifying and skeletonizing the anterior–medial aspect of the SCM, but sticking to principles of vascular surgery, to gain proximal and distal control of those thoracic inlet vessels, surgical approach can require a sternotomy, supra- or infra-clavicular incision.

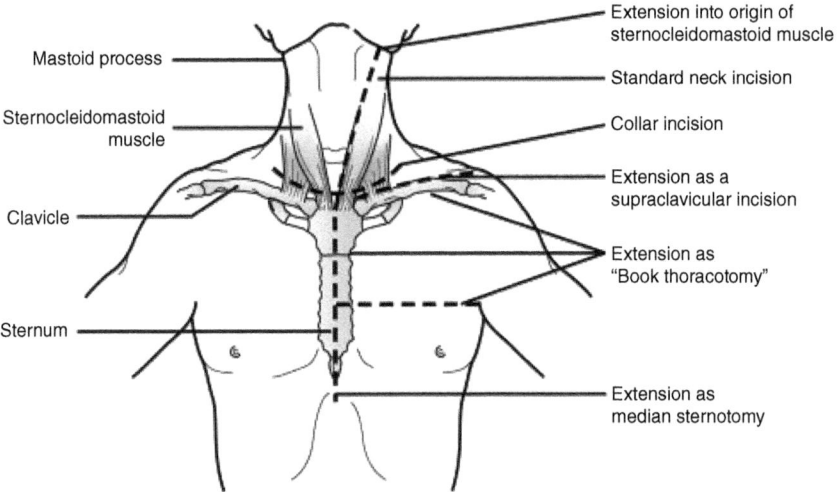

Fig. 20.3 Possible incisions that would allow access to the three zones of the neck [2]

- Furthermore, lower zone I injuries to the subclavian or innominate vessels may require a median sternotomy, disarticulation of the sternoclavicular joint, or anterolateral thoracotomy.

  - If there is strong clinical evidence of vascular or visceral injury in lower zone 1, surgical teams should consider early vascular or cardiothoracic surgery consultation.
- Proximal and distal control of the carotid artery can be obtained from the base of the skull to the clavicle.

  - High carotid injuries at or above the skull base (zone III) may require a vertical ramus mandibulotomy.
  - Exposure can be improved by dividing the digastric and stylohyoid muscles (distal) or dividing the SCM (proximal).
- In patients presenting with hemorrhage from a penetrating injury to the internal carotid artery in zone III, a balloon catheter can be passed through the wound in the skin in an attempt to tamponade the hemorrhage.

  - However, inadequate hemorrhage control should prompt urgent open exploration via ipsilateral incision along the SCM to allow exposure to the internal carotid artery, most likely to be followed by endovascular interventions.
- Use of a hybrid operating room may allow for simultaneous performance of advanced angiographic and operative procedures.

  - A hybrid room is a traditional operating room that also has advanced radiographic capabilities (e.g., fluoroscopy) to allow interventional radiologist (IR) to perform diagnostic and therapeutic procedures for hemorrhage control such as angiography, embolization, and stenting.
  - Thus, surgical and IR teams can jointly work on injured patients without having to move critically injured patient from one location to another.
  - The use of a trauma hybrid operating room is associated with earlier hemorrhage control and fewer early blood transfusions [10, 11].
  - This is especially important when there are inaccessible arterial injuries in zone III as these injuries are typically addressed with embolization or via covered stenting [5, 12].
  - There are case reports and case series reporting successful endovascular management of zone I arterial injuries, however, the standard open surgical technique—that is, sternotomy—is generally the most acceptable option.

Diagnostic Adjuncts

- CT angiography can be used to evaluate for arterial injury in penetrating trauma to any of the zones of the neck as well as *blunt* cerebrovascular injury (BCVI) to vertebral and carotid arteries.

- Patients must be hemodynamically stable and have a secure airway to go to the CT scanner.
- Laryngoscopy can be used to assess laryngeal injury.
- Bronchoscopy can be performed if tracheal injury is suspected.
- Esophagoscopy can be used to evaluate for esophageal injury.

  - Esophagoscopy and esophagram, in combination with physical exam, are highly sensitive in the diagnosis of esophageal injuries [2].

Types of Injuries

- Vascular injuries.

  - Vascular injuries are the most common injuries associated with penetrating neck trauma; 10% of vascular injuries involve the carotid artery.
  - Management strategies involve rapidly identifying the injury and preventing cerebral ischemia.
  - Operative strategies depend on type and severity of the injury, but include primary repair, bypass, ligation, or observation.

    - Observation is mostly utilized in the setting of blunt cerebrovascular trauma and sometimes includes antiplatelet therapy or anticoagulation.
    - Although endovascular repair was historically reserved for high zone III carotid and vertebral artery injuries, it has more recently emerged as an acceptable option for more proximal carotid injuries.
- Esophageal injuries.

  - Diagnosis of esophageal injuries requires a high index of suspicion as they present subtly, and delay in diagnosis is the most important contributor for mortality [1, 2].
  - The cervical esophagus, which is primarily a left-sided neck structure, should be repaired in a one-layer or two-layer fashion depending on whether the mucosa is intact.
  - To expose the esophagus one should dissect down to the cervical vertebrae and then lift the posterior wall of the esophagus off via careful blunt dissection with a finger.
  - Visualization of the esophagus can be maintained by looping it with a finger or Penrose drain and gently retracting laterally.
  - Muscle flaps constructed from the strap muscles or the SCM can be used to buttress the repair followed by liberal drainage.

- Laryngeal injuries.

  - Specific indications for operative management of laryngeal injury include large mucosal lacerations, lacerations involving the vibratory edge of the vocal cords, exposed cartilage, cartilage fractures, and injured arytenoids.
  - Operative strategies depend on the injury but can range from combination of suture of fractured segments, rigid internal fixation using miniplates, or placement of stents.
  - Laryngotracheal separation is the most severe form of laryngeal trauma.
  - It is useful to have otolaryngology (ear, nose, and throat [ENT] surgery) available if laryngeal trauma is suspected.

- Spinal cord injuries.

  - When a patient with neck trauma presents with neurological deficits such extremity paralysis or paresthesia, there should be high concern for spinal cord injury.
  - Spinal precautions should be maintained with prompt consultation with the orthopedic or neurosurgical spine surgery team.
  - CT can diagnose cervical vertebral fractures, whereas MRI can evaluate for spinal cord injury or ligamentous injury.

    - Those patients with cervical fractures should also have a CT angiogram to evaluate for BCVI [3].
  - Spinal cord injuries may present with hypotension; however, in the setting of trauma, one must rule out ongoing hemorrhage as the cause of shock [2].

Conclusion

- Initial evaluation of patients presenting with neck trauma includes the "ABCs" as outlined by ATLS with particular attention to assessing and securing the airway.
- Indications for immediate surgical exploration include refractory shock, expanding hematoma, airway compromise, and massive subcutaneous emphysema.
- Mandatory exploration of penetrating neck trauma to zone II will result in an unnecessary operation 50% of the time. CT angiography has allowed for a more selective approach in operative management of these cases.
- Surgical exposure is dictated by the zone of the presumed injury ranging from an ipsilateral oblique incision along the anterior border of the SCM, a high horizontal collar incision, median sternotomy (zone I), or vertical ramus mandibulotomy (zone III).

References

1. Rathlev NK, Medzon R, Bracken ME. Evaluation and management of neck trauma. Emerg Med Clin North Am. 2007 Aug;25(3):679–94.
2. Bagheri SC, Khan HA, Bell RB. Penetrating neck injuries. Oral Maxillofac Surg Clin North Am. 2008 Aug;20(3):393–414.
3. Tisherman SA, Bokhari F, Collier B, et al. Clinical practice guideline: penetrating zone II neck trauma. J Trauma. 2008;64:1392e405.
4. Shilston J, Evans DL, Simons A, Evans DA. Initial management of blunt and penetrating neck trauma. BJA Educ. 2021 Sep;21(9):329–35.
5. Sperry JL, Guardiani E, Snow G, Meenan K, Feliciano DV. Neck and larynx. In: Feliciano DV, Mattox KL, Moore EE, editors. Trauma, 9e. McGraw Hill; 2020. Accessed 5 Sept 2022. https://accesssurgery-mhmedical-com.ezproxy.bu.edu/content.aspx?bookid=2952&sectionid=249119537.
6. Monson DO, Saletta JD, Freeark RJ. Carotid vertebral trauma. J Trauma. 1969;9:987–99.
7. Driver BE, Prekker ME, Klein LR, Reardon RF, Miner JR, Fagerstrom ET, Cleghorn MR, McGill JW, Cole JB. Effect of use of a Bougie vs endotracheal tube and stylet on first-attempt intubation success among patients with difficult airways undergoing emergency intubation: a randomized clinical trial. JAMA. 2018;319(21):2179–89.
8. Hsiao J, Pacheco-Fowler V. Videos in clinical medicine. Cricothyroidotomy N Engl J Med. 2008;358(22):e25.
9. Mayglothling J, Duane TM, Gibbs M, McCunn M, Legome E, Eastman AL, Whelan J, Shah KH. Emergency tracheal intubation immediately following traumatic injury: an eastern association for the surgery of trauma practice management guideline. J Trauma Acute Care Surg. 2012;73(5):S333–40.
10. Loftus TJ, Croft CA, Rosenthal MD, Mohr AM, Efron PA, Moore FA, Upchurch GR Jr, Smith RS. Clinical impact of a dedicated trauma hybrid operating room. J Am Coll Surg. 2021;232(4):560–70.
11. Carver D, Kirkpatrick AW, D'Amours S, Hameed SM, Beveridge J, Ball CG. A prospective evaluation of the utility of a hybrid operating suite for severely injured patients: overstated or underutilized? Ann Surg. 2020;271(5):958–61.
12. Sperry J, Moore E, et al. Western trauma association critical decisions in trauma: penetrating neck trauma. J Trauma Acute Care Surg. 2013;75(6):936–40.

Chapter 21
Operative Approaches to the Chest

Caitlin A. Fitzgerald and Ryan P. Dumas

Introduction

Cardiothoracic trauma includes injuries to the airway, lungs, heart, great vessels, diaphragm, esophagus, and chest wall. Because these injuries are often life-threatening, being able to expose the injured structure through the appropriate incision is critically important [1].

Overview

- Choosing the correct incision for trauma to the chest depends on what structures are injured and whether the patient is hemodynamically stable or unstable.
- Management of these patients requires a multidisciplinary team effort and clear communication.
- Quick recognition and control of the injuries is extremely important as these patients can decompensate very quickly.

C. A. Fitzgerald · R. P. Dumas (✉)
Department of Surgery, Division of Burns, Trauma, Acute and Critical Care Surgery,
University of Texas Southwestern Medical Center, Dallas, TX, USA
e-mail: Ryan.Dumas@utsouthwestern.edu

T. S. Brahmbhatt, D. R. Scantling (eds.), *Trauma Surgery Clerkship*,
Contemporary Surgical Clerkships,
https://doi.org/10.1007/978-3-032-01412-2_21

Background and Principles

- Cardiothoracic trauma carries an overall mortality rate of 10%. Due to improvements in pre-hospital care, more patients are making it to the hospital alive; however, morbidity and mortality remain high [1].
- Immediate deaths are most often due to extensive injury to the lungs, heart, or great vessels, while later deaths are typically secondary to bleeding, tamponade, or airway obstruction.
- Regardless of presentation, a quick and methodical approach to the diagnosis and management of this patient population is important [2].
- The chest can be injured by both penetrating and blunt mechanisms. In penetrating trauma, gunshot wounds can cause both direct injury to structures along the trajectory of the bullet in addition to secondary blast injury to surrounding structures.
- Stab wounds are more predictable than gunshot wounds and tend to injure only structures along the trajectory of the blade.
- Blunt trauma can be more challenging to manage as the degree of external damage often does not predict the severity of internal injury [2].

- Initially, many life-threatening cardiothoracic injuries can be managed by Advanced Trauma Life Support principles including airway maintenance, establishing IV access, volume resuscitation, and tube thoracostomy [3].
- In some instances, patients present in extremis and require a resuscitative emergency department left anterolateral thoracotomy. In patients who are more hemodynamically stable, a planned operative approach can be performed.
- Once in the operating room, communication between the trauma surgeons, anesthesiologists, and nursing staff is key. Patients with chest trauma can quickly decompensate and successful management of this patient population depends on multidisciplinary teamwork.
- Choosing what exposure to perform depends on which structures are injured and need to be explored. Typical operative approaches include a subxiphoid pericardial window (often diagnostic rather than resuscitative anterolateral thoracotomy, posterolateral thoracotomy, and median sternotomy [4].

Current Practice

Median Sternotomy [5]

Indications

- Best incision for trauma within the cardiac box (parasternal) with tamponade present.

- Patient must be stable enough to be transported to operating room as a sternotomy requires more equipment and time.
- If patient too unstable, resuscitative left anterolateral thoracotomy is preferred given speed of entry and access to the descending aorta for cross-clamp placement.
- Provides access to heart, great vessels, and proximal exposure of the right subclavian artery. This incision provides limited exposure to left subclavian artery.

  - Injuries to ascending aorta and aortic arch are managed through a median sternotomy.
  - Innominate artery and vein are also well exposed.

- Consider early consultation to cardiothoracic surgery for cardiopulmonary bypass.

Technique

- Patient is positioned supine with arms out, prep from chin to thigh.
- Vertical midline incision with a knife centered over the sternum from sternal notch to xiphoid process (Fig. 21.1).
- Continue incision down through subcutaneous tissue, pectoralis fascia, onto sternum using electrocautery.

  - Mark midline on sternum with electrocautery.

- Incise interclavicular ligament and clear tissues deep to manubrium by bluntly removing attachments to bone with a finger.

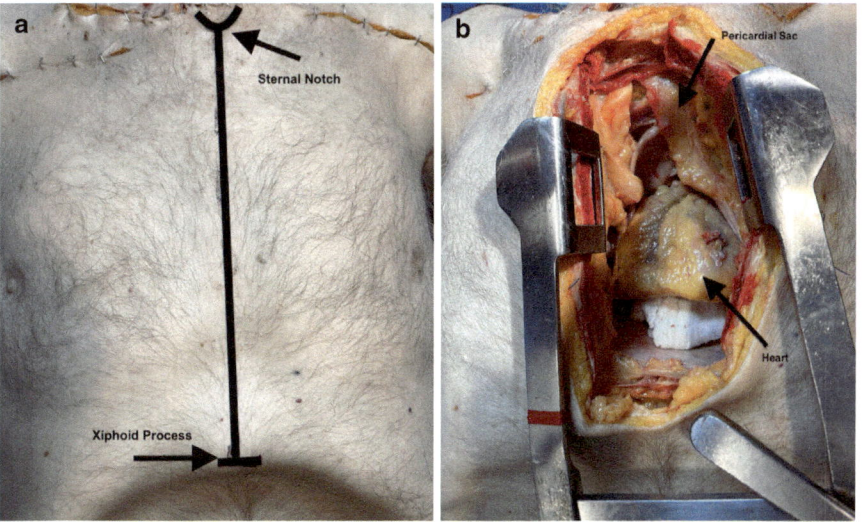

Fig. 21.1 (**a–b**). Median sternotomy incision landmarks (**a**). Completion sternotomy with pericardial sac open and heart elevated into field (**b**)

- Bluntly clear fat and peritoneum from under xiphoid process, cut xiphoid process in midline using heavy scissor.
- Use sternal saw to divide sternum in midline using previously placed line as a guide.

  - Point angled piece at the end of the saw blade upward to avoid injury heart and great vessels.

- If power saw not available, sternotomy can also be performed with Lebsche knife, Gigli saw, trauma shears, and/or a bone cutter.
- Once sternum is divided, place Finochietto retractor into chest.
- Divide pericardium with scissors from top to bottom to expose the heart, avoid injury to the phrenic nerve.
- Place pericardial stay sutures from edge of pericardium to the skin to elevate the heart and great vessels into the operative field and to move the pericardium out of the way (Fig. 21.1b).

Technical Considerations

- Cardiac injuries can be temporarily controlled with digital pressure, clamps, skin staples, or forceps.
- Atria are thin walled when compared to the ventricles and can tear when suturing.
- Suture cardiac injuries with 2–0 or 3–0 polypropylene sutures with or without pledgets.
- For injuries to great vessels, proximal and distal control is key.

  - Arteries can be temporarily shunted while planning definitive repair.
  - The majority of veins can be ligated.

- Definitive repair techniques for the great vessels include primary repair, interposition grafting, or jump grafts to the aorta.

Resuscitative Left Anterolateral Thoracotomy [5]

Indications

- Performed rapidly amid chaos of trauma bay, communication with team members is key.
- Indications vary based on both EAST and WEST guidelines (Figs. 21.2 and 21.3).
- Provides access to heart, descending thoracic aorta, left lung, distal esophagus, and left subclavian artery.
- Incision best used to quickly open the pericardium to perform cardiac massage, repair cardiac injuries, or cross clamp the descending aorta.

Question	Recommendation
PICO #1	In patients who present pulseless to the Emergency Department with signs of life after penetrating thoracic injury, we **strongly recommend** resuscitative Emergency Department thoracotomy. **Strong Recommendation**
PICO #2	In patients who present pulseless to the Emergency Department without signs of life after penetrating thoracic injury, we **conditionally recommend** resuscitative Emergency Department thoracotomy. **Conditional Recommendation**
PICO #3	In patients who present pulseless to the Emergency Department with signs of life after penetrating extra-thoracic injury, we **conditionally recommend** resuscitative Emergency Department thoracotomy. **Conditional Recommendation**
PICO #4	In patients who present pulseless to the Emergency Department without signs of life after penetrating extra-thoracic injury, we **conditionally recommend** resuscitative Emergency Department thoracotomy.[1] **Conditional Recommendation**
PICO #5	In patients who present pulseless to the Emergency Department with signs of life after blunt injury, we **conditionally recommend** resuscitative Emergency Department thoracotomy. **Conditional Recommendation**
PICO #6	In patients who present pulseless to the Emergency Department without signs of life after blunt injury, we **conditionally recommend against** resuscitative Emergency Department thoracotomy.[2] **Conditional Recommendation**

Fig. 21.2 The Eastern Association for the Surgery of Trauma guidelines for resuscitative thoracotomy [6]

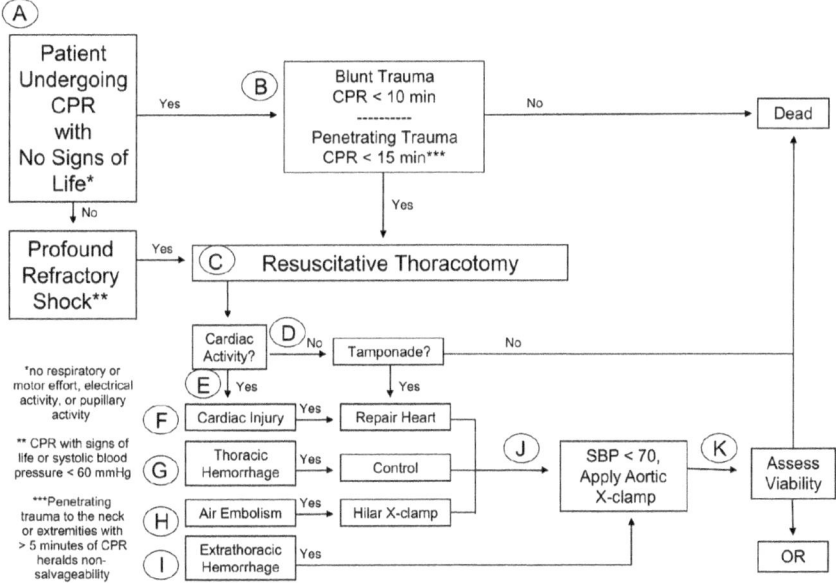

Fig. 21.3 The Western Trauma Association guidelines for resuscitative thoracotomy [7]

- A right-sided chest tube is typically placed to triage the right chest and evaluate if extension of the left anterolateral thoracotomy into a clamshell incision (bilateral anterolateral thoracotomies with transverse division of the sternum) is warranted.

Technique

- Position patient supine with left arm positioned above the patient's head, may need to use tape to keep arm elevated.
- Make an incision in fourth intercostal space, just superior to fifth rib with a scalpel (Fig. 21.4).

  - Incision made at nipple line in males and inframammary fold in females, similar to chest tube placement.

- Follow the curve of the rib (rather than a straight line from the sternum laterally) and extend incision from edge of sternum to posterior axillary line.
- Goal is to enter the chest just superior to the fifth rib (to avoid injury to the neurovascular bundle) in a little time as possible.
- Use scissors to divide the intercostal muscle.
- Insert Finochietto into rib space with handle facing toward bed.
- Upon entering the chest, open pericardium first with scalpel and then extend incision longitudinally with scissors avoiding injury to the phrenic nerve (Fig. 21.4b).
- Deliver the heart into the left chest to inspect it for injury or to perform cardiac massage.
- Divide inferior pulmonary ligament to retract left lung superiorly out of the chest.
- Palpate for aorta just anterior to the bony spine and posterior to the esophagus, using scissors or a Kelly clamp make anterior and posterior windows in the parietal pleura.

  - Palpation of the esophagus is better facilitated if there is a nasogastric tube in place.

- Once windows are made, place non-crushing aortic cross clamp.

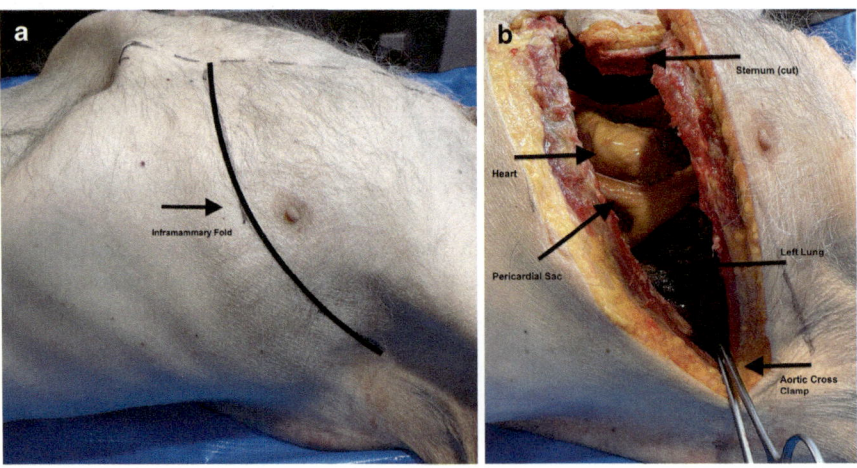

Fig. 21.4 (**a–b**). Resuscitative left anterolateral thoracotomy incision landmarks (**a**). Completion thoracotomy with pericardial sac opened and heart delivered into left side of chest (**b**)

Technical Considerations

- When performing resuscitative thoracotomy, place right-sided chest tube simultaneously to decompress the right chest.
- Lung parenchymal injuries are best managed with wedge resection or a tractotomy.

  - Injuries closer to the hilum may require non-anatomic resection or lobectomy.

- To perform tractotomy, place linear stapler into the wound and fire, once parenchyma is opened, oversew bleeding areas.
- A non-anatomic resection may require multiple staple loads.
- Hemorrhage from the central portion of the lung may require hilar control.

  - Hilum can be manually grasped to provide temporary control until an angled vascular clamp can be applied.
  - Hilum can also be controlled with a Rumel tourniquet.
  - Hilar twist can also be performed by gently rotating lung 180°.

- Trauma pneumonectomy is saved as a last effort to control bleeding.

Posterolateral Thoracotomy[5]

Indications

- Used in hemodynamically stable patients with no concern for life-threatening injuries to the abdomen, spine, or neck.
- Right posterolateral thoracotomy provides exposure to mid-esophagus, right lung, distal third of trachea, right main-stem bronchus, azygous vein, superior vena cava, and right atrium.
- Left posterolateral thoracotomy provides exposure to descending thoracic aorta, proximal left subclavian artery, distal esophagus, left lung, left main stem bronchus, and distal part of aortic arch.

Technique

- Position patient in lateral decubitus position.
- Make incision in fourth intercostal space, just superior to the fifth rib to avoid injury to the neurovascular bundle.
- Extend incision from anterior axillary line to the border of the scapula.
- Divide subcutaneous tissues and intercostal muscle with electrocautery.
- Place Finochietto retractor into rib space.

Technical Considerations

- In a stable patient, consider using a double lumen endotracheal tube to allow for deflation of one lung.
- To expose distal trachea, incise mediastinal pleura between trachea and esophagus (posterior structure).

  - Place nasogastric tube to better palpate esophagus.

- Divide azygous vein for complete exposure.
- Preserve tracheal length and minimize dissection, can devascularize trachea quickly.
- Routine tracheostomy is not necessary and most tracheal injuries can be repaired with simple interrupted sutures.
- Esophageal injuries can be repaired with a two layer closure, ensure that entirety of mucosal injury is exposed.

  - Buttress an esophageal repair with a muscle flap.

- In concomitant tracheal and esophageal injuries, place muscle flap between two structures.
- Destructive injuries to the esophagus are typically managed with a damage control cervical esophagostomy and wide drainage.

Subxiphoid Pericardial Window[5]

Indications

- Used to rule out cardiac injury in a hemodynamically stable patient.
- Can also be performed during trauma laparotomy to rule out pericardial fluid.
- It is diagnostic rather than therapeutic, and if the window is "positive," another procedure is needed.

Technique

- Patient is positioned supine with arms out, prepped from chest to knees.
- Make an incision midline over the xiphoid process, extend several centimeters down onto abdominal wall.
- Bluntly develop plane under the xiphoid and just above the peritoneum.
- Grasp central tendon of the diaphragm (lies directly over heart) with two Allis clamps and make a 1-cm window into the pericardium with scissors.

Technical Considerations

- If blood is encountered, proceed with median sternotomy.
- If there is no blood, irrigate pericardial sac with saline to look for a clot, if negative, cardiac injury is ruled out.

Less Common Exposures [5]

Clamshell Thoracotomy

- Indicated when access to both sides of the chest is needed.

  - Entire anterior mediastinum, both lungs, and great vessels are exposed through this incision.

- Extension of left resuscitative thoracotomy onto the right side.
- Perform right-side anterolateral thoracotomy.
- Use Lebsche knife to transect sternum to connect both sides of the incision.
- Place second Finochietto into right chest.

Supraclavicular Incision

- Used when distal control of subclavian artery or control of proximal axillary artery is indicated.
- Make longitudinal incision 1 cm above the medial half of the clavicle.
- Extend incision through platysma and divide sternocleidomastoid muscle at its attachments to the clavicle.

  - This will expose internal jugular vein and scalene fat pad.

- Expose anterior scalene muscle between subclavian vein and subclavian artery.

  - Identify and preserve phrenic nerve running obliquely across muscle.

- Divide anterior scalene 1 cm from clavicle to expose the subclavian artery.
- If exposure is not adequate, can divide and remove mid-portion of the clavicle.
- Best exposure of subclavian artery is achieved via median sternotomy with supraclavicular extension.

Take-Home Points

- Successful management of traumatic injuries to the chest requires quick decision-making, the appropriate exposure, rapid vascular control, and an effective repair.

- Patients presenting in extremis should undergo resuscitative thoracotomy, communication between participants is key to simultaneously manage the airway, obtain IV access, begin blood product resuscitation, and to avoid provider injury.
  - Goal is to gain access to the chest as quickly as possible to triage and manage any life-threatening cardiac or pulmonary injuries and to cross clamp the aorta.
- Place right chest tube while performing resuscitative thoracotomy to decompress and triage the right chest.
- For cardiac injuries, consider early consult to cardiothoracic surgery for consideration of cardiopulmonary bypass.
- Posterolateral thoracotomies are rarely utilized in a trauma setting as patients are often hemodynamically unstable with multiple injuries.
- During operative exposure of a thoracic injury, continuous communication with the anesthesia providers is key to a good patient outcome.
- Refer Table 21.1 for summary of operative approaches discussed.

Table 21.1 Operative approaches with landmarks and structures that are exposed

Incision	Key landmarks	Structures exposed
Median sternotomy	Sternal notch Xiphoid process	Heart Great vessels Proximal R subclavian artery Limited exposure to proximal L subclavian artery
Resuscitative thoracotomy	Fourth intercostal space Nipple line (males), inframammary fold (females) Edge of sternum Posterior axillary line	Heart Descending thoracic aorta Left lung Distal esophagus Left subclavian artery
Posterolateral thoracotomy	Fourth intercostal space Anterior axillary line Border of scapula	*Right:* Mid-esophagus, R lung, distal 1/3 of trachea, R mainstem bronchus, azygous vein, SVC, R atrium *Left:* Descending thoracic aorta, L subclavian artery, distal esophagus, L lung, L mainstem bronchus, distal aortic arch
Pericardial window	Xiphoid process	Pericardium
Clamshell thoracotomy	Bilateral anterolateral thoracotomies Connect through sternum with Lebsche knife	Entire anterior mediastinum Great vessels Both lungs
Supraclavicular incision	Superior border of clavicle Sternal notch	Distal subclavian artery Proximal axillary artery

References

1. Duan Y, Smith CE, Como JJ. Cardiothoracic trauma. In: Wilson W, Grande CM, Hoyt DB, editors. Trauma: emergency resuscitation, perioperative anesthesia, surgical management. 1st ed. New York: CRC Press; 2007. p. 469–99.
2. Farrier JM, Coimbra R, Lall R. Resuscitative thoracotomy. In: Wilson W, Grande CM, Hoyt DB, editors. Trauma: emergency resuscitation, perioperative anesthesia, surgical management. 1st ed. New York: CRC Press; 2007. p. 247–54.
3. Fagenholz P, Velmahos G. Surgical treatment of thoracic trauma: lung. In: Di Saverio S, et al., editors. Trauma surgery. 1st ed. Milan: Springer; 2014. p. 77–90.
4. Forti Pari SN, Boaron M. Surgical treatment of thoracic trauma: mediastinum. In: Di Saverio S, et al., editors. Trauma surgery. 1st ed. Milan: Springer; 2014. p. 91–8.
5. American College of Surgeons Committee on trauma. ASSET: exposure techniques when time matters. 2nd ed. American College of Surgeons; 2020.
6. Seamon MJ, et al. An evidence-based approach to patient selection for emergency department thoracotomy: a practice management guideline from the eastern association for the surgery of trauma. J Trauma Acute Care Surg. 2015;79(1):159–73.
7. Burlew CC, et al. Western trauma association critical decisions in trauma: resuscitative thoracotomy. J Trauma Acute Care Surg. 2012;73(6):1359–63.

Chapter 22
Operative Approaches to Abdominal Trauma

Sara Chiochetti and James P. Byrne

Overview

- The word "laparotomy" derives from Greek words "lapara" (*soft part of the body between the ribs and hip*, i.e., abdomen) and the suffix "-tomy" (*cut*).
- The decision to proceed to the OR for trauma laparotomy is made based on information gathered from initial assessment in the emergency department.
- The objectives of trauma laparotomy are to identify and treat intra-abdominal injuries in order from most-to-least life-threatening [1].
- The operative approach is systematic and adapted based on mechanism of injury (penetrating vs. blunt) and hemodynamic status of the patient (stable vs. unstable).
- The priorities are as follows [2]:

  1. Control of bleeding
  2. Control of contamination
  3. Definitive repair vs. damage control

- Laparoscopy has a diagnostic and therapeutic role in selected patients.

S. Chiochetti
Sinai Hospital of Baltimore, Baltimore, MD, USA

J. P. Byrne (✉)
Vancouver General Hospital, Vancouver, British Columbia, Canada

© The Author(s), under exclusive license to Springer Nature Switzerland AG 2025
T. S. Brahmbhatt, D. R. Scantling (eds.), *Trauma Surgery Clerkship*, Contemporary Surgical Clerkships,
https://doi.org/10.1007/978-3-032-01412-2_22

Indications for Trauma Laparotomy

Blunt Trauma

- In the *hemodynamically stable* patient, peritonitis is an indication for surgery as it suggests that hollow viscus injury is present. CT scan is often performed in stable patients to determine the specific complex of injuries. CT findings that are indications for abdominal exploration include free intraperitoneal air, diaphragmatic rupture, or evidence of hollow viscus injury.
- In the *hemodynamically unstable* patient, findings that suggest abdominal trauma such as peritonitis or positive FAST are indications to proceed to the OR for laparotomy. CT is often obtained preoperatively in patients that *durably* respond to initial resuscitation, with indications for surgery listed above.
- Severe pelvic fractures in hemodynamically unstable patients may present with a negative FAST but clinical or radiographic evidence of pelvic trauma. If such patients do not respond durably to transfusion, they may require emergent preperitoneal packing in the OR.

Penetrating

- In patients with penetrating abdominal injuries, the following are indications for abdominal exploration irrespective of hemodynamic stability: peritonitis, evisceration, free air on x-ray, bleeding from the GI tract, or positive FAST.
- Patients with gunshot wounds that clearly traverse the abdominal cavity typically require laparotomy as the rate of visceral injury is high (greater than 90%).
- Patients with isolated penetrating trauma to the right upper quadrant may be observed if hemodynamically stable, without peritonitis, or other evidence of injury to structures other than the liver and right-sided diaphragm. CT angiography should be performed to evaluate for active liver bleeding which may require angiographic intervention.
- In the *hemodynamically stable* patient with negative FAST, CT is useful to clarify trajectories of penetrating injuries and evaluate for peritoneal violation. Intraperitoneal air or fluid suggestive of visceral injury is an indication for laparotomy.
- *Hemodynamically unstable* patients with penetrating abdominal injuries should undergo urgent trauma laparotomy.

Rallying Your Resources: Communication and Preparation

- Once the decision for surgery has been made, it is the responsibility of the surgeon to mobilize resources for success.

- Effective communication between the trauma, anesthesia, and OR teams is critical to minimize delay and prevent gaps in care. All teams should be made aware of the operative plan. Specific equipment should be requested early.
- Preparation includes a warmed OR, informed anesthesia and OR teams, trauma operative equipment (laparotomy, thoracotomy, and vascular trays), and any addition equipment necessary for the unique scenario.

Essential Equipment for Trauma Laparotomy

- Scalpel (10 blade)
- Bovie Cautery
- Two suction devices
- Abdominal packing sponges
- Laparotomy tray (includes multiple types of forceps, scissors, clamps, needle drivers, retractors, and suction tips)
- Thoracotomy tray in the event that supra-celiac cross clamp becomes necessary (includes rib spreader retractor, aortic clamp)
- Retractor system (Bookwalter, Thompson, or Omni)
- Surgical staplers
- Hemostatic adjuncts (QuikClot® Combat Gauze, Surgicel, etc.)
- Irrigation

Positioning and Preparing the Patient

- The patient is positioned supine with arms outstretched to allow for access by the anesthesia team for line placement and blood draws.
- Skin is prepped from neck-to-knees to provide surgical access to any cavity, to the groin for line placement, and to the thighs for saphenous vein harvest if a vascular graft is needed.

The Systematic Trauma Laparotomy

- An incision is made from xiphoid to pubis using the 10 blade scalpel. When a patient is in extremis, the abdomen is entered sharply with only a knife and curved Mayo scissors.
- Eviscerate the small intestine and systematically pack all quadrants of the abdomen with sponges. This is done in a coordinated manner by surgeons standing on both sides of the operating table: one surgeon retracts, the other packs. Packing

serves to tamponade hemorrhage and helps to evacuate hemoperitoneum when the sponges are removed.

- Caveat: When a major life-threatening source of hemorrhage is identified upon entering the abdomen, this should be controlled directly prior to packing. This is most common in *penetrating trauma.*
- Packing is removed in a systematic manner, beginning with areas least concerning for injury.
- As injuries are identified, they are treated with the following priorities:

  1. Control of bleeding
  2. Control of contamination

- The three Zones of the Retroperitoneum are next evaluated carefully.
- Zone 1: The midline retroperitoneum. Contains the intra-abdominal aorta and inferior vena cava extending inferiorly to their bifurcation (level of the sacral promontory). Both the supra-mesocolic (above the colon mesentery) and infra-mesocolic (below the colon mesentery) Zone 1 retroperitoneum must be inspected. A Zone 1 hematoma must be explored in both *blunt* and *penetrating trauma* to evaluate for for major vascular injury.
- Zone 2: The lateral retroperitoneum. Extends from the renal hilum to the paracolic gutter on both sides. Contains the kidneys, ureters, and adrenal glands. In *blunt trauma*, Zone 2 hematomas are typically observed unless they are expanding. In *penetrating trauma*, Zone 2 hematomas are typically explored.
- Zone 3: The pelvic retroperitoneum. The retroperitoneum inferior to bifurcation of the intra-abdominal aorta and inferior vena cava (level of the sacral promontory). Contains the common, internal, and external iliac arteries and veins. In the setting of *blunt trauma*, Zone 3 hematomas are usually observed as they most often represent contained venous bleeding due to pelvic fractures. However, in the setting of hemodynamic instability pre-peritoneal packing is performed as a temporizing hemorrhage control technique (described below). In the setting of *penetrating trauma,* Zone 3 hematomas are explored out of concern for iliac vessel injury.
- When major bleeding due to pelvic fractures is suspected to be the cause of hemodynamic instability, pre-peritoneal packing is commonly performed. In this maneuver, the extraperitoneal space (of Retzius) is accessed between the pubic symphysis and bladder. Typically, three rolled surgical sponges are then packed posteriorly toward the sacrum on either side. When done correctly, this compresses bleeding from major venous, and lesser arterial, branches. When more significant arterial hemorrhage is present, this serves as a temporizing measure until angioembolization can be performed.
- The large solid organs (liver and spleen) are inspected. Where injuries are present, deliberate packing is an effective temporizing measure. Injuries are then treated as described in following chapters.
- Careful evaluation of the GI tract is then performed from top to bottom. This begins with the gastroesophageal junction and anterior stomach. A Sweetheart or Deever retractor can help to visualize the most proximal intra-abdominal esophagus at the hiatus.

- When there is concern for injury to the posterior stomach or lesser sac (e.g., as indicated by a *penetrating injury* to the anterior stomach) the lesser sac must be explored. To achieve this, the gastrocolic ligament is divided, allowing the posterior stomach and pancreas to be inspected.
- The duodenum, in its retroperitoneal position, can only be partially visualized initially. This is typically adequate to identify overt signs of injury. When there is concern for *penetrating injury* on basis of trajectory, or hematoma is present, the duodenum should be exposed and Kocherized.
- The small intestine is run in its entirety from the ligament to Treitz to the cecum (terminal ileum). This is done carefully and deliberately, 2–3 inches at a time, such that all participants are able to inspect for injury to the bowel or mesentery.
- The colon is then visualized from cecum to the proximal rectum at the peritoneal reflection in the pelvis.
- Any full-thickness injuries identified in the GI tract can be controlled temporarily using a 3–0 silk suture, Babcock forceps, or atraumatic clamp. In a stable patient, more definitive repair or resection can be performed. In a hemodynamically unstable patient, initial temporary control by suture is best.

Commonly Encountered Injuries

- In the setting of blunt trauma, the spleen (40%–55%), liver (35%–45%), and small intestine or mesentery (5%–10%) are the most commonly injured organs [3].
- Stab wounds are associated with injuries directly along the trajectory of the penetrating instrument although the depth and orientation of penetration may not be obvious. Organs most commonly injured by stab wounds are the liver (40%), small intestine (30%), diaphragm (20%), and colon (15%) [3].
- Gunshot wounds cause injury both directly, by energy transfer along the trajectory of the bullet, and indirectly, by cavitation and energy transfer to adjacent structures. The trajectories of gunshot wounds are frequently not predictable and bullet fragmentation adds to complexity when assessing for injuries. The most common injuries found with gunshot wounds are small intestine (50%), colon (40%), liver (30%), and abdominal blood vessels (25%) [3].

Definitive Repair Versus Damage Control

- Once control of bleeding and control of contamination has been achieved, the surgeon must decide whether definitive repair of injuries is feasible at the index operation. This decision is based on the physiologic status of the patient and complexity of injuries.
- The alternative to definitive repair at the index operation is called damage control [4]. Damage control entails temporary abdominal closure and transfer to an ICU

where resuscitation, correction of coagulopathy, and correction of physiologic abnormalities are prioritized.

- Expert consensus recommends damage control in the setting of [5]:

    1. Severe physiologic abnormalities

        - Hypothermia
        - Coagulopathy
        - Acidosis

    2. Massive transfusion of blood products (>10 units)
    3. Inability to control bleeding surgically (i.e., requiring angioembolization)
    4. Injury pattern requiring staged repair

- Wide drainage of injuries to specific organs should be performed, including pancreas, genitourinary, and liver.
- Temporary abdominal closure can be performed using skin only closure techniques, commercially available negative pressure systems (i.e., ABTHERA™), or assembly of other available equipment [6].
- Return to the OR is appropriate once patient physiology has improved and the necessary resources are gathered. This should be no later than 48 h following the index operation.

Maneuvers and Mobilizations

Intra-abdominal Aortic Control

- Performed when a patient is in extremis from major arterial hemorrhage below the diaphragm.
- The supra-celiac aorta can be accessed through the gastro-hepatic (lesser) omentum. The left triangular ligament of the liver can be divided to allow upward reflection of the left lobe out of the way. The supra-celiac aorta can be compressed using fingers, the smooth surface of a Richardson retractor, or clamped.
- The infra-renal aorta can be controlled for more distal injuries (such as iliac vessel injuries). This can be compressed directly, or fully exposed via Cattell-Braasch maneuver to allow clamping.

Pringle Maneuver

- Performed to control major hemorrhage from liver trauma. Occludes the hepatic inflow from hepatic artery and portal vein.

- To achieve this, the surgeon's fingers are passed through the foramen of Winslow into the lesser sac and the lesser omentum is opened. This allows the gastro-hepatic ligament, containing the portal structures, to be encircled.
- Occlusion is performed using a vessel loop, Rumel tourniquet, or vascular clamp.
- While there is no evidence to dictate the maximum duration of occlusion, Pringle time should be recorded and minimized given the sensitivity of the liver to ischemia.
- It is important to note that the Pringle maneuver does not stem bleeding from the hepatic veins or inferior vena cava. The presence of hemorrhage from a retrohepatic venous injury is indicated by ongoing bleeding despite application of the Pringle maneuver.

Kocher Manuever

- Performed to fully inspect the first, second, and third portions of the duodenum and head of pancreas for injury.
- The right colon and hepatic flexure are medialized. Gentle medial traction is then applied to the anterior aspect of the duodenum as the lateral peritoneal and retroperitoneal attachments are divided. This allows the duodenum to be reflected upward from the retroperitoneum. The limit to this mobilization is reached when the superior mesenteric artery (which passes posterior to the neck of the pancreas) is palpable with the fingertips.

Cattell-Braasch Maneuver (Right-Sided Medial Visceral Rotation)

- Performed to gain exposure of the entire infra-mesocolic retroperitoneum including the infrarenal aorta and IVC, usually for the purpose of exploring a zone 1 hematoma.
- Begins with Kocher maneuver and full mobilization of the right colon. The line of fusion between the small bowel mesentery and the posterior peritoneum is then divided in the direction of the ligament of Treitz. This allows the entire length of the small bowel and right colon to be reflected upward, out of the abdomen, or packed out of the way.
- This is the exposure of choice when there is concern for infra-mesocolic major vascular injury, including the aorta, inferior vena cava, renal, and iliac vessels.

Mattox Maneuver (Left-Sided Medial Visceral Rotation)

- Performed to gain access to the supra-mesocolic aorta and its branches. This portion of the aorta is otherwise very difficult to access due to its position posterior to the stomach, pancreas, and other major blood vessels.
- Begins with mobilization of the left colon by incising the white line of Toldt. This is carried superiorly to release the retroperitoneal attachments of the spleen, and inferiorly to the sigmoid colon. The plane of dissection then carries posterior to the left kidney, such that the spleen, tail of pancreas, and left kidney are reflected upward from the muscles of the posterior abdominal wall.
- With these structures medialized, the aorta is accessible anterior to the spinal column. The proximal superior mesenteric artery is also accessible by this approach.
- This is the exposure of choice when a supra-mesocolic zone 1 hematoma is present, raising concern for proximal major vascular injury.

Aird Maneuver

- Performed to mobilize and inspect the body and tail of the pancreas for injury.
- Best achieved with exposure to the lesser sac by dividing the gastrocolic ligament. The splenic flexure of the colon is mobilized and the retroperitoneal attachments of the spleen are divided. This allows the spleen to be lifted anteriorly, bringing with it the tail and body of the pancreas.
- This is the mobilization of choice when there is concern for high grade injury to the body or tail of the pancreas. Sets the stage for distal pancreatectomy with splenectomy.

The Role of Laparoscopy in Trauma

- Laparoscopy has both diagnostic and therapeutic roles in selected patients that are hemodynamically stable [7].
- Use of laparoscopic approaches in trauma requires that the surgeon performing the procedure is sufficiently experienced.
- Diagnostic laparoscopy is helpful for the purpose of evaluating for specific injuries based on high index of suspicion. Common uses are:
  1. Determining whether penetrating injury caused peritoneal violation.
  2. Evaluating for bowel injury in the setting of low energy (stab) penetrating trauma.

3. Evaluating for hollow viscus or mesenteric injury in blunt trauma, indicated by peritoneal fluid not explained by solid organ injury.
4. Evaluating for presence of diaphragmatic injury in the setting of penetrating trauma [8].

- Therapeutic laparoscopy is most commonly performed for repair of diaphragmatic injury caused by penetrating trauma. Other roles, such as repair of penetrating hollow viscus injury, are less common and case specific.
- Laparoscopy is typically contraindicated in the setting of hemodynamic instability, concomitant life-threatening injuries (e.g., traumatic brain injury), large volume hemoperitoneum, or when the trajectory of penetrating injuries is unclear.

References

1. Bowman JA, Jurkovich JG. Trauma laparotomy: principles and techniques. In: Feliciano DV, Mattox KL, Moore EE, editors. Trauma. 9th ed. New York: McGraw-Hill; 2021. p. 629–44.
2. Hirshberg A, Mattox KL. The crash laparotomy. In: Allen MK, editor. Top knife: the art and craft of trauma surgery. 1st ed. TFM Publishing Limited; 2005. p. 53–70.
3. American College of Surgeons Committee on Trauma. Abdominal and pelvic trauma. In: Advanced trauma life support: student course manual. 10th ed. American College of Surgeons; 2018. p. 82–101.
4. Rotondo MF, Schwab CW, McGonigal MD, Phillips GR 3rd, Fruchterman TM, Kauder DR, et al. 'Damage control': an approach for improved survival in exsanguinating penetrating abdominal injury. J Trauma. 1993;35(3):375–82.
5. Roberts DJ, Bobrovitz N, Zygun DA, Ball CG, Kirkpatrick AW, Faris PD, et al. Indications for use of damage control surgery in civilian trauma patients: a content analysis and expert appropriateness rating study. Ann Surg. 2016;263(5):1018–27.
6. Cirocchi R, Birindelli A, Biffl WL, Mutafchiyski V, Popivanov G, Chiara O, et al. What is the effectiveness of the negative pressure wound therapy (NPWT) in patients treated with open abdomen technique? A systematic review and meta-analysis. J Trauma Acute Care Surg. 2016;81(3):575–84.
7. Wang J, Cheng L, Liu J, Zhang B, Wang W, Zhu W, et al. Laparoscopy vs. laparotomy for the management of abdominal trauma: a systematic review and meta-analysis. Front Surg. 2022;9:817134.
8. Murray JA, Demetriades D, Asensio JA, Cornwell EE 3rd, Velmahos GC, Belzberg H, et al. Occult injuries to the diaphragm: prospective evaluation of laparoscopy in penetrating injuries to the left lower chest. J Am Coll Surg. 1998;187(6):626–30.

Chapter 23
Lower Extremity Vascular Injury

Emmanuel C. Nwachuku and Alik Farber

Peripheral Vascular Injury

Overview

- The lower extremity is a common location for vascular injury, particularly the superficial femoral artery (SFA)
- The mechanism of the injury, whether blunt or penetrating, often dictates patient presentation
- Patients presenting with a vascular injury resulting from blunt force tend to have worse outcomes
- The presence or absence of hard and soft signs of vascular injury dictate the management and work up of patients
- Knowledge of vascular anatomy is important for proper management of vascular injuries
- Key tenets of vascular surgery, such as obtaining proximal and distal control, are very important in the management of these patients

E. C. Nwachuku (✉)
Department of Vascular and Endovasular Surgery, Boston Medical Center, Boston University School of Medicine, Boston, MA, USA
e-mail: Emmanuel.Nwachuku@bmc.org

A. Farber
Division of Vascular and Endovascular Surgery, Department of Surgery, Boston Medical Center, Surgery and Radiology, Boston University School of Medicine, Boston, MA, USA
e-mail: Alik.Farber@bmc.org

T. S. Brahmbhatt, D. R. Scantling (eds.), *Trauma Surgery Clerkship*, Contemporary Surgical Clerkships,
https://doi.org/10.1007/978-3-032-01412-2_23

Epidemiology and Pathophysiology

Trauma to the lower extremity is very common, accounting for 1–2% of all injuries in the non-military population [1]. When looking at the location of injury as it relates to the mechanism, the common femoral artery (CFA) and the superficial femoral artery (SFA) are mostly commonly injured in the setting of penetrating trauma, while the popliteal artery is frequently injured as a result of blunt trauma. Due to anatomical relationships, many musculoskeletal injuries have an associated vascular injury. For example, popliteal vessels can be injured when the knee is dislocated posteriorly, while iliac vessels are most injured in the setting of a pelvic fracture. Recognizing this association allows the physician to have a high index of suspicion during patient evaluation. As previously mentioned, vascular injury can result from either blunt or penetrating trauma. The mechanism of injury can influence patient outcomes. According to Urrechaga et al., the odds of poor outcomes are increased in patients with blunt trauma associated with fractures and/or extensive soft tissue injury [2]. Additionally, when associated with a vascular injury, lower extremity trauma carries a 10% risk of mortality or limb loss.

Injury to an artery can manifest in multiple ways and a patient can present with either ischemia hemorrhage, or both, depending on the pattern of injury. An occlusive injury is an injury that results in complete or partial cessation of blood flow distal to the site of injury. The pathophysiology is such that damage to the intima of an artery activates the clotting cascade which promotes platelet activation and aggregation, leading to thrombus formation. Additionally, intimal dissection or intramural hematoma can lead to a vascular stenosis or occlusion. This injury pattern, depending on the vessel involved and presence of collateral circulation, often results in acute limb ischemia characterized by pain, pulselessness, pallor, and impaired motor or sensory function. Conversely, injury to an artery can also manifest with bleeding. The "hard signs" of bleeding include active hemorrhage, pulsatile mass in area of injury, expanding hematoma and a palpable thrill in the suspected area of injury (Table 23.1).

In the literature, there are very few accounts of isolated traumatic venous injury. Most venous injuries occur in the setting of an arterial injury. According to Kurtoglu et al., approximately 20% of patients with extremity vascular trauma had isolated venous injury, while the rest were associated with an arterial injury [3]. Concomitant venous injuries are mostly seen in the setting of complex traumatic injuries

Table 23.1 Hard and soft signs of vascular injury

Hard signs	Soft signs
Active arterial bleeding	Neurologic injury in proximity to vessel
Absent distal pulses	Unexplained hypotension
Expanding or pulsatile hematoma	Large blood loss at the scene
Distal ischemia (6 Ps)	ABI <0.9
Bruit or thrill	Unequal pulse

involving the SFA. Just like arterial injuries, venous injuries can present with significant hemorrhage but there is no consensus on the right way to manage these injuries.

Options for treatment of a vascular injury include primary repair, repair with a patch, interposition bypass graft, and ligation. Given recent advances in endovascular technology, endovascular interventions with use of stent-grafts and embolization have become part of the armamentarium of the vascular surgeon in addressing traumatic arterial injuries.

Regardless of presentation, traumatic vascular injuries require an efficient and timely approach in order to increase the chance of limb salvage. Therefore, it is important to understand the nuances of properly managing these injuries. Proper management of any patient with a vascular injury requires a profound knowledge of anatomy. For example, knowing the location and path of an artery or vein and their relationship to surrounding structures allows the surgeon to quickly expose and control injured vessels.

Anatomy

The infra-renal abdominal aorta usually bifurcates into the right and left common iliac arteries at the level of the fourth lumbar vertebrae. Each common iliac artery then gives rise to the external and internal iliac arteries. The CFA is a continuation of the external iliac artery as it passes underneath the inguinal ligament along with the femoral vein. The common femoral vessels are found within the femoral triangle, which is bounded superiorly by the inguinal ligament, medially and laterally by the adductor longus and sartorius, respectively. In the femoral triangle, the femoral nerve is the most lateral structure, followed by the femoral artery, the femoral vein, and lymphatics. This association can be easily remembered with the mnemonic NAVEL (lateral to medial: nerve, artery, vein, lymphatics). The CFA overlies the head of the femur, varies in length, and eventually bifurcates into the SFA and the deep femoral artery (Fig. 23.1). The deep femoral artery, also known as the profunda femoris artery, takes a course lateral and posterior in the thigh, while the SFA continues down the thigh, travels through the adductor canal, and exits the at the adductor hiatus posteriorly, giving rise to the popliteal artery. The popliteal artery courses behind the knee and usually bifurcates into the anterior tibial artery and the tibioperoneal trunk. The anterior tibial artery courses through the anterior compartment of the leg and continues as the dorsalis pedis artery in the foot. The tibioperoneal trunk then divides into the peroneal artery (fibular artery) and the posterior tibial artery. The posterior tibial artery usually comes off approximately 2 cm distal to takeoff of anterior tibial artery and then travels in the posterior compartment, eventually giving rise to plantar arteries of the foot.

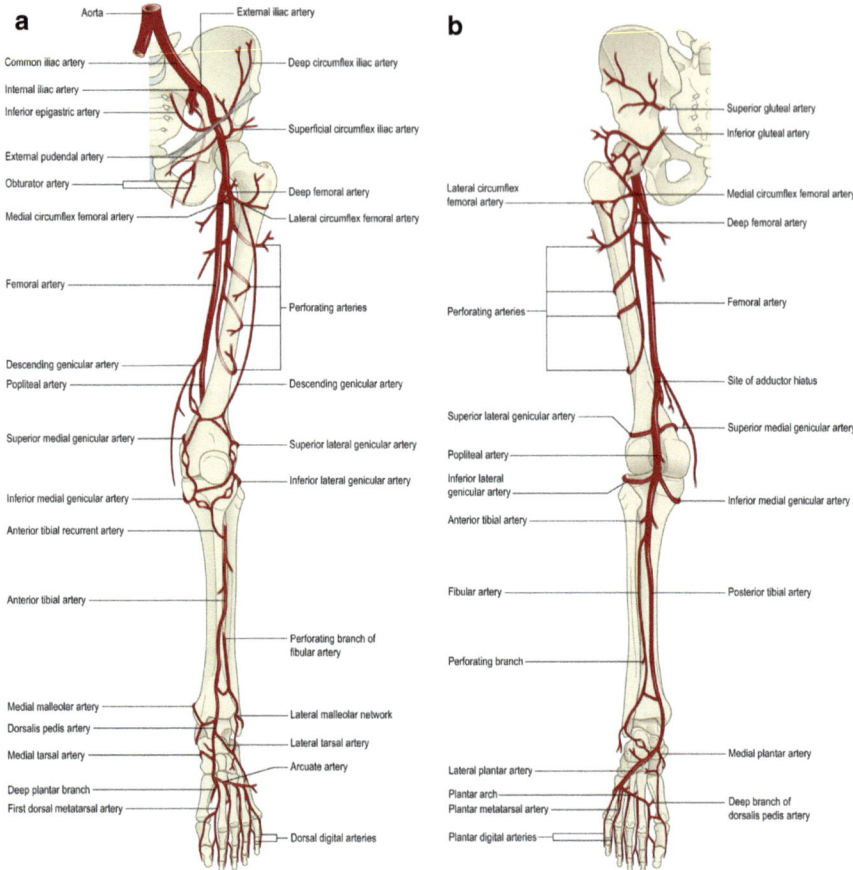

Fig. 23.1 Lower extremity vascular anatomy. (**a**) Anterior aspect. (**b**) Posterior aspect. (*Note*: From *Gray's Surgical Anatomy*. Forsythe et al. Published December 31, 2019. Pages 577–583. e2. © 2020)

Current Management Practices

- *Pre-hospital*
    - Pre-hospital management of vascular injury includes direct manual pressure and the use of tourniquets.
    - The use of tourniquets is associated with a reduction in prehospital death from 23.3 deaths per year to 3.5 deaths per year [4].
- *Trauma bay*

- Vascular injuries can be distracting; therefore, it is important to examine the patient in a systematic fashion by following advance trauma life support (ATLS) algorithms.
- Often, patients will arrive to the trauma bay with a tourniquet already in place. It is important to ensure appropriate equipment and personnel are available before removing the tourniquet. Ideally, the tourniquet should be removed in the operating room after the patient is prepped and draped and the surgeons are ready to address the vascular injury.
- Proper work-up begins with a good physical exam which includes checking for hard and soft signs of vascular injury.
- If pulses cannot be palpated, then a Doppler should be used to listen for signals of blood flow.
- In patients with suspected vascular injury an ankle-brachial index (ABI) is an invaluable tool. ABI is calculated by dividing the blood pressure measured at the ankle by the blood pressure measured in the arm. A number below 0.9 is abnormal and warrants further investigation such as a CT angiogram (CTA).
- Palpable thrill or audible bruit should raise concern for an arterial-venous fistula.
- Arterial injuries are often associated with musculoskeletal injuries. Misaligned bony structures can compress blood vessels resulting in diminished or absent pulses. In these situations, reduction of the fracture, followed by re-examination is recommended.
- In a patient who is hemodynamically stable, it is prudent to obtain basic imaging to guide operative management. Hence, patients with soft signs of vascular injury should undergo a CTA (Fig. 23.2) which helps to fully assess the nature of the injury and plan the revascularization should it be indicated.

Fig. 23.2 CTA of the left lower extremity showing active extravasation after a stab wound (blue arrow)

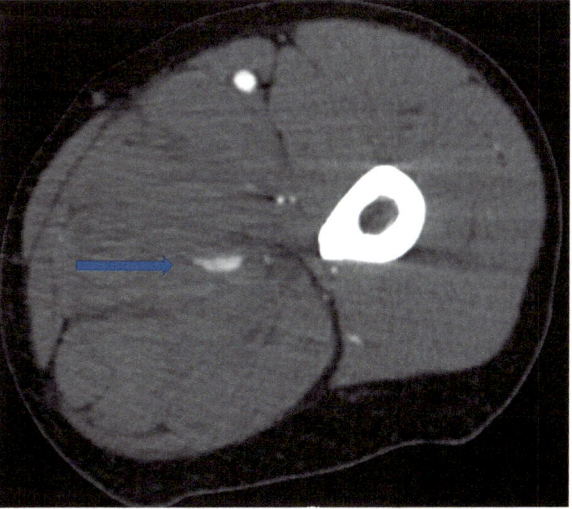

– Patients with hard signs of vascular injury should be taken to the operating room for further management.

• *The operating room*

– If operative intervention is necessary, the patient should be ideally taken to a hybrid operating room with endovascular capabilities, if possible. Otherwise, an operating room with a radiolucent table and a portable C-arm can be used.
– The patient should be positioned supine on the operating table and prepared widely according to distribution of injuries. If the patient has injuries isolated to the lower extremity, the umbilicus, the groin, and the entire leg should be exposed and incorporated within the sterile field. This ensures that the surgeon can obtain control at a more proximal location to the site of injury and have access to the entire limb.
– *Principles of vascular repair*

• Obtain proximal and distal exposure.
• Debride back to healthy tissue.
• Administer systemic heparin if there are no contraindications, namely head trauma. Otherwise, localized heparinized saline flushes can be used.
• If the patient is floridly unstable and is unable to tolerate ongoing blood loss or operative time, an intravascular shunt may be used as a temporizing manner until definitive repair can be performed.
• Perform proximal and distal thrombectomy before repair.
• Reversed saphenous vein from the unaffected limb is the preferred conduit, if available. Otherwise, ipsilateral saphenous vein or polytetrafluoroethylene graft (PTFE) can be used.
• After repair, check for pulse/listen for signals before leaving the operating room.
• Conversely, in a patient with severely mangled extremity and irreparable damage, the limb should be amputated.

– *Repair based on level of injury*

• Femoral vessels

– Approached via a vertical incision in the groin.
– Depending on how proximal the injury is, a retroperitoneal approach through the lower abdomen may be necessary in order to achieve proximal control.
– The SFA is approached through an oblique incision over the sartorius muscle.
– Sometimes, an occlusion balloon can be used to achieve proximal control in difficult to expose areas or in the setting of heavily calcified vessels that cannot be clamped.
– Depending on the degree and location of the injury, primary repair, patch repair, or an interposition graft can be used.

- Popliteal artery

  - Placing a bump under the thigh and abducting/everting the thigh helps to facilitate exposure.
  - For injuries above the knee, proximal control can be achieved by exposing the mid-thigh SFA. For injuries below the knee, the above knee popliteal can be exposed distal to the adductor canal.
  - Distal exposure is through a medial incision located 4–5 cm distal to the knee.
  - Depending on the degree and location of the injury, primary repair, patch repair, or an interposition graft can be used. Given the difficulty in accessing the mid-knee popliteal artery from the medial approach, bypass and interval ligation around the zone of injury is commonly used in this setting.

- Tibial vessels

  - If there is transection of a single artery at the level of the calf, the injured vessel can be ligated if the remaining two vessels are patent to the ankle or one is patent to the foot.

- *Venous injuries*

  - If patient is hemodynamically stable, femoral and popliteal veins should be repaired.
  - Repair of tibial veins are usually not pursued because of poor outcomes following repair. Hence, small tibial veins can be ligated.
  - Ligation of deep veins can result venous congestion leading to compartment syndrome and the need for fasciotomy.

- *Instruments and tools*

  - Fogarty thrombectomy catheters.
  - Occlusive balloons.
  - Vascular clamps.
  - Polypropylene sutures.
  - Prosthetic patches and grafts.

- *Endovascular management*

  - Vascular injuries located in difficult to expose vascular beds are better managed with endovascular technique.
  - For example, injuries to branches of the internal iliac artery from pelvic fractures can be managed using embolization.
  - Additionally, an injury to a perforator branch of the profunda femoris artery can be seen on an angiogram (Fig. 23.3) and this branch in turn can be selected and coil embolized (Fig. 23.4) to achieve hemostasis.

- *Compartment syndrome*

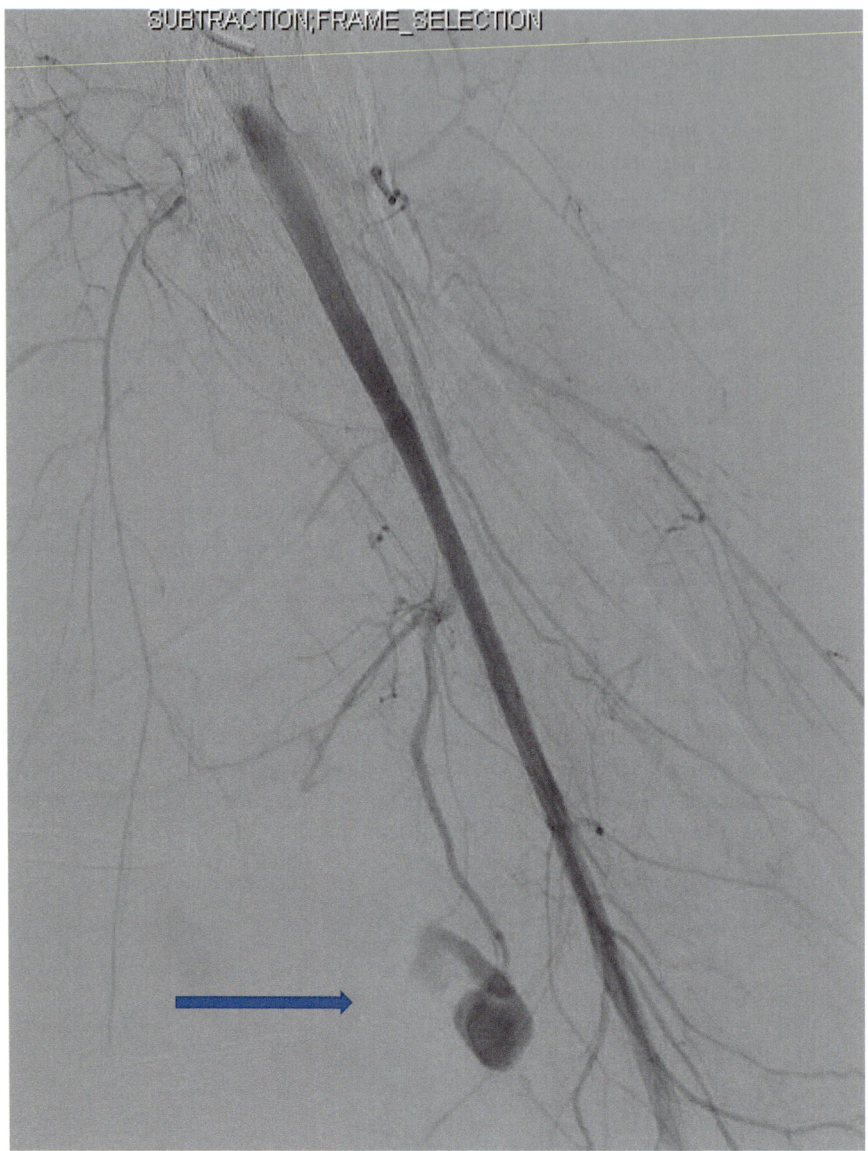

Fig. 23.3 Angiogram showing active extravasation from a profunda femoris branch (blue arrow)

- There are four compartments in the lower leg (anterior, lateral, superficial posterior, and deep posterior).
- Compartment syndrome occurs in the setting of hematoma, edema from muscle injury, or reperfusion after prolonged ischemia.
- This insult results in increased compartment pressure within a confined space, and as a result, venous outflow is obstructed.

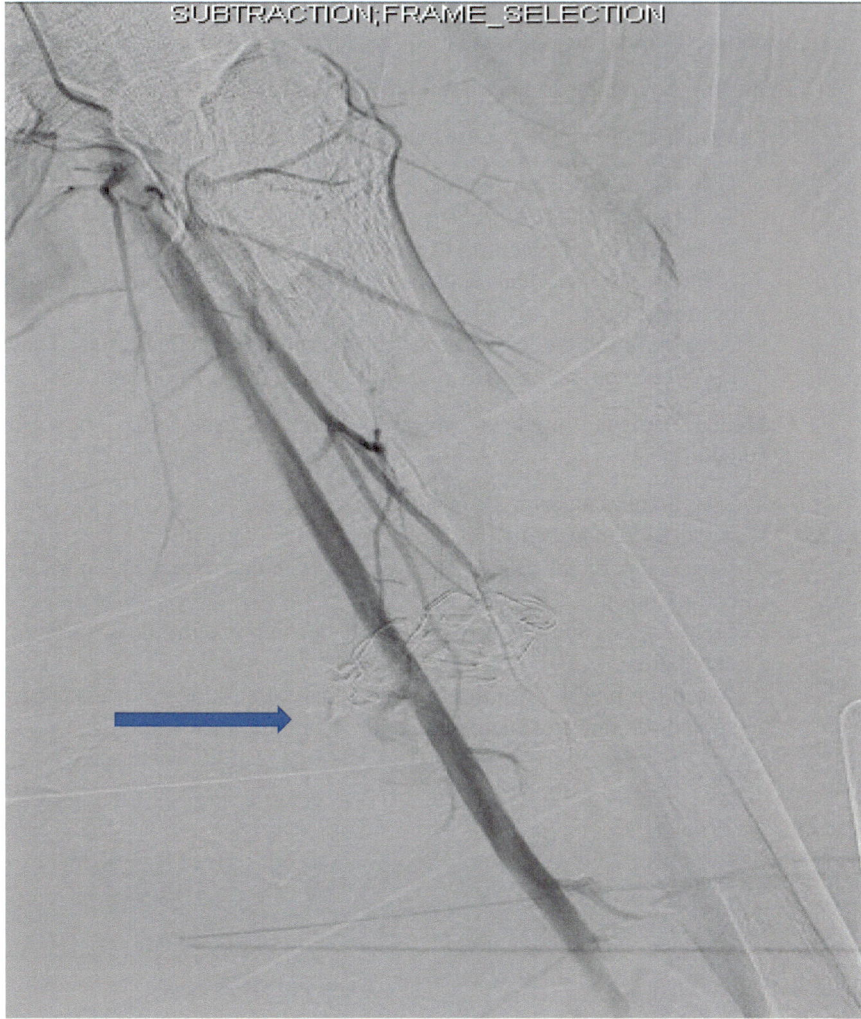

Fig. 23.4 Angiogram showing successful coil embolization of profunda femoris branch (blue arrow)

- The anterior compartment is the most frequently affected.
- Physical exam should focus on the 6 Ps (pain, pallor, paresthesia, poikilothermia, paralysis, and pulselessness).
- Pain with passive movement is a sensitive physical exam finding.
- Although compartment pressures can be measured, this is a clinical diagnosis and intervention should not be delayed to obtain compartment pressures.
- If there is concern for acute limb ischemia of a duration approaching 4–6 h prophylactic fasciotomies should be considered. Patients with collateral

circulation due to coexisting peripheral artery disease may tolerate longer periods of ischemia related to an injury to a specific vessel.

- Treatment: Four-compartment fasciotomies (Fig. 23.5)

  - Lateral incision used to release anterior and lateral compartments.

    - Longitudinal incision 3 cm lateral and parallel to the tibia.
    - Avoid superficial peroneal nerve.
    - Incise fascia and decompress anterior compartment.
    - Identify intermuscular septum and ensure lateral compartment is decompressed.
    - Avoid limiting the length of the incision in the skin and fascia. These should be completed across the entire length of the lower leg.

  - Medial incision used to release superficial and deep posterior compartments

    - Longitudinal incision 2 cm medial to the tibia.
    - Avoid saphenous vein.
    - Incise superficial fascia and decompress the superficial posterior compartment.
    - Incise soleus muscle to expose and decompress the deep posterior compartment.
    - Avoid limiting the length of the incision in the skin and fascia. These should be completed across the entire length of the lower leg.

Fig. 23.5 Incisions for four-compartment lower extremity fasciotomy. (*Note*: From *Atlas of Vascular Surgery and Endovascular Therapy*. Rasmussen et al. Published January 1, 2014. Pages 617–625. © 2014)

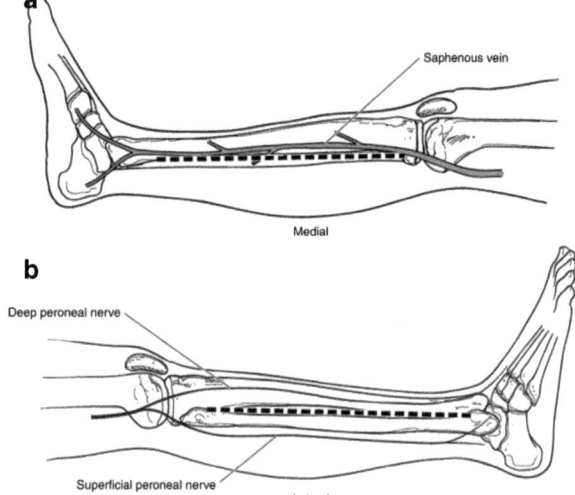

- *Postoperative care*
  - Depending on the severity of injury, most of these patients should be admitted to surgical intensive care unit for close monitoring.
  - Frequent neurovascular checks should be performed.
  - Continued resuscitation and management of complex injuries.

Take-Home Points for Patient Care

- Lower extremity vascular injuries if not adequately managed can result in limb loss.
- Knowledge of anatomy is essential to the care of a patient with vascular injury.
- In general, patients with softs signs of vascular injury should undergo further workup, while patients with hard signs of vascular injury should be taken directly to the operating room.
- Before administering systemic heparin, ensure that the patient has no contraindications.
- Understand when to employ damage control maneuvers in the operating room.
- Endovascular intervention can be utilized in some patients with vascular injuries.
- Compartment syndrome is a clinical diagnosis and four-compartment fasciotomies should be performed in situations where there is a high index of suspicion.

References

1. Konstantinidis A, Inaba K, Dubose J, et al. Vascular trauma in geriatric patients: a national trauma databank review. J Trauma Acute Care Surg. 2011;71:909–16.
2. Urrechaga E, Jabori S, Kang N, Kenel-Pierre S, Lopez A, Rattan R, Rey J, Bornak A. Traumatic lower extremity vascular injuries and limb salvage in a civilian urban trauma center. Ann Vasc Surg. 2022;82:30.
3. Kurtoglu M, Yanar H, Taviloglu K, Sivrikoz E, Plevin R, Aksoy M. Serious lower extremity venous injury management with ligation: prospective overview of 63 patients. Am Surg. 2007;73(10):1039–43. https://doi.org/10.1177/000313480707301026.
4. Eastridge BJ, Mabry RL, Seguin P, et al. Death on the battlefield (2001–2011): implications for the future of combat casualty care. J Trauma Acute Care Surg. 2012;73:S431–7.

Chapter 24
Damage Control Surgery

Dane R. Scantling and Tony Xia

Introduction

As damage control surgery does not aim to correct all existing surgical problems, the strategy involves a planned re-operation when the patient has improved or emergently needs further operation. Patients often develop substantial edema from resuscitation or may need more durable repairs than initially performed or further exploration to identify injuries not initially seen, and definitive closure of the body cavity is not typically performed in order to facilitate re-operation and to allow for swelling. The operative course of critically injured patients undergoing damage control surgery is thus divided into three stages: the initial damage control operation, the resuscitative phase, and the re-exploration.

Goals of Initial Damage Control Surgery

- Explore injured body cavity
- Control of hemorrhage
- Limit contamination
- Prevent ischemia

D. R. Scantling (✉)
Division of Acute Care Surgery, Boston Medical Center/Boston University Chobanian and Avedisian School of Medicine, Boston, MA, USA
e-mail: Dane.Scantling@bmc.org

T. Xia
Southcoast Health, New Bedford, MA, USA
e-mail: Tony.xia@southcoasthealth.org

© The Author(s), under exclusive license to Springer Nature   213
Switzerland AG 2025
T. S. Brahmbhatt, D. R. Scantling (eds.), *Trauma Surgery Clerkship*,
Contemporary Surgical Clerkships,
https://doi.org/10.1007/978-3-032-01412-2_24

• Temporary closure of the body cavity

Surgical Considerations and Techniques

• The surgeon and team should be prepared for the worst-case scenario. The operating room team should be informed of the situation and plan, as well as potential back-up plans or concurrent procedures. This includes positioning the patient and the operating room to facilitate any potential surgical access, widely preparing the skin surface as time permits. Vascular access and advanced monitoring should be obtained or remain accessible when needed. The appropriate surgical trays should be selected, hemostatic agents available, and blood products made ready to transfuse. Consideration should be taken between the patient's potential injuries and the vascular access through which resuscitative fluids, blood products, and medications are given through.

  – Wide skin preparation
  – Adequate vascular access and advanced monitoring
  – Equipment available
  – Blood products available

• The operative field should be extended as much as needed to access the site of injury. This is done to achieve the goal of intervening on a life-threatening wound with minimal struggle. Packing a cavity can tamponade bleeding effectively, but may only remain for a temporary period of time. This is done to allow resuscitation to occur prior to the worsening of any hemorrhagic shock. It is also particularly useful when an alternate therapeutic modality such as angioembolization is required for surgically difficult or inaccessible areas, such as major hepatic bleeding.

• Injuries should be dealt with in order of life-threatening nature. Hemorrhagic shock should be assessed and controlled promptly. Consideration should also be made for cardiogenic or obstructive etiologies of shock such as cardiac injury, tamponade, or tension pneumothorax. These can be assessed and intervened upon with relative ease should shock continue despite control of hemorrhage and appropriate resuscitation. Hemorrhagic shock is often accompanied by vascular injury which must be addressed. In the damage control setting, complex major vascular injuries may be temporized by shunting if the patient is unstable and difficult repair is anticipated, specialty equipment is needed, or contamination concerns arise. Finally, evaluation and temporization of hollow viscus injury should be rapid. This can be achieved by simple ligation, stapling, or simple closure of a damaged structure, rather than spending time restoring enteric continuity.

• Temporary closure techniques should be employed to protect the visceral structures if a re-operation is planned or severe edema is expected. Typically, this is most relevant to temporary abdominal closure. Many systems exist, ranging

Fig. 24.1 A typical open abdomen negative pressure wound therapy system

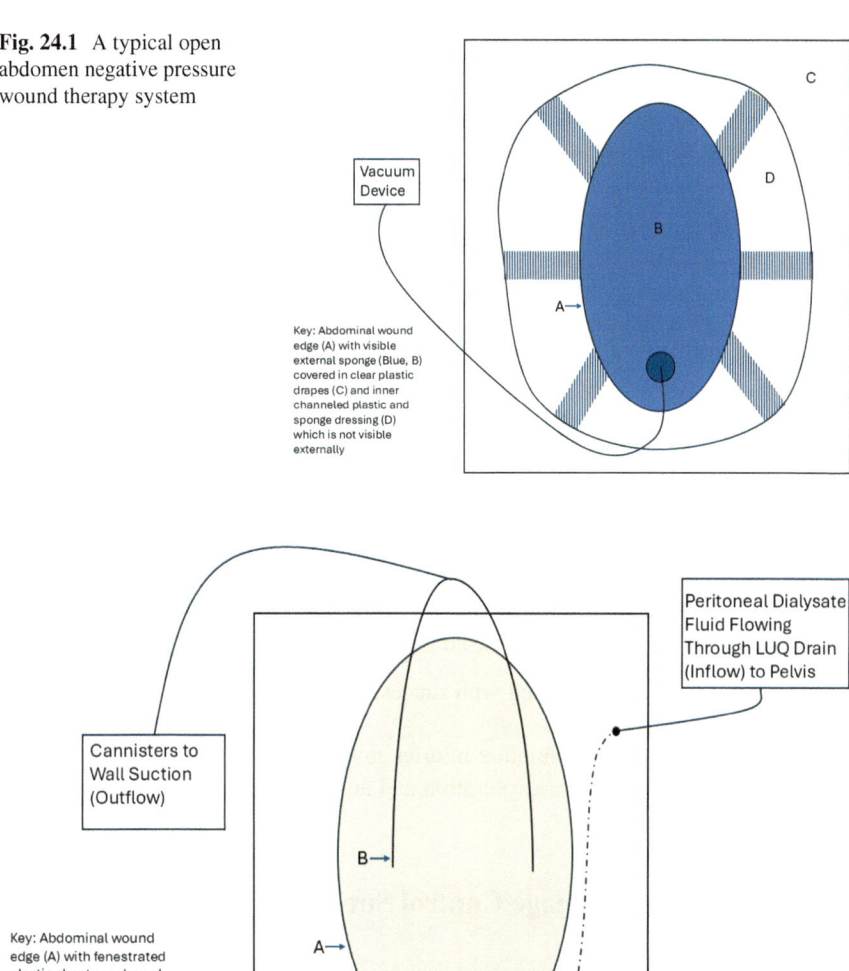

Vacuum Device

Key: Abdominal wound edge (A) with visible external sponge (Blue, B) covered in clear plastic drapes (C) and inner channeled plastic and sponge dressing (D) which is not visible externally

Peritoneal Dialysate Fluid Flowing Through LUQ Drain (Inflow) to Pelvis

Cannisters to Wall Suction (Outflow)

Key: Abdominal wound edge (A) with fenestrated plastic sheet over bowel covered by radiolucent surgical towels (both not shown) and two drain lines above the fascia (B) covered in Ioban (light yellow)

Fig. 24.2 Direct peritoneal resuscitation—a catheter is used to instill peritoneal dialysis fluid while two suction catheters evacuate excess fluids

from skin-only closures to the more common method consisting of plastic-lined drapes to protect underlying structures (Fig. 24.1). Perforations in these drapes or separate drains are used to facilitate fluid removal. Direct peritoneal resuscitation (DPR) in temporary abdominal closure may improve microvascular perfusion, decrease edema, and shorten time to definitive abdominal closure (Fig. 24.2). Closure technique should prevent abdominal hypertension and facilitate re-exploration of the cavity with ease.

Resuscitative Stage

- The goal of the resuscitative stage is to correct physiologic derangements, most importantly coagulopathy, acidosis, and hypothermia (termed the lethal triad).
- Blood product resuscitation is used to correct coagulopathy.

  - Massive transfusion should be done in a balanced fashion of packed red blood cells, plasma, and platelets in a 1:1:1 fashion or with whole blood as local protocols allow.
  - Transfusion of cryoprecipitate should be given if fibrinogen is low.
  - Correction of acidosis typically occurs with blood product and fluid resuscitation.

- All efforts should be made to keep the patient warm, beginning in the trauma bay and operating room.

  - The ambient temperature of the operating room and the intensive care setting should be kept elevated.
  - Resuscitative fluids, blood products, and any input into the patient such as the air in the ventilator circuit should be warmed to physiologic temperatures.
  - Warming blankets should be used liberally.

- Acidosis is typically corrected with successful resuscitation and maintenance of good perfusion.
- Additional work-up of traumatic injuries may be done during the resuscitative phase in preparation for re-exploration and definitive fixation.

Complications of Damage Control Surgery

- Damage control surgery is an effective tool used to temporize the critically injured trauma patient, but is associated with a number of complications. These include a high rate of organ space and surgical site infections [3] and fluid shifts and losses from an open body cavity. In addition, complications may arise from the open cavity itself. Within the abdomen, this can result in abdominal compartment syndrome, loss of abdominal domain, incisional hernias, and enteric fistulas.
- Given the potential for such catastrophic complications, the decision to implement a damage control surgery strategy should be carefully undertaken. Elements of the lethal triad are classically used as indicators that a damage control approach should be used, though no specific criteria are universally accepted [4]. The benefits of damage control may diminish as physiologic derangements worsen, and thus early implementation should be considered upon identification of a declining clinical trajectory.

Re-exploration

- After adequate resuscitation and physiologic stabilization, re-exploration of the injured body cavity is undertaken. Many surgeons will opt to have CT imaging completed after stabilization but before re-exploration if the patient did not have imaging completed before the index operation. This facilitates the identification of occult injuries and may further guide re-exploration and reconstruction efforts. In the repeat operation, laparotomy pads used for packing are removed and the field assessed for hemostasis, the surgical site can be carefully inspected for any missed injuries, and injured structures are definitively repaired or resected. All attempts should be made to close the cavity if possible, although alternative means such as mesh implantation or grafting are often required.

Conclusion/Take-Home Points

- The lethal triad of trauma can rapidly progress to mortality if not promptly intervened upon.
- Damage control surgery aims to correct only life-threatening injuries and limit operative time in order to address more rapid resuscitation of the patient.
- Temporary closure of the explored cavity is used to facilitate re-operation.
- A damage control approach has significant associated complications and should only be used for select patients.

References/Further Reading

1. Rotondo MF, Schwab CW, McGonigal MD, Phillips GR 3rd, Fruchterman TM, Kauder DR, Latenser BA, Angood PA. 'Damage control': an approach for improved survival in exsanguinating penetrating abdominal injury. J Trauma. 1993;35(3):375–82. discussion 382–3.
2. Schreiber MA. Damage control surgery. Crit Care Clin. 2004;20(1):101–18. https://doi.org/10.1016/s0749-0704(03)00095-2.
3. George MJ, Adams SD, McNutt MK, et al. The effect of damage control laparotomy on major abdominal complications: a matched analysis. Am J Surg. 2018;216(1):56–9. https://doi.org/10.1016/j.amjsurg.2017.10.044.
4. Roberts DJ, Bobrovitz N, Zygun DA, et al. Evidence for use of damage control surgery and damage control interventions in civilian trauma patients: a systematic review. World J Emerg Surg. 2021;16:10. https://doi.org/10.1186/s13017-021-00352-5.

Chapter 25
Nutrition for Trauma Patients

Allan E. Stolarski, Lorraine Young, and Peter A. Burke

Trauma surgery patients are unique in that they are thrust into highly catabolic states with high energy and protein demands while their gastrointestinal tract may be compromised and nutritional intake is limited. A solid understanding of their pre-existing nutritional status, risk factors, and methods to deliver nutritional interventions is necessary to optimize outcomes for surgical patients.

Trauma patients, particularly those who suffer significant injury burden requiring admission to the surgical intensive care unit, concurrently have high nutritional and metabolic demands while complicated by frequent contra-indications to enteral delivery. Trauma patients frequently require multiple trips to/from the operating theater requiring "nothing by mouth" (aka NPO) status for prolonged periods of time despite high protein and caloric requirements to promote injury response and healing.

Why

The provision of nutritional support following trauma is important, as it is a way we can prevent the development of complications associated with malnutrition that are prone to develop in post-operative trauma patients. Malnutrition is a risk factor for post-operative complications such as surgical infections, increased hospital length of stay, re-admission, and even death. A surgical patient's nutritional status is a

A. E. Stolarski (✉) · P. A. Burke
Boston Medical Center, Boston University – Department of Surgery, Boston, MA, USA
e-mail: Allan.Stolarski@bmc.org; Peter.Burke@bmc.org

L. Young
Boston Medical Center, Boston University – Department of Medicine, Boston, MA, USA

T. S. Brahmbhatt, D. R. Scantling (eds.), *Trauma Surgery Clerkship*, Contemporary Surgical Clerkships,
https://doi.org/10.1007/978-3-032-01412-2_25

modifiable risk factor. Accurate assessment and optimization of nutrition has observable positive impacts on patient care [1–4].

What

Malnutrition is defined as "a state resulting from lack of intake or uptake of nutrition that leads to altered body composition (decreased fat free mass) and body cell mass leading to diminished physical and mental function and impaired clinical outcome from disease [5]." The American Society for Parenteral and Enteral Nutrition (ASPEN) outlines six different criteria, two of which that need to be met to diagnose malnutrition [2]:

ASPEN criteria for malnutrition (≥2 criteria must be met to diagnose malnutrition)
1. Low energy intake
2. Weight loss
3. Loss of muscle mass
4. Loss of subcutaneous fat
5. Fluid accumulation
6. Decreased hand grip strength

The American Society for Parenteral and Enteral Nutrition (ASPEN) outlines six different criteria, two of which that need to be met to diagnose malnutrition [2]

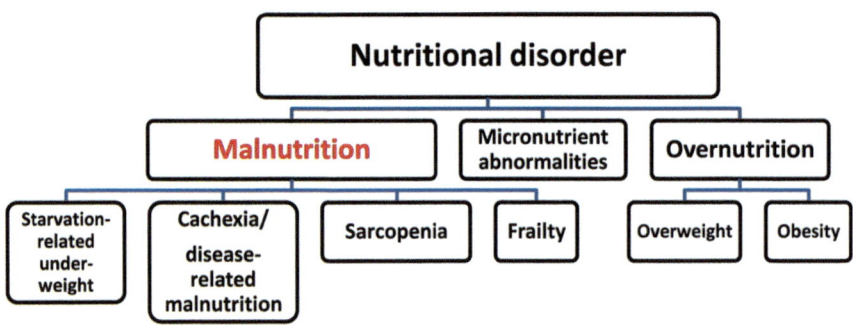

Diagnostic criteria for malnutrition—An ESPEN consensus statement [5]

Calorie and protein requirements vary by the patient's degree of catabolic stress. Immediately after significant traumatic injury, patients are highly stressed. This highly active catabolic state requires more energy and protein intakes than they would in a non-injured state. As a general rule, protein requirements for critically ill patients are approximately 1.5 g protein/day with suggested higher intakes (2–2.5 g protein/day) for those with increased stress, such as severe burns [6, 7]. Calorie requirements vary widely depending on sex, weight, height, and degree of stress. As a general rule for critically ill patients, it is recommended that the caloric goals can be estimated using 25 kcal/kg ideal body weight [8]. However, this must be used cautiously with attention to catabolic state and BMI.

Who

Nutrition is essential for all surgical patients but is critical for patients with established malnutrition or who are risk of developing malnutrition during their surgical stay. Trauma patients are unlike other surgical patients in that a large proportion of patients that suffer catastrophic injuries are younger and well-nourished at the time of injury. However, trauma is a disease that spans all populations and as such early recognition of trauma patients with malnutrition is essential to reducing the associated morbidity and mortality. Risk factors for malnutrition can be subdivided into patient characteristics, disease, and treatment [3, 9–12]:

Patient Risk Factors:

- Age over 70 years old.
- Comorbidities (diabetes, obesity, cognitive disorders, organ dysfunction, immune suppressive conditions, delirium, dementia, depression).
- Prior surgery of gastrointestinal tract.

Disease Risk Factors:

- Cancer of the oropharynx, esophagus, stomach, pancreas, and biliary system.
- High cancer stage.
- Nausea, vomiting, diarrhea, diminished appetite.

Treatment Risk Factors:

- Chemotherapy
- Radiation therapy
- Corticosteroid use
- Polypharmacy

Review of these risk factors reveal that they are often intertwined and co-exist. This further increases the risk for nutritional deficiencies and the development of the complications of malnutrition. This has been clinically recognized and published in numerous studies that demonstrate that over 50% of surgical patients suffer from some degree of malnutrition. This is even higher for those with cancer of the gastrointestinal tract, and again exacerbated by chemotherapy or radiation therapy for these already at-risk patients [13–16]. This is a true clinical challenge that warrants early recognition because neoadjuvant chemotherapy and/or radiation often precede the surgical management of many types of cancer.

An additional population that has classically been nutritionally neglected are critically ill trauma patients. Following significant traumatic injury, patients are often admitted to the surgical intensive care unit, directly from the emergency department or after surgery. These patients commonly require multiple procedures, requiring frequent pausing of feeds or have significant injury to their gastrointestinal tract precluding enteral feeding leaving them significantly malnourished and in a metabolically demanding state [4].

When

Nutrition screening is so important that the Joint Commission on Accreditation of Healthcare Organizations requires all patients to be screened for nutritional deficits within 24 h of admission. This is a key aspect that should be incorporated in the workup of all patients after traumatic injury. Assessment of a patient's nutritional status involves a thorough history, physical exam, laboratory tests, and possibly imaging studies. Body mass index (BMI) combined with anthropometry (i.e., arm or leg circumference) are useful aspects of the physical exam. A thorough history collected from a patient can reveal a history of weight loss. It is essential to specify if this weight loss was intentional or unintentional to qualify the amount lost over a specified time period. A complete history will also explore any recent history of appetite changes and self-reported food intake. Patients with a history of 10–15% unintentional weight lose over a period of 2–4 weeks should be considered to be at risk of malnutrition. Laboratory analysis such as measurement of albumin may be useful, especially if measured prior to resuscitation and surgery. However, no lab test at present can reliably predict the presence of malnutrition. More recently, there have been many novel applications of imaging techniques to assess for nutritional status such as measurement of psoas muscle volume and density which correlates strongly with nutritional status [17]. This technique to identify sarcopenia, a marker of malnutrition, is particularly applicable for trauma patients as the majority undergo axial imaging studies to assist in diagnosis of traumatic injuries.

Historically, patients have been made NPO at midnight the evening prior to a planned operation or procedure due to fear of aspiration and associated pulmonary complications. However, there is strong evidence that the risk of aspiration remains low when patients are allowed to drink clear liquids up to 2 h before surgery and solid food up to 6 h before. Carbohydrate-rich liquid consumed 2 h prior to surgery has been demonstrated to improve surgical outcomes. Post-operatively, oral intake should be encouraged immediately depending on the patient's post-operative status and the type of surgery that was performed [3]. These recommendations have been adapted to a surgery specific protocol called *Enhanced Recovery After Surgery (ERAS)* [2, 3, 6, 11].

When to start nutritional support is an important variable in the care of surgical patients. This should be discussed on admission and every day forward for trauma patients regardless of their admission nutritional state due to the uniquely high catabolic demands they will endure. Patients who present in a malnourished state should have nutritional support started as soon as feasible. Well-nourished surgical patients can tolerate periods of up 2 weeks of minimal caloric intake before developing malnutrition. The tolerance of a prolonged state of minimal nutrition is patient-specific and is influenced in many respects by the individual patient reserves and the levels of stress that they are exposed to. In general, well-nourished patients who are critically ill (those requiring ICU level care) should be considered for supplemental nutritional support within 5 days of hospitalization and those who levels of stress are lower, such as those being cared for on the floor, will require active nutritional support after at 7–10 days of hospitalization.

Where

Nutrition can be delivered in a number of ways. The ideal delivery method is utilizing the gastrointestinal tract, called enteral nutrition. Feeding patients by mouth is the natural and preferred method; however, it is not always possible due to various surgical procedures or surgical pathologies that may be contra-indications to enteral nutrition. Consequently, parenteral nutrition delivered via established peripheral intravenous access (peripheral parenteral nutrition (PPN)) or via central venous access (total parenteral nutrition (TPN)) may be utilized. Both PPN and TPN deliver essential nutrients including amino acids, carbohydrate (dextrose), lipids, micronutrients, and macronutrients while bypassing the gastrointestinal tract. Parenteral nutrition requires close monitoring of glucose, electrolytes, triglyceride levels, and hepatic function to prevent injury. In addition to possible end organ injury, parenteral nutrition places the patient at an increased risk of infections, particularly bacteremia. This can be minimized with protocolized sterile technique and routine sterile care of venous catheters.

Summary

The provision of nutritional support can help prevent and treat the complications of malnutrition. Malnourished patients require nutritional support as early as feasible. Well-nourished patients do not all need early nutritional support due to adequate reserves. However, those with significant levels of stress, such as those with traumatic injury, and those who are at risk for prolonged periods of minimal caloric/protein intake, need a plan for nutritional support to prevent the development of malnutrition complications. When possible, enteral nutrition support is preferred, but when unfeasible, parenteral nutritional support is critical. The provision of nutritional support should be tailored to the individual patients but a caloric intake of 20–25 kcal/kg/day and 1.5 g/kg/day of protein are reasonable goals to start.

References

1. Bistrian BR, Blackburn GL, Sherman M, Scrimshaw NS. Therapeutic index of nutritional depletion in hospitalized patients. Surg Gynecol Obstet. 1975;141:512–6.
2. White JV, Guenter P, Jensen G, et al. Consensus statement: Academy of Nutrition and Dietetics and American Society for Parenteral and Enteral Nutrition: characteristics recommended for the identification and documentation of adult malnutrition (undernutrition). JPEN J Parenter Enteral Nutr. 2012;36:275–83.
3. Weimann A, Braga M, Carli F, et al. ESPEN practical guideline: clinical nutrition in surgery. Clin Nutr. 2021;40:4745–61.
4. Stolarski AE, Young L, Weinberg J, et al. Early metabolic support for critically ill trauma patients: a prospective randomized controlled trial. J Trauma Acute Care Surg. 2022;92:255–65.
5. Cederholm T, Bosaeus I, Barazzoni R, et al. Diagnostic criteria for malnutrition – an ESPEN consensus statement. Clin Nutr. 2015;34:335–40.
6. McClave SA, Taylor BE, Martindale RG, et al. Guidelines for the provision and assessment of nutrition support therapy in the adult critically ill patient: Society of Critical Care Medicine (SCCM) and American Society for Parenteral and Enteral Nutrition (A.S.P.E.N.). JPEN J Parenter Enteral Nutr. 2016;40:159–211.
7. De Waele E, Jakubowski JR, Stocker R, Wischmeyer PE. Review of evolution and current status of protein requirements and provision in acute illness and critical care. Clin Nutr. 2020;40:2958.
8. Casaer MP, Mesotten D, Hermans G, et al. Early versus late parenteral nutrition in critically ill adults. N Engl J Med. 2011;365:506–17.
9. Singer P, Blaser AR, Berger MM, et al. ESPEN guideline on clinical nutrition in the intensive care unit. Clin Nutr. 2019;38:48–79.
10. Chambrier C, Sztark F, (SFNEP) SFdncem, (SFAR) Sfdaer. French clinical guidelines on perioperative nutrition. Update of the 1994 consensus conference on perioperative artificial nutrition for elective surgery in adults. J Visc Surg. 2012;149:e325–36.
11. Compher C, Bingham AL, McCall M, et al. Guidelines for the provision of nutrition support therapy in the adult critically ill patient: The American Society for Parenteral and Enteral Nutrition. JPEN J Parenter Enteral Nutr. 2022;46:12–41.
12. Benoist S, Brouquet A. Nutritional assessment and screening for malnutrition. J Visc Surg. 2015;152(Suppl 1):S3–7.
13. Hébuterne X, Lemarié E, Michallet M, de Montreuil CB, Schneider SM, Goldwasser F. Prevalence of malnutrition and current use of nutrition support in patients with cancer. JPEN J Parenter Enteral Nutr. 2014;38:196–204.
14. Correia MI, Waitzberg DL. The impact of malnutrition on morbidity, mortality, length of hospital stay and costs evaluated through a multivariate model analysis. Clin Nutr. 2003;22:235–9.
15. Williams DGA, Molinger J, Wischmeyer PE. The malnourished surgery patient: a silent epidemic in perioperative outcomes? Curr Opin Anaesthesiol. 2019;32:405–11.
16. Wie GA, Cho YA, Kim SY, Kim SM, Bae JM, Joung H. Prevalence and risk factors of malnutrition among cancer patients according to tumor location and stage in the National Cancer Center in Korea. Nutrition. 2010;26:263–8.
17. Jones KI, Doleman B, Scott S, Lund JN, Williams JP. Simple psoas cross-sectional area measurement is a quick and easy method to assess sarcopenia and predicts major surgical complications. Color Dis. 2015;17:O20–6.

Chapter 26
Wound Management, Dressings, and Vacuum Devices

Sophia M. Smith and Kathryn Twomey

Overview

- Wounds can be largely classified as surgical, pressure, or traumatic
- Normal wound healing progresses through three stages: inflammation, proliferation, and remodeling
- Chronic wounds are associated with a lack of progression through normal wound healing physiology
- Wound closure options include primary intention, delayed primary closure, and secondary intention
- Wound dressing choices depend on wound characteristics, including size, infection status, presence of nonviable tissue, and exudate/drainage
- Common dressing options include impregnated dressings, gauze, film, hydrogels, hydrocolloid, foam, alginate, and hydrofiber
- Negative pressure wound therapy is an option to reduce edema, promote granulation tissue formation, and facilitate later wound closure or secondary intention healing

S. M. Smith
Department of Surgery, Boston Medical Center, Boston University School of Medicine, Boston, MA, USA
e-mail: sophia.smith@bmc.org

K. Twomey (✉)
Boston Medical Center, Boston University Chobanian & Avedisian School of Medicine, Boston, MA, USA
e-mail: kathryn.twomey@bmc.org

© The Author(s), under exclusive license to Springer Nature Switzerland AG 2025
T. S. Brahmbhatt, D. R. Scantling (eds.), *Trauma Surgery Clerkship*, Contemporary Surgical Clerkships, https://doi.org/10.1007/978-3-032-01412-2_26

Background

Wound Classifications

Here, we classify the most common wounds encountered on a surgical service, however, it is by no means an exhaustive list.

Surgical wounds are classified as clean (without infection or inflammation), clean-contaminated (controlled entry into the respiratory, gastrointestinal, urinary, or genital tracts), contaminated (non-sterile wounds or uncontrolled leakage from the gastrointestinal tract), or dirty (infected or devitalized tissue). Pressure wounds (sometimes termed "bedsores" or "decubitus ulcers") are found in chronically ill or immobile patients, frequently in the skin and soft tissue overlying the sacrum, the ischial spines, and heel. However, these can occur in any area of pressure, including extremity casts/braces and cervical collars.

Pressure wounds can be classified in four stages. Stage 1 is intact skin with non-blanching erythema, stage 2 is partial thickness epidermal injury, stage 3 is a full thickness skin injury with involvement of subcutaneous tissue, and stage 4 includes involvement of deeper structures (muscle, tendon, bone). Some wounds have an overlying eschar or necrotic tissue that prevents staging; these wounds are termed "unstageable."

Traumatic wounds are typically obtained in a non-sterile environment; their management is individualized based on the patient, mechanism, wound characteristics, and underlying injuries.

Certain wound types should prompt consideration of surgical subspecialist evaluation, including wounds to the face, scalp, ear, mucous membranes, hands, nail beds, and deep wounds overlying major joints [1, 2].

Wound Healing

Wound healing progresses in three phases: inflammation, proliferation, and remodeling [3]. During the inflammation phase (days 1–10), a platelet plug is formed and the coagulation cascade is initiated. Neutrophils are the dominant cell type during this phase [1]. During the proliferation phase (5 days–3 weeks), epithelialization occurs. Macrophages are the predominant cell type during this stage. During the final phase of wound healing, remodeling (3 weeks–1 year), fibroblasts are the dominant cell type. Maximum tensile strength occurs at about 8 weeks, and the scar is considered mature after 1 year [1]. Wound healing can be inhibited by a variety of factors, such as smoking and peripheral vascular disease (which lead to poor tissue oxygenation), diabetes, and malnutrition [1].

Wound Closure

Primary intention is immediate closure of a wound within 24 h, ideal for clean, tension-free wounds [1, 2]. Methods of primary closure are sutures or staples. An alternative that is frequently used over sutured wounds, but can be used independently, is Steri-Strips™, which are equivalent to staple and suture closures in tensile strength and cosmesis [2]. Wounds closed via primary intention do not necessarily require dressings; however, if a dressing is desired, the standard recommended dressing is simple or adhesive, left in place for 24–72 h [4]. Surgical skin glue (e.g., Dermabond™, SkinAffix™) can be used instead of a dressing—it is either used as a standalone closure method or over suture closures [2].

Delayed primary closure refers to wound closure that occurs after 24 h and is preferred for a variety of wound types, including some contaminated wounds (particularly those from penetrating trauma to the colon, such as stab and gunshot wounds), poorly circumscribed wounds, and wounds with delayed presentation [1, 2].

Secondary intention refers to the practice of allowing a wound to close by itself, from inside out, promoting drainage and minimizing exudate accumulation [1, 4]. Indications for allowing wounds to heal via secondary intention include tension on wound edges, dirty or infected wounds, partial thickness avulsions, and small contaminated wounds [1, 2]. Wounds healing via secondary intention can either be packed be left open to air [1, 4].

Wound Healing Complications

Infection

Before becoming frankly infected, wounds are contaminated. Organisms in the wound proliferate, colonizing the wound. Once a critical threshold of organisms is present (typically, 10^5 bacteria per high power field), the wound is infected. Signs of wound infection include warmth, erythema, edema, increasing pain, purulent drainage, and wound dehiscence or tissue breakdown [5]. Management of wound infection includes systemic antibiotics and debridement of nonviable tissue [6].

Dehiscence

Wound dehiscence is a failure of wound healing in which a previously approximated tissue separates. The risk for wound dehiscence increases in wounds that are under tension, infected, and in patients with malnutrition or other conditions that affect wound healing (steroid use, diabetes, etc.). Of note, this refers to separation of the superficial tissues, rather than fascial dehiscence, which is a separation of deeper fascial layers, a complication that can occur particularly after open abdominal operations.

Chronic Wounds

Chronic wounds do not progress through the expected phases of wound healing. The etiology of chronic wounds is multifactorial. Chronic wounds characteristically have persistent inflammation, failure of epithelialization, and a defective extracellular matrix [7]. Risk factors for chronic wounds include diabetes, immunosuppression, smoking, and obesity, in addition to innumerable other patient and wound-related factors [8]. Management of chronic wounds can be challenging. Underlying conditions should be optimized and any exacerbating factors (such as undue pressure on the wound) should be remedied. Simultaneously, nonviable tissue should be debrided, exudate removed, and infection treated [7, 9].

Current Practice

Wound Management

- Debridement of nonviable and infected tissue in the wound bed [2, 6]
  - Surgical debridement: sharp excisional debridement or the use of electrocautery
  - Enzymatic debridement (Santyl™): digests collagen, reduces wound exudate
  - Mechanical debridement: blunt debridement of nonviable tissue, typically done with gauze [9]

Dressings

- Factors in choosing dressings: wound characteristics, supply availability, pain, cost, and patient-related factors (Fig. 26.1) [4, 5]
- Ideal dressing: inert, cost-effective, maintains a moist environment, absorbs drainage, facilitates debridement [5]

Impregnated Dressings

- Indications: Superficially infected or colonized wounds [6]
- Contraindications: None
- Dressing change: 1–2 days

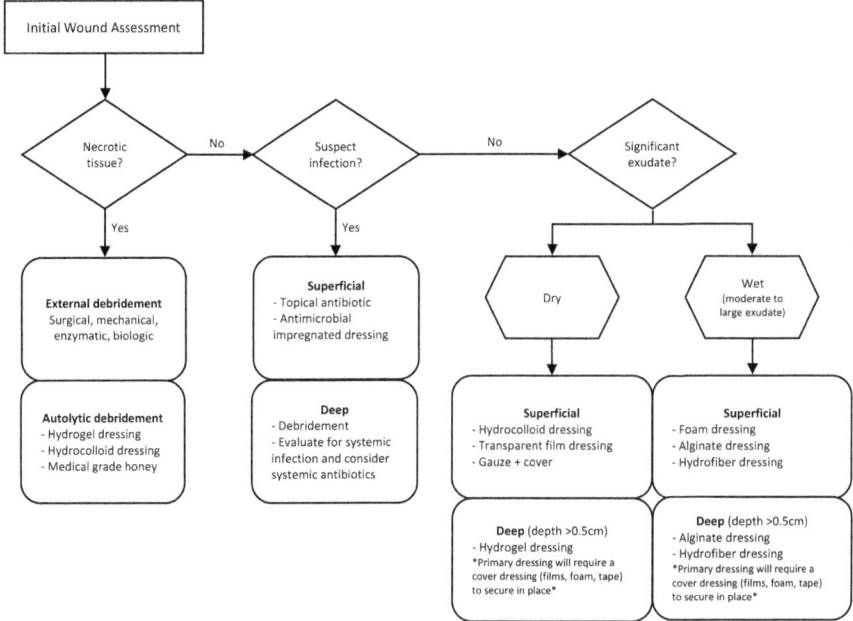

Fig. 26.1 Wound assessment and management [5]

- Details: Antibiotics and antimicrobial agents can be impregnated into dressings, usually gauze.
- Examples:
  - Silver-impregnated dressings: broad-spectrum antimicrobial activity [5, 10]
  - Iodine: antimicrobial properties but can be locally caustic to healthy tissue, and systemically absorbed through the wound bed [5, 10]
  - Medihoney®: most common in burn wounds [5]

Gauze Dressings

- Indications: Wounds closed by primary intention [4]
- Contraindications: None
- Dressing change: 1–2 days
- Details: Plain gauze does not retain moisture and can adhere to the wound bed, which can function as a source of mechanical debridement when removed [5]
- Examples: plain gauze, wet-to-dry dressings, Xeroform™

Film Dressings

- Indications: superficial, partial thickness wounds, wounds closed by primary intention, skin graft donor sites, minor abrasions, IV access sites, first degree burn wounds, stage 1 pressure ulcers, secondary dressings secure other dressings [4, 5]
- Contraindications: Exudative wounds, macerated wound edges [5, 9, 10]
- Dressing change: 2–3 days [5]
- Details: Occlusive, maintain moisture, provide visualization of the wound bed [5]
- Examples: Tegaderm™, Mepore®

Hydrogels

- Indications: dry gangrene, calciphylaxis, warfarin-induced skin necrosis, painful non-exudative wounds [4, 5, 9, 10]
- Contraindications: exudative wounds [5]
- Dressing change: 1–3 days [5]
- Details: Cross-linked starch polymer, with limited absorptive ability [5]
- Examples: Tegagel™, FlexiGel™

Hydrocolloid

- Indications: wounds over joints, abrasions, superficial ulcers, diabetic wounds, partial thickness burns, skin graft donor sites, mild to moderately exudative wounds, dry necrotic wounds [4, 5]
- Contraindications: Exudative or infected wounds [10]
- Dressing change: 2–4 days [5]
- Details: Starch polymers, absorb fluid, and form a gel-like dressing [5]. Self-adhesive, waterproof, maintain moisture [5, 9]
- Examples: Duoderm®, Tegasorb™

Foam Dressing

- Indications: wounds over bony prominences, skin graft donor sites, mildly exudative wounds, superficial partial thickness wounds [4, 5]
- Contraindications: dry necrotic wounds
- Dressing change: 1–3 days
- Details: Maintain moisture, some absorptive capacity [5, 9, 10].
- Examples: Aquacel®, Mepilex®

Alginate Dressings

- Indications: Deep, exudative wounds, pyoderma gangrenosum, diabetic wounds, bleeding wounds, skin graft donor sites, contaminated wounds, heavily exudative wounds [4, 5, 10]
- Contraindications: heavy bleeding, dry wounds, minimal exudate
- Dressing change: 1–3 days
- Details: Made of seaweed or kelp, retain moisture [5, 9].
- Examples: Melgisorb®

Hydrofiber

- Indications: deep, exudative wounds, pyoderma gangrenosum, diabetic wounds, traumatic wounds, partial thickness wounds, contaminated wounds [4, 5, 10]
- Contraindications: Allergy to product
- Dressing change: 3 days [5]
- Details: Absorptive, form a gel upon contact with wound bed.
- Examples: Aquacel®

Vacuum Devices

- Indications: diabetic foot ulcers, pressure wounds, skin grafts, flap salvage, burns, crush injuries, sternal/abdominal wound dehiscence, fasciotomies, extravasation wounds, animal bites, frostbite [11]
- Contraindications: malignant wounds, untreated osteomyelitis, fistulas, necrotic wounds, exposed arteries, nerves, or anastomoses, blood dyscrasias (relative), actively bleeding wounds, anticoagulation (relative) [11]
- Mechanism of action: Promotes granulation tissue formation, increases local blood flow to the wound bed, maintains a moist wound bed, reduces wound area and edema, promotes wound contraction, and reduces risk of wound infection (Fig. 26.2) [1, 11]
- Technical considerations:
  - Wound vacuum kit: vacuum container, tubing, two sponges (white and black), film dressing. Foam is cut to size and placed over the wound bed. Do not overlap the foam with skin. Foam choice depends on the wound—white foam has smaller pores, black foam has larger pores [11]. White sponges are used when there are vulnerable structures nearby (bone, tendon, hardware, etc.), or in tunneled wounds. After the sponge is placed, film is placed over the sponge and the surrounding skin, with a skin border overlap of 3–5 cm [11].

Fig. 26.2 Negative
pressure wound
therapy [12]

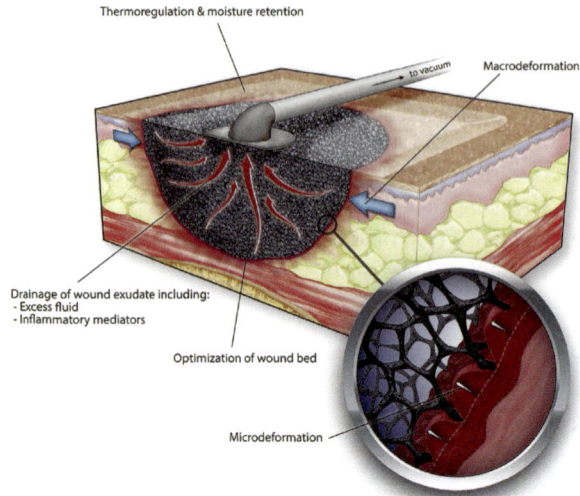

– A hole is created in the center of the film over the wound, exposing the underlying foam. The pad of the vac tubing is placed over the hole, and the circuit
  is connected.

• Dressing change: 2–3 days [11]

Take-Home Points for Patient Care

• Wounds should be managed and dressed according to their mechanism and
  classification.
• Pay particular attention to exudate, infection, and non-viable tissue, as this will
  guide choice of dressing.
• NPWT can be used for large wounds to reduce edema, promote granulation tissue formation, and facilitate wound closure.

References

1. Childs DR, Murthy AS. Overview of wound healing and management. Surg Clin N Am.
   2017;97(1):189–207. https://doi.org/10.1016/j.suc.2016.08.013.
2. Moreira ME, Markovchick VJ. Wound management. Crit Care Nurs Clin N Am.
   2012;24(2):215–37. https://doi.org/10.1016/j.ccel.2012.03.008.
3. Gurtner GC, Werner S, Barrandon Y, Longaker MT. Wound repair and regeneration. Nature.
   2008;453(7193):314–21. https://doi.org/10.1038/nature07039.
4. Foster L, Moore P. Acute surgical wound care 3: fittin the dressing to the wound. Br J Nurs.
   1999;8(4):200–10. https://doi.org/10.12968/bjon.1999.8.4.6694.

5. Broussard KC, Powers JG. Wound dressings: selecting the most appropriate type. Am J Clin Dermatol. 2013;14(6):449–59. https://doi.org/10.1007/s40257-013-0046-4.
6. Daeschlein G. Antimicrobial and antiseptic strategies in wound management. Int Wound J. 2013;10(Suppl 1):9–14. https://doi.org/10.1111/iwj.12175.
7. Schultz GS, Sibbald RG, Falanga V, Ayello EA, Dowsett C, Harding K, et al. Wound bed preparation: a systemic approach to wound management. Wound Rep Reg. 2003;11(Supply 1):S1–28. https://doi.org/10.1046/j.1524-475x.11.s2.1.x.
8. Park H, Copeland C, Henry S, Barbul A. Complex wounds and their management. Surg Clin North Am. 2010;90(6):1181–94. https://doi.org/10.1016/j.suc.2010.08.001.
9. Powers JG, Higham C, Broussard K, Phillips TJ. Wound healing and treating wounds: chronic wound care and management. J Am Acad Dermatol. 2016;74(4):607–725. https://doi.org/10.1016/j.jaad.2015.08.070.
10. Yao K, Bae L, Yew WP. Post-operative wound management. Aust Fam Physician. 2013;42(12):867–70.
11. Agarwal P, Kukrele R, Sharma D. Vacuum assisted closure (VAC)/negative pressure wound therapy (NPWT) for difficult wounds: a review. J Clin Orthop Trauma. 2019;10(5):845–8. https://doi.org/10.1016/j.jcot.2019.06.015.
12. Huang C, Leavitt T, Bayer LR, Orgill DP. Effect of negative pressure wound therapy on wound healing. Curr Probl Surg. 2014;51(7):301–31. https://doi.org/10.1067/j.cpsurg.2014.04.001.

Chapter 27
An Introduction to Surgical Tubes, Lines, and Drains

Andrea Alonso and Sheina Theodore

Introduction

- The tubes, lines, and drains are frequently used in the management of surgical patients. A fundamental understanding of these tools is crucial in the care of surgical patients.
- These are used in an array of surgical pathologies and are the first-line treatment for surgical diseases, such as pneumothorax and small bowel obstructions. Other indications include nutritional support and respiration.
- In the postoperative period, surgical tubes and drains are used to minimize dead space and to monitor internal spaces for postoperative complications including postoperative leak or abscess, hematoma, and lymph leakage [1].

Tubes

- Tubes can be placed in natural orifices of the body, such as the oral cavity, and in surgical incisions, such as incisions in the chest cavity.
- Common uses include enteral feeding in the setting of dysphagia, for respiration, pulmonary pathologies, and colonic decompression.
- *Historical fun fact*: Artificial enteral feeding via a tube system has its origin as early as the 1800s. In 1846, John Hunter, a Scottish surgeon and comparative

A. Alonso · S. Theodore (✉)
Department of Surgery, BU Chobanian & Avedisian School of Medicine, Boston, MA, USA

Division of Trauma, Acute Care Surgery & Surgical Critical Care, Boston Medical Center, Boston, MA, USA
e-mail: Andrea.Alonso@bmc.org; Sheina.Theodore@bmc.org

© The Author(s), under exclusive license to Springer Nature Switzerland AG 2025
T. S. Brahmbhatt, D. R. Scantling (eds.), *Trauma Surgery Clerkship*, Contemporary Surgical Clerkships,
https://doi.org/10.1007/978-3-032-01412-2_27

anatomist, described one of the earliest orogastric tubes made with whalebone covered with eel skin. In 1846, the French surgeon Charles Sedillot was the first to describe a gastrostomy tube. The first gastrostomy with long term survival was performed by Dr Staton in the United States in the 1870s. In 1894, M. Stamm published his description of the gastrostomy tube, which is still used today with slight modifications [2].

Enteric Tubes

- In the surgical patient, enteral tubes are used for either nutritional support or for decompression of the gastrointestinal tract.
- Common enteral indications: poor oral intake in the setting of dysphagia due to mechanical or physiologic diseases, or for malnutrition.
- Common surgical pathologies requiring decompression: Small bowel obstructions (SBO), ileus, gastrointestinal anastomosis requiring diversion of gastric contents.
- *Types of enteric tubes:* Enteral tubes can be categorized into short-term and long-term tubes, or permanent tubes.
- Short-term tubes (less than 4 weeks) include orogastric and nasoenteric tubes.

  – Nasoenteric tubes can terminate in the stomach (nasogastric tube, see Fig. 27.1) and in post-pyloric regions, such as the duodenum (nasoduodenal) and jejunum (nasojejunal). Figure 27.2 describes the steps for NG tube placement.
  – Types: large bore tubes, such as Ryle's tube, and fine bore tubes, such as the Dobhoff tube.

Fig. 27.1 Illustration of NG tube [3]

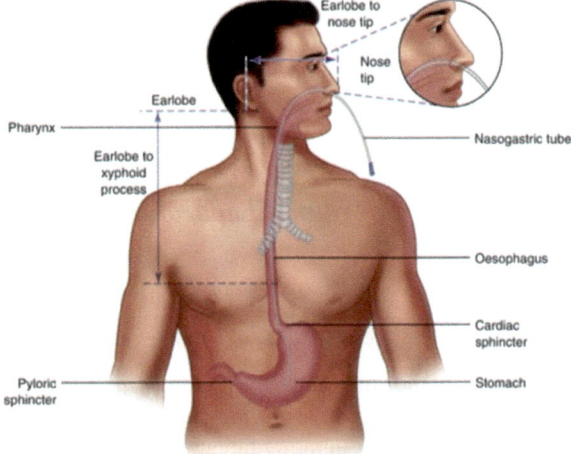

Fig. 27.2 How to confirm
successful ETT placement

1. **Good color change of the end-tidal CO2 detector.**
2. **Auscultate bilateral lung fields and ensure bilateral breath sounds.**
3. **Check pulse oximetry for constant wave form.**
4. **CXR confirmation.**

- Long-term tubes (greater than 4 weeks) include g-tubes and j-tubes. These are used in chronic medical or surgical diseases impacting oral intake. The g-tube can be placed endoscopically, open, laparoscopically, or by interventional radiology [4].

Respiratory Tubes

- The endotracheal tube (ETT) is a tube constructed of polyvinylchloride placed between the vocal cords through the trachea and serves as a conduit to provide oxygen and inhaled gases to the lungs.
- The ability to place an ETT, otherwise known as intubation, is a lifesaving skill.
- The ETT has a length and a diameter. Diameter is measured in millimeters, such as "pass me a 7.0 tube" means an ETT with an inner diameter of 7 mm. The narrower the tube, the higher the resistance to flow. Figure 27.3 describes methods to confirm successful ETT placement.
- Indications: secure a definitive airway.
- Relative contraindications: severe airway trauma or obstruction, severe cervical spine injury who requires strict immobility [6].

Tracheostomy

- A tracheostomy is a surgically placed airway (see Fig. 27.3). It is typically performed in a planned fashion, as opposed to an emergent cricothyroidotomy.
- A tube is placed directly into the trachea through an incision in the neck.

Fig. 27.3 Illustration of tracheostomy appliance [5]

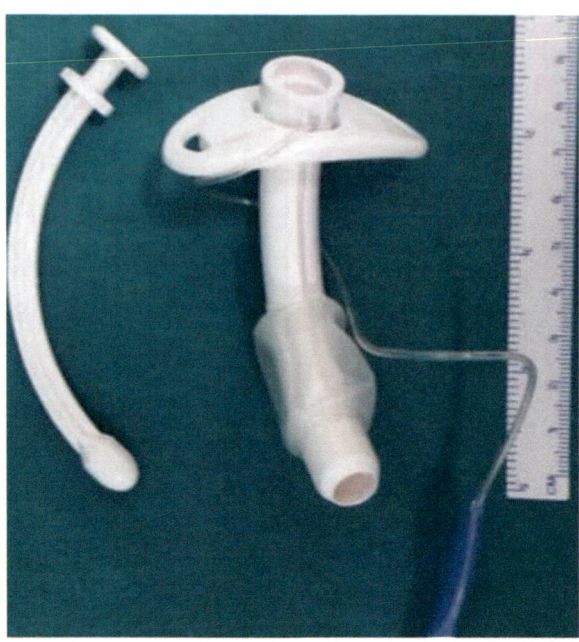

- Placement of a tracheostomy tube is indicated in patients with acute respiratory failure who classically require mechanical ventilation for 7 days or more, and who are expected to have a meaningful recovery. For patients who have incurred traumatic brain injuries and require intubation, earlier tracheostomy placement is indicated.
- Other indications include upper airway obstructions, vocal cord paralysis, large amounts of secretions requiring frequent pulmonary hygiene, and debilitating neurologic disease or traumatic brain injury (TBI).
- The benefits of a tracheostomy, as compared to an ETT, include decreased sedation requirements, improved suctioning ability and improved weaning from a ventilator with a reduced intensive care unit length of stay.
- No absolute contraindications to open tracheostomies.
  Relative contraindications: difficult anatomy, severe respiratory disease resulting in inability to withstand periods of apnea or loss of positive-pressure ventilation. Below is a figure of the percutaneous tracheostomy procedure [7].

Chest Tubes

- The thoracostomy tube, known as the chest tube, is used in a variety of clinical settings and can be lifesaving. *Please see the chest tube chapter for more in-depth information regarding chest tube types, insertions, and indications.*

- This tube is inserted into the space between the visceral and parietal pleura of the lung, a potential space that can fill with abnormal air, causing a pneumothorax, or fluid, causing a hemothorax or pleural effusion.
- Abnormal air or fluid in this space causes mass effect on the lung and can result in life-threatening conditions, such as a tension pneumothorax. Chest tubes are used to evacuate this space and aid in re-expansion of the lung [8, 9].

Rectal Tubes

- Rectal tubes are inserted into the rectum and allow for decompression of the colon.
- These are the initial treatment attempt for surgical diseases, such as sigmoid volvulus.
- The passage of a well-lubricated rubber rectal tube allows for decompression of the segment of bowel. This allows for bowel detorsion.
- The tube is typically left in place for 48 h. These rectal tubes are placed after colonic decompression by our GI colleagues.
- These tubes differ from fecal diversion tubes (common brand name, flexiseals) as fecal diversion tubes are placed at the bedside into the upper anus/lower rectum and held in place with a balloon [10].

Lines

- Vascular access is critical in patient care and in the critically ill patient.
- Common indications include administration of fluids, medications, such as antibiotics and vasoactive agents, blood laboratory draws, and blood pressure monitoring.
- *Historical fun fact*: In 1885, experiments on cardiac catheterizations in animals was being recorded by French physiologist, Claude Bernard. In the same era, the first hypodermic needle and syringe were introduced. In 1900s, sterile needles, tubing, and continuous IV fluid infusions became commonplace. Soon after, the "catheter through the needle" became the first long term IV device, followed by "cannula over the needle [11]."

Intravenous Catheters

- IV catheters, or cannulas, are indwelling single, double, or triple lumen catheters that serve as conduits for fluids, medications and blood products, as well as for blood draws.

Table 27.1 IV gauge and
flow rates

Gauge	Approximate flow rate (mL/min)
14G	250
16G	150
18G	100
20G	60
22G	35
Interosseous (IO)	80
Cordis	130
Triple lumen	70

- These are measured in gauge (G) of the needle, or the inner diameter of the needle. The number G is inversely related to diameter of the needle. The higher the number, the narrower the catheter (as observed in Table 27.1 and Fig. 27.4) [12]. The larger the diameter of the needle (i.e., the smaller the G), the faster the flow rates. This becomes relevant in the management of unstable patients, such as the trauma patient, who require rapid infusion of crystalloids and colloids, such as blood products.
- Two broad categories of IV catheters: peripheral intravenous (PIV) access and central venous catheters.
- Central venous catheters:

  - Large IVs placed in major veins (such as internal jugular vein, femoral vein, subclavian vein). Figure 27.5 illustrates placement of internal jugular line.
  - Indications: volume replacement, emergent access, dialysis, chemotherapy, long-term antibiotics, frequent blood draws.
  - Contraindications: infection, trauma to ipsilateral side (subclavian only), distorted anatomy [13].

Arterial Catheters

- Arterial catheterization, or arterial lines (a-line), involves the placement of a catheter in an artery, rather than a vein.
- Commonly employed in critically ill patients for serial arterial blood gas sampling, and real-time blood pressure monitoring.
- Common sites include radial artery and femoral artery. Always check for complete palmar arch prior to placement of a-line (Fig. 27.6).
- Contraindication: circulatory compromise in extremity, third-degree burns, Raynaud's syndrome, thromboangiitis obliterans.
- Complications of this line include hematomas, catheter-related infection, embolic or thrombotic events, amputation for ischemic injury [1].

Fig. 27.4 Illustration of PIV by gage (G). The smaller the number, the larger the diameter [12]

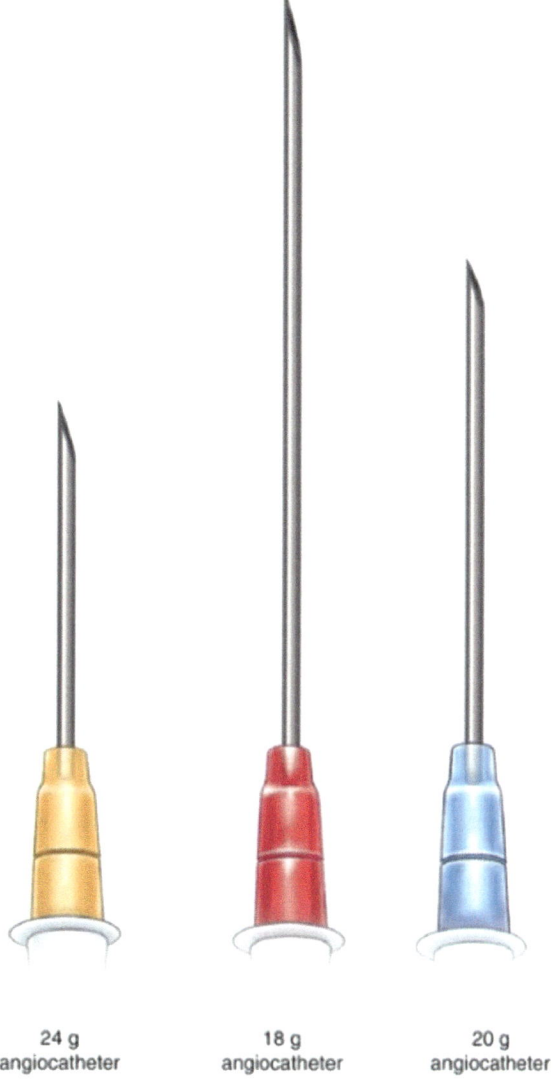

24 g
angiocatheter

18 g
angiocatheter

20 g
angiocatheter

Fig. 27.5 Placement of central line in internal jugular vein [13]

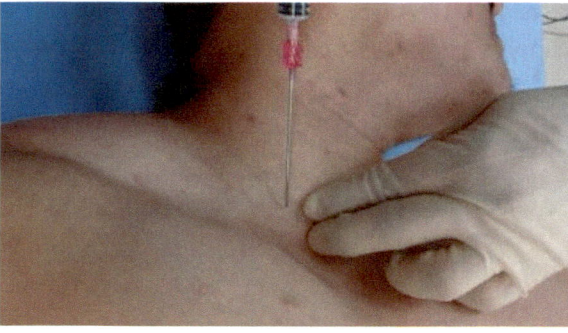

Fig. 27.6 Assessment of complete palmar arch. Picture on left shows occlusion of radial and ulnar arteries with blanching of palm. Picture on right shows release of ulnar artery with reperfusion of entire hand [14]

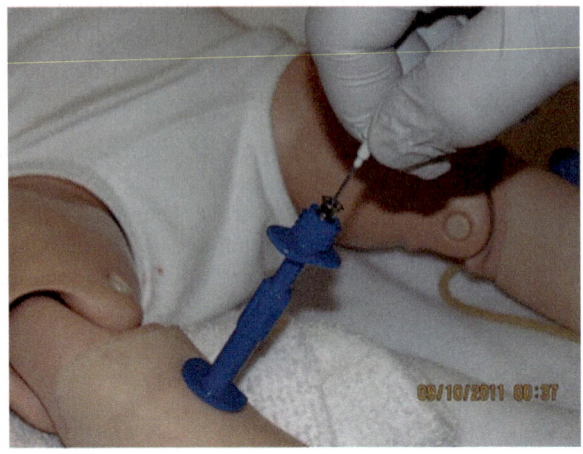

Pulmonary Artery Catheter

- The pulmonary artery catheter (PAC), commonly referred to as a Swan-Ganz catheter, is a catheter that is placed in the internal jugular vein, through the right atrium, into the right ventricle and wedged in the pulmonary artery.
- Because of its location, it gives important information on cardiac function.
- Indications: evaluation and/or management of patients with complicated myocardial infarction, unexplained or unknown volume status in shock, severe cardiogenic shock, and suspected or known pulmonary artery hypertension (PAH). They are also used peri-operatively in patients undergoing open-heart surgery, such as coronary artery bypass graft (CABG) surgery, and in patients with congenital heart disease [15].

Intraosseous Access

- Intraosseous (IO) infusion is an alternative mode of vascular access in the injured, such as a trauma patient, or critically ill patient. These are placed in long bones, such as the humerus, on the principle that medullary veins of long bones remain patent during hypovolemia.
- Common locations for placement: proximal tibia (Fig. 27.7), distal tibia, distal femur, proximal humerus, sternum.
- The fluid and blood infusion through an IO is equivalent to a 21G IV catheter, thus the fluid or blood should be given under pressure.
- Indication: Failure to obtain vascular access in acute, life-threatening situations.
- Contraindications: long bone fracture [16].

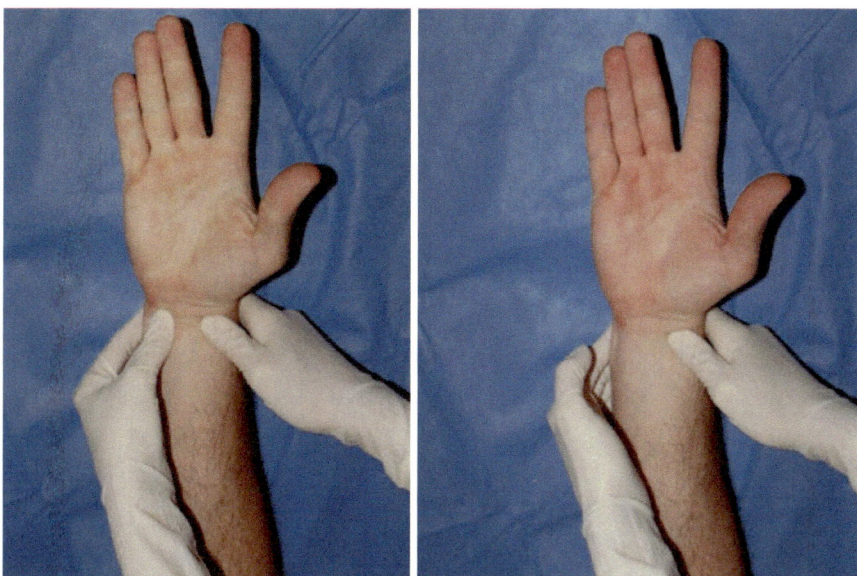

Fig. 27.7 Illustration of IO placement on proximal tibia [16]

Drains

- Drains serve as a tract for fluids to leave the body, such as purulent material, blood, lymph, bile, pancreatic juices.
- Drains can provide therapeutic benefits, such as providing egress for intra-abdominal fluids, or for prophylactic benefits.
- Disadvantages of drains include increased risk for infection, discomfort, and pain. Below is a chart of the various different forms of drains.
- Drains can work passively, such as gravity-dependent, or actively, such as suction-dependent. These can be an open system or a closed system [17]. (please see Fig. 27.8 for different surgical drains).
- *Historical fun facts*: The first written descriptions of drains dates back to Hippocrates, who described using linens and small tubes to drain infection from empyemas. Present-day adaptations of closed drain have their origin in onco-logic breast surgery, particularly the radical mastectomy. By the mid-twentieth century, the use of closed suction negative-pressure drains to prevent seromas became routine. This led to the creation of the closed-system drainage, including the Jackson Pratt (JP) drain and the Blake drain [19].

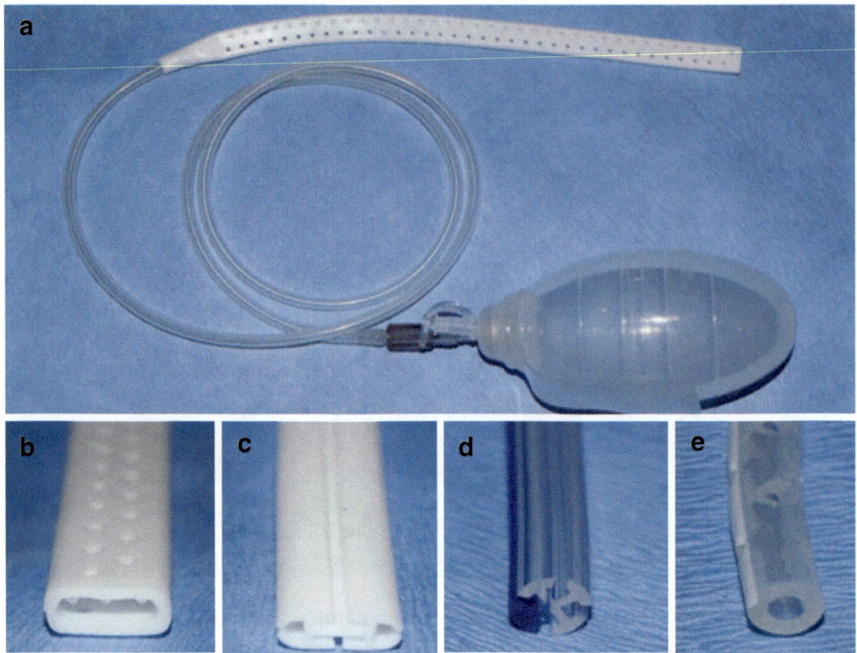

Fig. 27.8 Illustration of closed suction drains (**a**) Jackston Pratt drain, (**b**) flat Jackson-Pratt, (**c**) BLAKE drain, (**d**) Round BLAKE, (**e**) Round perforator drain [18]

Negative Pressure Wound Therapy

- Negative pressure wound therapy (NPWT), also known as vacuum-assisted wound closure (VAC), is a wound-healing technique that employs open-cell foam dressing over a wound cavity through which evenly distributed negative pressure is applied over a wound bed to suck fluid from the wound with the intention of accelerating wound healing.
- WV affects wound healing through various mechanisms including the following: (1) macrodeformation or wound shrinkage, (2) microdeformation at the wound base, (3) fluid removal, (4) creation of a favorable wound environment that promotes granulation [20].
- Wound VACs should be applied to wounds after they have been debrided and cleaned (see Fig. 27.9).
- These are often placed at −125 mm Hg of pressure. Dressings are often left in place for 48–72 h before being replaced.
- Benefits of wound VAC therapy include accelerated wound-healing time and decreased tissue edema, protection from contamination, and reduced need for complex wound changes.

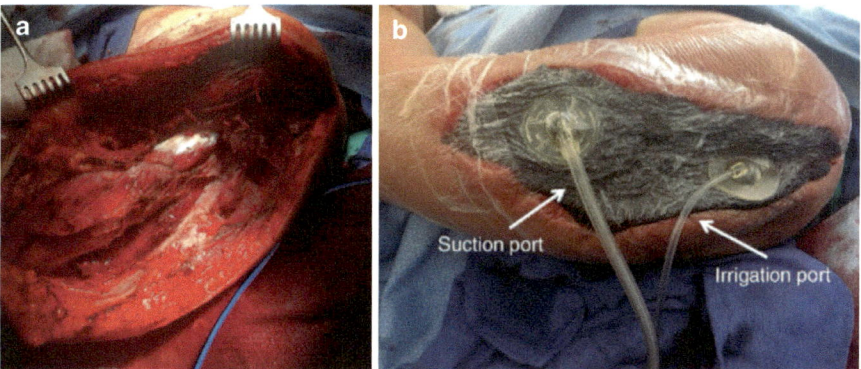

Fig. 27.9 Large upper extremity wound after debridement with wound vac placement [21]

- These are used in a range of surgical pathology including ulcers, open abdomens, sternal wounds, traumatic wounds, burns, wound dehiscence, and skin graft recipient sites.
- Contraindications: severely ischemic wounds, dry wounds, necrotic wounds, over malignancies, exposed organs, osteomyelitis, bleeding wounds, or infection [21].

Urinary Catheters

- Indwelling urinary catheters allow passage of urine from the urinary system into a drainage device.
- Common indications for urinary drainage include obstruction, incomplete bladder emptying, prolonged operative times, operations in the lower abdomen or in the pelvis where bladder decompression lowers the risk of bladder injury, and in critically ill patients necessitating strict intake and outputs.
- The risks of urinary catheters include urinary tract infections (UTI).
- Different types of catheters:

  - Urethral catheter—used to pass urine from the bladder through the urethra. Most commonly used catheter is the Foley catheter (Fig. 27.10). Foley catheters are measured in French gauge (Fr).
  - Suprapubic catheter—empties bladder through the abdominal wall. Indications include prolonged need for bladder decompression.
  - Ureteral catheters—placed in the operating room within the urethra to stent these open.
  - Renal catheters (nephrostomy tube)—placed in the renal calyces and empty externally to skin. These are typically placed for hydronephrosis due to a downstream urinary obstruction, such as a ureteral stone, nephrolithiasis, or for urological reasons [23].
  - See Fig. 27.11 for steps for Foley placement.

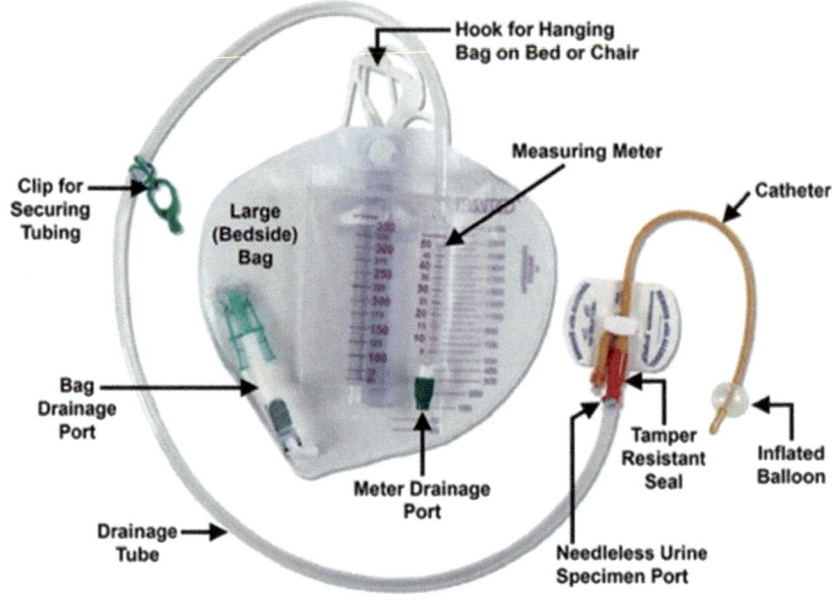

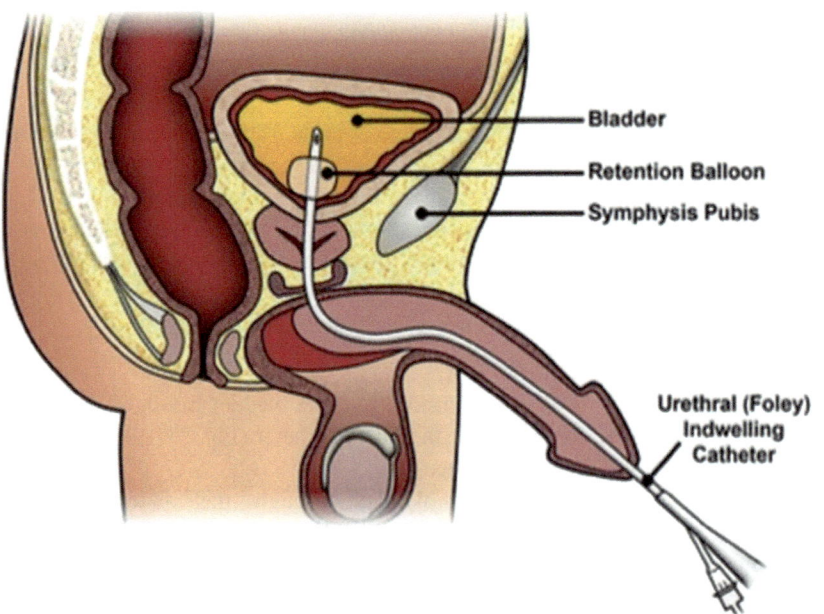

Fig. 27.10 Picture above is a foley catheter parts. Picture below is an illustration of a foley catheter placement in the male patient [22]

Fig. 27.11 Indwelling
urinary catheter placement

Fig 11: Indwelling Urinary Catheter Placement

Equipment: sterile pack for catheterization, sterile gloves, cleansing fluid, syringe and sterile water (about 10 mL), sterile lubrication gel, appropriate catheter size, drainage system.

1. Discuss the procedure with the patient
2. Position the patient: Help the patient into a supine position. For female patients, the legs should be bent and knees apart. Do NOT perform these maneuvers if patient has pelvic or femur fractures.
3. Use a standard indwelling urinary catheter kit.
4. Open the kit in a sterile fashion.
5. Wash your hands. Put on sterile gloves.
6. Lubricate tip of catheter. Connect a 10mL saline syringe to the catheter hub to inflate the balloon. Balloon must be deflated prior to insertion
7. Clean the urethral meatus with your dominant hand using sterile solution. For female patients, hold the labia open with your non-dominant hand. Clean in downward movements towards the anus using single strokes. For male patients, hold the penile shaft with your non-dominant hand. Clean area with dominant hand.
8. Holding the catheter in your dominant hand, introduce the tip into the urethral orifice and advance. Insert the catheter. In females, urethral length is 3-4cm. In males, urethral length 15-20cm or longer.
9. Once urine begins to drain, inflate the balloon. Inflation of the balloon in the bladder is painless. If you elicit pain, stop and deflate the balloon. Remove the catheter.

References

1. Cooper ZA, Ashley S. Chapter 47. Surgical tubes and drains. In: McKean SC, Ross JJ, Dressler DD, Brotman DJ, Ginsberg JS, editors. Principles and practice of hospital medicine [Internet]. New York: McGraw-Hill; 2012. Available from: https://accessmedicine.mhmedical.com/content.aspx?bookid=496&sectionid=41304011.
2. Minard G. The history of surgically placed feeding tubes. Nutr Clin Pract [Internet]. 2006;21(6):626–33. Available from: https://doi.org/10.1177/0115426506021006626.
3. Nguyen DP, Nickels LC, De Portu G. Nasogastric tube placement. In: Atlas of emergency medicine procedures [Internet]. New York: Springer; 2016. p. 411–3. Available from: http://dx.doi.org/https://doi-org.ezproxy.bu.edu/10.1007/978-1-4939-2507-0_72.
4. Welbank T, Kurien M. To PEG or not to PEG that is the question. Proc Nutr Soc [Internet]. 2021;80(1):1–8. Available from: https://doi.org/10.1017/S002966512000703X.
5. de Almeida Vital JM, Dias FL, da Trindade Meira Henriques MEG, da Trindade Meira Henriques MAG, de Moura MEL, de Farias TP. Tracheostomy tube types. In: Tracheostomy [Internet]. Cham: Springer International Publishing; 2018. p. 23–46. Available from: http://dx.doi.org/https://doi-org.ezproxy.bu.edu/10.1007/978-3-319-67867-2_3.
6. Ahmed RA, Boyer TJ. Endotracheal tube [Internet]. National Center for Biotechnology Information. U.S. National Library of Medicine; 2022. Available from: https://pubmed.ncbi.nlm.nih.gov/30969569.
7. Hashimoto DA, Axtell AL, Auchincloss HG. Percutaneous Tracheostomy. N Engl J Med. 2020;383(20):e112. https://doi.org/10.1056/NEJMvcm2014884. Epub 2020 Oct 28. PMID: 33113296.
8. Anderson D, Chen SA, Godoy LA, Brown LM, Cooke DT. Comprehensive review of chest tube management: a review: a review. JAMA Surg [Internet]. 2022;157(3):269–74. Available from: https://doi.org/10.1001/jamasurg.2021.7050.
9. Chawla R, Jain A, Bali RK. Chest tube placement. In: ICU protocols [Internet]. Singapore: Springer; 2020. p. 475–86. Available from: https://doi.org/10.1007/978-981-15-0902-5_47.
10. Tuech JJ, Pessaux P, Arnaud JP. Obstruction of the colon (benign pathology). In: Holzheimer RG, Mannick JA, editors. Surgical treatment: evidence-based and problem-oriented. Munich: Zuckschwerdt; 2001.
11. Gow KW, Tapper D, Hickman RO. Between the lines: the 50th anniversary of long-term central venous catheters. Am J Surg. 2017;213(5):837–48. Available from: https://doi.org/10.1016/j.amjsurg.2017.03.021. Epub 2017 Mar 24.
12. Smith DN, Lucas JK. Peripheral venous catheterization. In: Ganti L, editor. Atlas of emergency medicine procedures. New York: Springer; 2016. https://doi-org.ezproxy.bu.edu/10.1007/978-1-4939-2507-0_120.
13. Ergle KD, Kramer ZB, Jones J, Patel RP. Central venous line placement: internal jugular vein, subclavian vein, and femoral vein. In: Ganti L, editor. Atlas of emergency medicine procedures. New York: Springer; 2016. https://doi-org.ezproxy.bu.edu/10.1007/978-1-4939-2507-0_3.
14. Kile J, John K, Aghera A. Arterial cannulation (radial and femoral). In: Ganti L, editor. Atlas of emergency medicine procedures. New York: Springer; 2016. Available from: https://doi-org.ezproxy.bu.edu/10.1007/978-1-4939-2507-0_1.
15. Patel RP, Elie MC. Pulmonary artery catheter. In: Ganti L, editor. Atlas of emergency medicine procedures. New York: Springer; 2016. Available from: https://doi-org.ezproxy.bu.edu/10.1007/978-1-4939-2507-0_4.
16. Lucas JK. Intraosseous access. In: Ganti L, editor. Atlas of emergency medicine procedures. New York: Springer; 2016. Available from: https://doi-org.ezproxy.bu.edu/10.1007/978-1-4939-2507-0_122.
17. Petrowsky H, Wildi S Principles of drainage. In: Clavien PA, Sarr MG, Fong Y, Georgiev P, editors. Atlas of upper gastrointestinal and Hepato-Pancreato-biliary surgery. Berlin, Heidelberg: Springer; 2007. Available from: https://doi-org.ezproxy.bu.edu/10.1007/978-3-540-68866-2_5.

18. Chevrollier GS, Rosato FE, Rosato EL. Fundamentals of drain management. In: Palazzo F, editor. Fundamentals of general surgery. Cham: Springer; 2018. Available from: https://doi-org.ezproxy.bu.edu/10.1007/978-3-319-75656-1_11.
19. Meyerson JM. A brief history of two common surgical drains. Ann Plast Surg. 2016;77(1):4–5. Available from: https://doi.org/10.1097/SAP.0000000000000734.
20. Argenta LC, Morykwas MJ. Vacuum-assisted closure: a new method for wound control and treatment: clinical experience. Ann Plast Surg. 1997;38(6):563–76. discussion 577.
21. Benjamin ER, Demetriades D. Negative pressure wound therapy for soft tissue infections. In: Demetriades D, Inaba K, Lumb P, editors. Atlas of critical care procedures. Cham: Springer; 2018. Available from: https://doi-org.ezproxy.bu.edu/10.1007/978-3-319-78367-3_29.
22. Newman DK, Cumbee RP, Rovner ES. Indwelling (transurethral and suprapubic) catheters. In: Clinical application of urologic catheters, devices and products. Cham: Springer; 2018. Available from: https://doi-org.ezproxy.bu.edu/10.1007/978-3-319-14821-2_1.
23. Carruthers RK. Catheters. In: First on call for urology. London: Palgrave Macmillan; 1991. Available from: https://doi-org.ezproxy.bu.edu/10.1007/978-1-349-12258-5_1.

Chapter 28
Venous Thromboembolism in Trauma Patients

Katherine Florecki and Elliott R. Haut (ID)

Introduction

Venous thromboembolism (VTE) comprising deep vein thrombosis (DVT) and pulmonary embolism (PE), is a common complication in the trauma population and is associated with significant morbidity and mortality. VTE affects up to 900,000 individuals, killing more than 100,000, with one-third of patients dying within 30 days of diagnosis each year in the United States. The incidence of VTE in trauma patients ranges from 5% to 63%, depending on patient risk factors, modality of prophylaxis, and methods of detection. Trauma patients, many of whom are critically ill and/or undergo major surgery are at inherently high risk for VTE. Therefore, understanding risk assessment, prevention, diagnosis, and treatment is fundamental to reduce morbidity and mortality [1–3].

K. Florecki
Division of Acute Care Surgery, Department of Surgery, The Johns Hopkins University School of Medicine, Baltimore, MD, USA
e-mail: kflorec1@jhmi.edu

E. R. Haut (✉)
Division of Acute Care Surgery, Department of Surgery, The Johns Hopkins University School of Medicine, Baltimore, MD, USA

Department of Anesthesiology and Critical Care Medicine, Department of Emergency Medicine, The Johns Hopkins University School of Medicine, Baltimore, MD, USA

The Armstrong Institute for Patient Safety and Quality, Johns Hopkins Medicine, Baltimore, MD, USA

Department of Health Policy and Management, The Johns Hopkins Bloomberg School of Public Health, Baltimore, MD, USA
e-mail: ehaut1@jhmi.edu

© The Author(s), under exclusive license to Springer Nature Switzerland AG 2025
T. S. Brahmbhatt, D. R. Scantling (eds.), *Trauma Surgery Clerkship*, Contemporary Surgical Clerkships, https://doi.org/10.1007/978-3-032-01412-2_28

251

Risk Factors

- While all hospitalized patients are at risk for VTE, trauma patients are at an especially high risk.
- In the absence of pharmacologic prophylaxis, those with severe injuries have a risk of DVT and pulmonary embolism that surpasses 50% and 11%, respectively.
- Spinal cord injury, traumatic brain injury, pelvic and long bone fractures, need for major surgery, or multiple transfusions have all been identified as independent high-risk factors for VTE after trauma.
- Virchow's triad of venous stasis, endothelial injury, and hypercoagulability increase the risk of VTE and all of these components are common after trauma.

Prevention and Prophylaxis

Given the high incidence and potential complications of VTE, all trauma patients should be evaluated for risk factors and prescribed appropriate prophylaxis. Pharmacologic prophylaxis remains the most effective modality at preventing VTE. Pharmacologic prophylaxis medications primarily include low-molecular-weight heparin (LMWH) and unfractionated heparin (UFH). Sequential compression devices remain important and effective adjuncts to pharmacologic prophylaxis and should be applied to all trauma patients without contraindication (i.e., casts, external fixation devices, wounds). Ambulation is often recommended as VTE prophylaxis, although there is no data to suggest its effectiveness. This misconception often leads to erroneously omitting appropriate pharmacologic or mechanical options [4–7].

- In terms of which pharmacologic agent should be prescribed to trauma patients, this has been well studied and described in the literature [8].
- Trauma and orthopedic literature have demonstrated that subcutaneous injections of LMWH are superior to subcutaneous heparin at reducing VTE in trauma patients. This is the first-line agent recommended by most VTE prevention guidelines. Heparin, a naturally occurring polysaccharide, augments the activity of antithrombin III, a potent, naturally occurring inhibitor of activated factor X (Xa) and thrombin, which results in an interruption of both the intrinsic and extrinsic pathways of the coagulation cascade. UFH is administered in 5000 units subcutaneously two or three times daily (or at higher doses for obese patents). UFH has relatively little proven efficacy of preventing VTE after trauma. However, in patients with a contraindication to LMWH, UFH is the best alternative [9, 10].
- LMWH is derived from depolymerization of UFH resulting in molecular weight that is on average one-third of UFH. Given its smaller size, LMWH is less capable of inhibiting thrombin and more specifically acts as a factor Xa inhibitor. Enoxaparin dosed at 30 mg subcutaneous every 12 h has been widely accepted

as the standard regimen in trauma patients. However, newer data regarding dose adjustment for a more personalized medicine approach now exist. Some trauma centers routinely use the 40 mg twice daily dosing regimen. Some studies now suggest adjusting the dose based on patient weight, anti-factor Xa levels, thromboelastography, or renal function (creatinine clearance) [11].

- Pharmacologic prophylaxis should be initiated as early as possible and continue throughout hospitalization while avoiding missed doses for procedures. Historically, VTE prophylaxis was withheld from certain trauma patient populations, particularly patients with solid organ injury (SOI) or traumatic brain injury (TBI), due to concern for the risk of exacerbating bleeding. However, newer data shows safety and efficacy in many of these patient populations [12]

- A 2-year retrospective analysis of American College of Surgeons Trauma Quality Improvement (ACS TQP) program studied the impact of early initiation of pharmacological prophylaxis in patients with blunt SOI. A total of 36,187 patients with blunt SOI undergoing non-operative management were divided based on timing of initiation of chemoprophylaxis, early ≤48 h, late >48 h, and no prophylaxis. The study found no increase in failure of non-operative management, transfusion requirements after pharmacologic prophylaxis administration, or mortality in patients when comparing early vs. late initiation of VTE prophylaxis. Early prophylaxis was associated with decreased DVT (1.9% vs. 4.1%) and PE (1.0% vs. 1.8%) rates compared with late prophylaxis.

Patients with TBI represent another special population for consideration of timing of initiation of VTE prophylaxis given concern for intracranial hemorrhage expansion. A large retrospective study of 3634 patients with severe TBI found that early initiation of pharmacologic VTE prophylaxis within 72 h of injury was associated with lower rates of both pulmonary embolism (OR = 0.48; 95% CI = 0.25–0.91) and DVT (OR = 0.51; 95% CI = 0.36–0.72) without an increased risk of new or expanding intracranial hemorrhage, neurosurgical intervention, or mortality [13]. The modified Berne-Norwood criteria, a tiered approach to guide VTE chemoprophylaxis initiation in patients with TBI has shown efficacy in VTE prevention and safety and is outlined in ACS TQP best practice guidelines (Table 28.1).

Direct Oral Anticoagulants and Aspirin

- Direct oral anticoagulants (DOACs) include dabigatran, a direct thrombin inhibitor, and factor X inhibitors including edoxaban, apixaban, rivaroxaban, and betrixaban. Aspirin, an irreversible cyclooxygenase inhibitor, blocks formation of thromboxane A2 resulting in decreasing platelet aggregation and vasoconstriction. While these medications are routinely used for VTE prophylaxis in certain non-trauma populations, their role in trauma has been relatively limited. However, new data published in 2023 will likely change practice dramatically as aspirin has been shown to be non-inferior to LWMH in preventing death in trauma patients with fractures [10].

Table 28.1 Recommendations for venous thromboembolism prophylaxis in patients with traumatic brain injury based on the Berne-Norwood criteria

Low risk	No moderate or high-risk criteria	Initiate pharmacologic prophylaxis if repeat head CT stable at 24 h
Moderate risk	Subdural or epidural hematoma >8-mm contusion or intraventricular hemorrhage >2-cm multiple contusions per lobe Subarachnoid hemorrhage with abnormal CT angiogram Evidence of progression at 24 h	Initiate pharmacologic prophylaxis if repeat head CT stable at 72 h
High risk	ICP monitor placement Craniotomy Evidence of progression at 72 h	Consider surveillance duplex Delay pharmacologic prophylaxis until CT stable Consider IVCF

IVC Filter (IVCF) Placement

- Prophylactic IVCF placement in trauma patients was a commonly accepted practice for many years, yet their role is now less utilized, likely because of the safety of early prophylaxis as reviewed above. The past thinking was that an IVCF would be considered as primary prophylaxis in trauma patients that are at high risk and cannot receive prophylaxis for a prolonged period. Studies now show only a relatively small benefit which is likely outweighed by the complications of filter placement. Even when filters are planned to be retrieved, many were left in place, as many patients were lost to follow-up. Filters still have a role in treatment of VTE when diagnosed in trauma patients with relative contraindications to treatment dose anticoagulation. If placed, these patients must be closely followed to monitor for any complication, anticoagulation should be resumed when safe, and the filter retrieved.

Diagnosis of VTE

- Diagnosis of VTE in trauma patients can be quite challenging as there are often many confounding variables (i.e., critically ill patient, cast, wounds). Maintaining a high index of suspicion is key to early detection. Symptoms that should raise suspicion for DVT are acute swelling, tenderness, and/or erythema of an extremity. Hypoxia, tachycardia, shortness of breath, and/or chest pain can be symptoms of PE [2, 3].

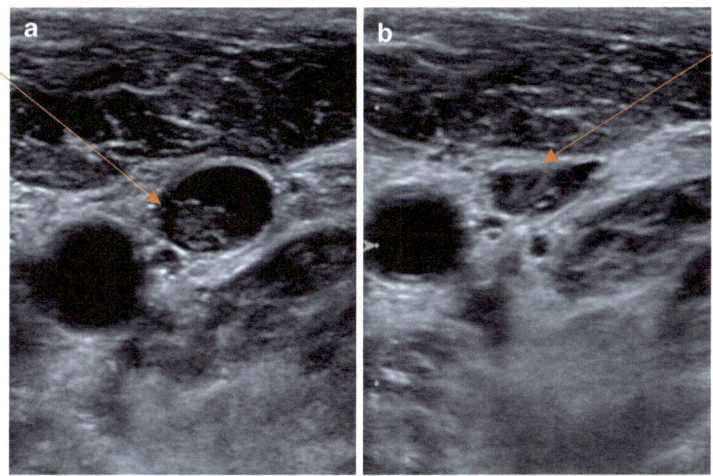

Fig. 28.1 (**a**) Vein with echogenic thrombus. (**b**) Incomplete vein compressibility

Duplex Ultrasonography

- Duplex ultrasonography is the diagnostic test of choice for detection of DVT. It is an inexpensive and noninvasive test that can be rapidly performed. Routine screening for DVT in all trauma patients is not recommended as it has not been shown to influence rate of symptomatic DVT or PE. However, screening duplex can be considered in high-risk trauma patients (i.e., pelvic, long bone fractures). Positive duplex will demonstrate an echogenic thrombus in a vein which is non-compressible (Fig. 28.1).

Computed Tomography Pulmonary Angiography

- Computed tomography pulmonary angiography (CTPA) is the gold standard imaging modality for evaluation of PE. CTPA is a minimally invasive test; however, it requires transport of an often critically ill patient from the intensive care unit and the injection of iodine-contrast agent to highlight the pulmonary vessels. Contrast-filled pulmonary vessels will appear as bright white and any filling defect, such as a PE, will appear dark (Fig. 28.2).

Alternative Diagnostic Modalities

- The D-dimer is a relatively simple blood draw which may help in VTE diagnosis. D-Dimer is a degradation product of cross-linked fibrin, which increases in VTE. Since D-dimer is known to be elevated in inflammatory states, after sur-

Fig. 28.2 Computed tomography pulmonary angiography demonstrating pulmonary artery embolism

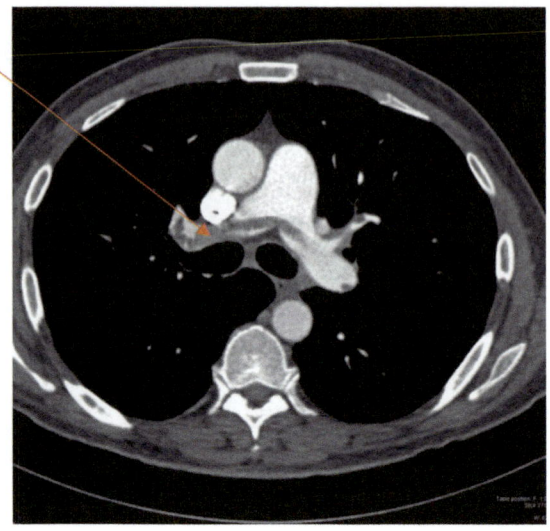

gery, and in many hospitalized patients (even without VTE, an elevated D-dimer does not rule in VTE. On the contrary, a negative D-dimer can definitively rule out VTE and negate the need for imaging in a patient when VTE is on the differential diagnosis list.

- In certain patient populations, other modalities must be used to evaluate for PE. In patients who cannot receive contrast dye because of an allergy or a ventilation/perfusion (V/Q), scan can be performed. This is a nuclear medicine test that uses radioactive material to examine ventilation and perfusion of the lungs. The scan consists of inhalation of radioactive material, analysis of ventilation followed by injection of radioactive material, and evaluation of lung perfusion. Although not the gold standard, its sensitivity and specificity have been reported between 80–85% and 93–97%, respectively, when compared to CTPA.
- The presence of renal insufficiency has often been suggested as a reason to avoid IV contrast; however, data show that contrast is not associated with worsening renal failure and should be given if needed for diagnostic purposes. In critically ill patients with hemodynamic instability, point-of-care ultrasound (POCUS) can be used to examine the heart and may help diagnose PE with findings such as a dilated right ventricle compared to the left, a flattened interventricular septum, and/or a distended inferior vena cava. McConnell's sign on echocardiogram (segmental right ventricular wall-motion abnormality with apical sparing) is pathognomonic for PE.

Treatment

Treatment of DVT

- Treatment for DVT is primarily focused on anticoagulation therapy. For hospitalized patients, most protocols involve the rapid initiation of heparin, either weight-based intravenous unfractionated heparin or subcutaneous LMWH. Therapy duration is dependent on patient characteristics and the circumstances surrounding DVT.
- In general, 3 months of therapy is recommended for provoked DVT (i.e., trauma-related, post-operative). Therapy should be continued for 3–6 months in spontaneous DVT and indefinitely in high-risk patients (i.e., inherited hypercoagulable state, recurrent, cancer). Patients are transitioned to oral anticoagulation (i.e., DOAC, warfarin) or continued on LMWH to complete long-term therapy (Fig. 28.3).
- For patients with isolated below-knee DVT, there are different treatment options. High-risk patients can be treated with anticoagulation, while low-risk patients might receive compression stockings and close follow-up with repeat duplex performed within 2 weeks after diagnosis to ensure the DVT has resolved. If propagation has occurred, anticoagulation should be initiated. Patients with a contraindication to anticoagulation should be considered for IVCF placement. While mechanical treatments (i.e., catheter-based mechanical thrombectomy and/or lysis) by vascular surgeons or interventional radiologists is possible, it is not recommended for all patients. However, patients with large, symptomatic iliofemoral DVT may benefit from this approach.

Treatment of PE

- Treatment of PE depends on the clinical stability of the patient.
- Patients who are hemodynamically stable should have similar initial treatment algorithm to that of DVT.
- Patients with or impending cardiopulmonary compromise secondary to submassive or massive PE should be treated more aggressively. Assuming there is no contraindication and there is an acceptable bleeding risk, these patients should receive systemic lytic therapy. If patients are not candidate for systemic lytic therapy, surgical or catheter-based embolectomy is an alternative option. In some cases, extracorporeal membrane oxygenation (ECMO) may be needed. One potential algorithm is shown in Fig. 28.4. Some hospitals have created dedicated pulmonary embolism response teams (PERTs) that can rapidly bring together a multidisciplinary group of physicians (i.e., intensivists, hematologists, cardiologists, cardiac surgeons, vascular surgeons, interventional radiologists) to discuss options and quickly offer optimal treatment.

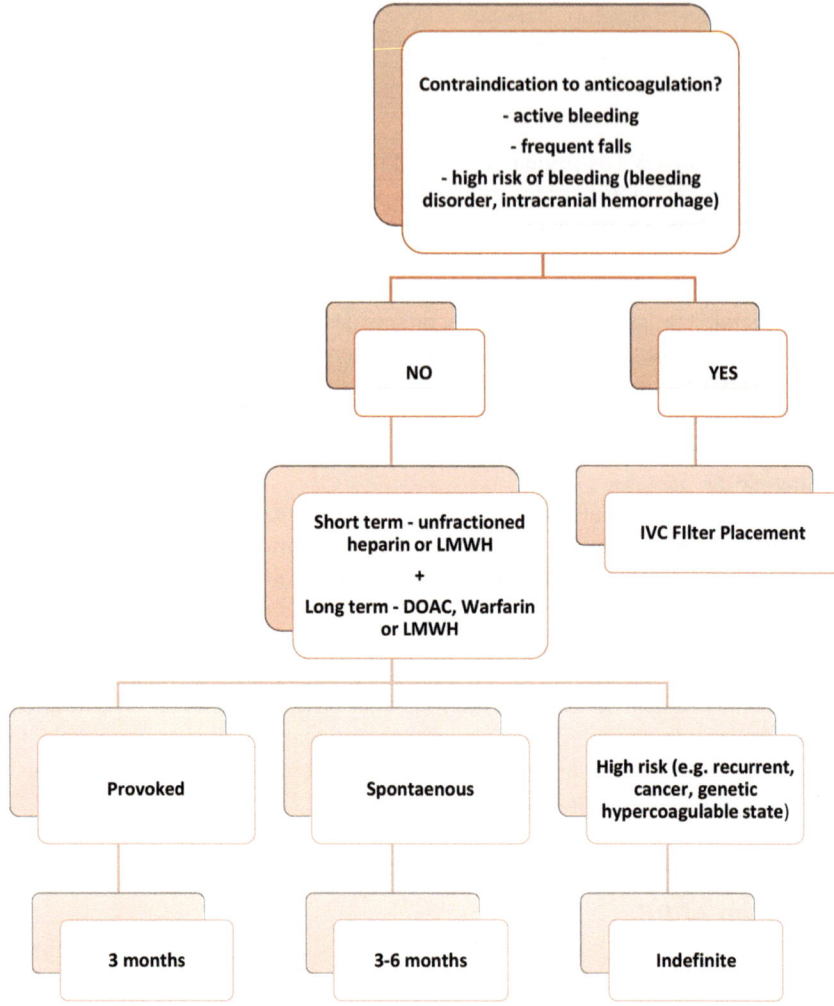

Fig. 28.3 VTE treatment algorithm

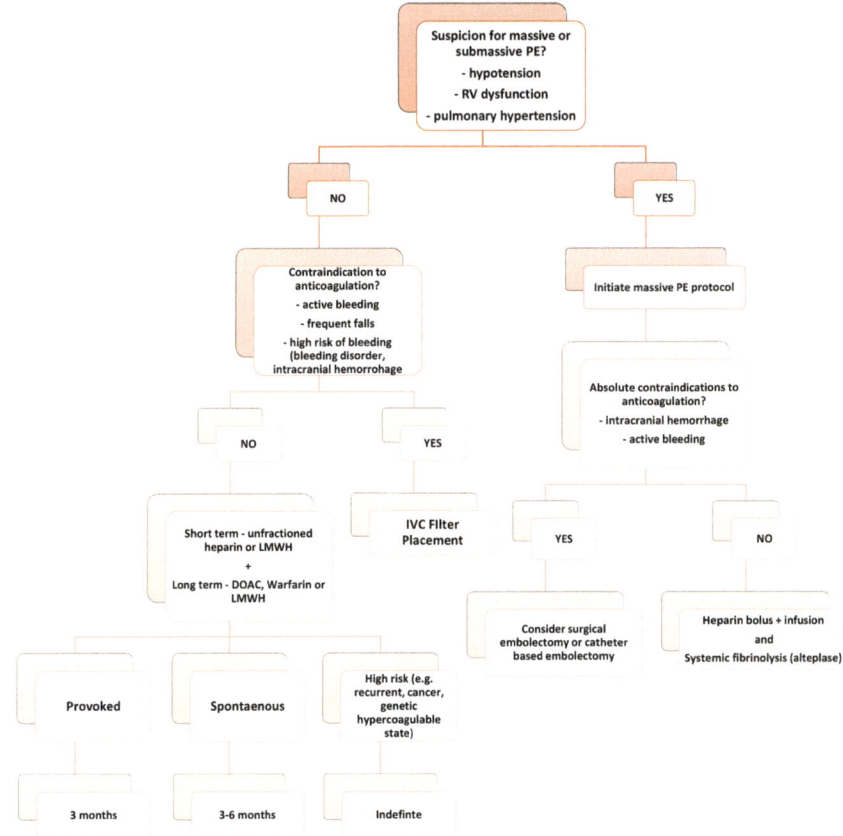

Fig. 28.4 PE treatment algorithm

Conclusion

VTE remains a common source of morbidity and mortality in trauma patients. Prophylaxis should be initiated as soon as possible and continued throughout hospitalization. Early diagnosis and prompt treatment are crucial to prevent mortality and long-term morbidity.

References

1. Lau BD, Haut ER. Practices to prevent venous thromboembolism: a brief review. BMJ Qual Saf. 2014;23(3):187–95.
2. Torres C, Haut ER. Prevention, diagnosis, and management of venous thromboembolism in the critically ill surgical and trauma patient. Curr Opin Crit Care. 2020;26(6):640–7.

3. Velopulos CG, Haut ER. In: Cameron JL, Cameron AM, editors. "Venous thromboembolism: prevention, diagnosis and treatment" in current surgical therapy. 11th ed. Philadelphia: Elsevier, Inc; 2014.

4. Yorkgitis B, Berndtson A, Cross A, Kennedy R, Kochuba M, Tignanelli C, Tominaga G, Jacobs D, Marx W, Ashley D, Ley E, Napolitano L, Costantini T. American Association for the Surgery of Trauma/American College of Surgeons-Committee on Trauma Clinical Protocol for inpatient venous thromboembolism prophylaxis after trauma. J Trauma Acute Care Surg. 2022;92(3):597–604.

5. Haut ER, Byrne JP, Price MA, Bixby P, Bulger EM, Lake L, Costantini T. Proceedings from the 2022 consensus conference to implement optimal venous thromboembolism prophylaxis in trauma. J Trauma Acute Care Surg. 2023;94(3):461–8.

6. Ratnasekera A, Geerts W, Haut ER, Price M, Costantini T, Murphy P. Implementation science approaches to optimizing venous thromboembolism prevention in patients with traumatic injuries: findings from the 2022 consensus conference to implement optimal venous thromboembolism prophylaxis in trauma. J Trauma Acute Care Surg. 2023;94(3):490–4.

7. Ley EJ, Brown CVR, Moore EE, Sava JA, Peck K, Ciesla DJ, Sperry JL, Rizzo AG, Rosen NG, Brasel KJ, Kozar R, Inaba K, Martin MJ. Updated guidelines to reduce venous thromboembolism in trauma patients: a Western Trauma Association critical decisions algorithm. J Trauma Acute Care Surg. 2020;89(5):971–81.

8. Schellenberg M, Costantini T, Joseph B, Price MA, Bernard AC, Haut ER. Timing of venous thromboembolism prophylaxis initiation after injury: findings from the consensus conference to implement optimal VTE prophylaxis in trauma. J Trauma Acute Care Surg. 2023;94(3):484–9.

9. Dhillon NK, Haut ER, Price MA, Costantini TW, Teichman AL, Cotton BA, Ley EJ. Novel therapeutic medications for venous thromboembolism prevention in trauma patients: findings from the consensus conference to implement optimal venous thromboembolism prophylaxis in trauma. J Trauma Acute Care Surg. 2023;94(3):479–83.

10. Major Extremity Trauma Research Consortium (METRC), O'Toole RV, Stein DM, O'Hara NN, Frey KP, Taylor TJ, Scharfstein DO, Carlini AR, Sudini K, Degani Y, Slobogean GP, Haut ER, Obremskey W, Firoozabadi R, Bosse MJ, Goldhaber SZ, Marvel D, Castillo RC. Aspirin or low-molecular-weight heparin for thromboprophylaxis after a fracture. N Engl J Med. 2023;388(3):203–13.

11. Teichman AL, Cotton BA, Byrne J, Dhillon NK, Berndtson AE, Price MA, Johns TJ, Ley EJ, Costantini T, Haut ER. Approaches for optimizing venous thromboembolism prevention in injured patients: findings from the consensus conference to implement optimal venous thromboembolism prophylaxis in trauma. J Trauma Acute Care Surg. 2023;94(3):469–78.

12. Skarupa D, Hanna K, Zeeshan M, Madbak F, Hamidi M, Haddadin Z, Northcutt A, Gries L, Kulvatunyou N, Joseph B. Is early chemical thromboprophylaxis in patients with solid organ injury a solid decision? J Trauma Acute Care Surg. 2019;87(5):1104–12.

13. Byrne JP, Mason SA, Gomez D, et al. Timing of pharmacologic venous thromboembolism prophylaxis in severe traumatic brain injury: a propensity- matched cohort study. J Am Coll Surg. 2016;223:621–631.e5.

Chapter 29
Principles of Pain Management in Trauma Patients

Robert Canelli and Nicole Spence

Epidemiology

- Often, a single patient presents with multiple injuries to different parts of the body simultaneously.

  - In one study, 338 motor vehicle drivers presented with a total of 2566 injuries, averaging 7.6 injuries per patient [1].
  - Different types and locations of pain may require different management.
  - Acute pain after trauma can have major clinical implications, such as impaired ventilation and the potential for intubation (or re-intubation) and all of the sequela arising from this.

- The prevalence of pain in the trauma patient is high on admission and at discharge. Most trauma patients report moderate or severe pain at discharge [2].

Pain Management Options

The underlying principle of pain management in the trauma victim is to provide adequate analgesia while minimizing side effects to allow for mobilization and enhanced recovery. Components of multimodal analgesia include the following: regional analgesia techniques, pain medication, and non-pharmacologic therapy.

R. Canelli (✉) N. Spence
Department of Anesthesiology, Boston University School of Medicine, Boston, MA, USA
e-mail: Robert.Canelli@bmc.org; Nicole.Spence@bmc.org

© The Author(s), under exclusive license to Springer Nature Switzerland AG 2025
T. S. Brahmbhatt, D. R. Scantling (eds.), *Trauma Surgery Clerkship*, Contemporary Surgical Clerkships,
https://doi.org/10.1007/978-3-032-01412-2_29

- Regional Analgesia Techniques

  - Provides superior analgesia while minimizing opioid-related adverse effects on respiration and bowel function
  - Increases tissue blood flow and perfusion
  - May be especially useful depending on injury location

    - Approximately 60% of polytrauma patients have an extremity injury [3]
    - Extremity injuries may affect post-injury functional outcome and quality of life
    - Peripheral nerve blocks are well suited to provide analgesia to extremities with little systemic side effects

  - Single-shot nerve block (SSNB) vs. continuous peripheral nerve blockade (CPNB):

    - Local anesthetic, i.e., bupivacaine or ropivacaine delivered directly to nerve bundle, providing analgesia for the duration of the local anesthetic
    - SSNB may provide up to 24+ h of analgesia; however, pain intensity associated with trauma often outlasts SSNB
    - CPNB can provide continuous infusion of local anesthetic via catheter that can remain in place for days to weeks
    - Multiple CPNB catheters can be placed; however, local anesthetic is limited by total dosage to avoid local anesthetic systemic toxicity

  - Examples: epidural, paravertebral, erector spinae plane, serratus anterior, transversus abdominis plane, femoral, among others (Fig. 29.1)
  - Concerns and contraindications to regional analgesia

    - Acute compartment syndrome: osseofascial compartment pressure increases to threshold that decreases tissue perfusion, causing tissue hypoxia, cell death, irreversible muscle, and nerve damage

      - Diagnosis generally based on clinical suspicion:

        - Pain out of proportion of clinical scenario
        - Pulselessness is a late clinical finding

      - Regional anesthesia may mask symptoms of compartment syndrome such as worsening pain, altered sensory, or motor exam leading to delay in diagnosis [4]
      - Best practice: reduce local anesthetic volumes and concentrations and follow clinically with frequent examinations

    - Acute peripheral nerve injury: potential risk of worsening nerve injury from needle trauma or local anesthetic
    - Infection at site of regional blockade needle insertion, overall incidence is very low (0–3%):

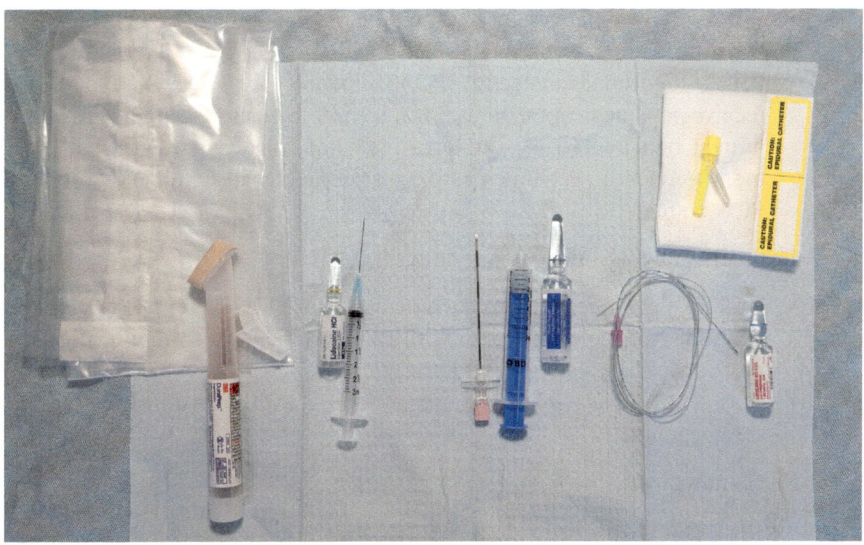

Fig. 29.1 Epidural Kit: Contents of an epidural catheter kit which can also be used for continuous peripheral nerve blockade

- Factors associated with catheter site infection:
  - Duration of indwelling catheter
  - Catheter insertion location, i.e., femoral or axillary
  - Frequent dressing changes.

- Coagulation status: hematoma formation from regional analgesia procedure can be detrimental depending on anatomic location, i.e., epidural hematoma

  - Patient's use of anticoagulant medications may limit options for regional analgesia (follow *American Society of Regional Anesthesia* anticoagulation guidelines for regional analgesia techniques)

- Pain medication

  - Opioids:
    - Oral, parenteral, or neuraxial: oxycodone (oral only), morphine, hydromorphone, among others, can all be used. For patients on chronic opioids, opioid rotation may be helpful. Converting between opioids can easily be accomplished using conversion tables and appropriate dose reductions for cross tolerance. Patients using high doses of opioids, chronic opioids, or on maintenance therapies for opioid use disorder may require higher doses of opioids.
    - Parenteral opioids are most common approach to providing analgesia for trauma patients.

- Adverse effects: respiratory depression, addiction, nausea, delirium, constipation, immunosuppression.
- Patient-controlled analgesia (PCA): Patients press the PCA button to receive pain medication bolus. PCA is safer than nurse-administered intermittent bolusing because boluses are often in lower dosages but timed more frequently. Patients must be awake and aware in order to press the PCA button.

– Non-steroidal anti-inflammatory drugs (NSAIDs):

- Oral or parenteral: ketorolac (non-specific NSAID) or COX-2-specific NSAIDS, i.e., celecoxib. Use with caution in patients with kidney injury, gastric ulcer, or history of bariatric surgery.
- May potentiate bleeding, especially with coadministration of anticoagulants.

– Acetaminophen:

- Oral, parenteral, rectal: well tolerated. Adjust daily maximum doses for patients with liver injury
- Few side effects but efficacy may be limited if high pain intensity

– NMDA-receptor antagonists, i.e., ketamine:

- Intravenous (bolus or continuous infusion)
- Decreases opioid consumption
- Hallucinations occur more frequently with bolus dosing
- Limited effects on hemodynamics unlike many other medications

- Non-pharmacologic Therapy

– Integrative medicine options generally have limited adverse effects and may work synergistically to provide analgesia
– Virtual reality

- Various studies have reported the use of immersive virtual reality to reduce pain scores and pain medication use in a variety of clinical scenarios [5–7]

– Hypnosis
– Massage and acupuncture
– Aromatherapy

Rib Fractures

- Epidemiology

– >300,000 patients with rib fractures admitted to trauma centers yearly
– Approximately 10% will die

- Incidence of 12% of all trauma admissions [8]
- Greater than one-third have pulmonary complications
- Elderly patients with rib fractures have five times mortality risk
- Mortality increases with increased number of rib fractures [9]

  - 5% for one to two ribs
  - 15% for three to five ribs
  - 34% for greater than six ribs fractured

- Most common complication: pneumonia
- Large healthcare expenditure burden

• Regional analgesia

  - Minimize respiratory depression, optimize respiratory function
  - *Epidural*: Fig. 29.2

    • Gold standard, robust data reduces paradoxical chest wall movement, may decrease number of days on mechanical ventilation
    • Contraindications: depending on anticoagulant use, epidural may not be an option. Head or spinal injury, sepsis, hypovolemia/hypotension
    • Adverse effects: systemic vasodilation, hypotension
    • Eastern Association for the Surgery of Trauma: considered preferred analgesic modality and may improve clinically significant outcomes [10]

  - *Paravertebral:* Unilateral coverage or bilateral if two catheters are placed [11, 12].

    • Similar limitations as epidural but no concerns about spinal cord trauma
    • Risks: contralateral spread of local anesthetic, pneumothorax, hypotension

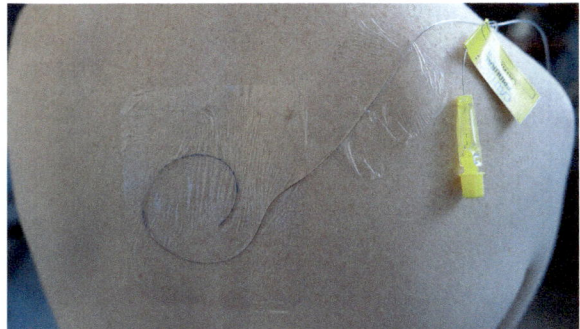

Fig. 29.2 Epidural Placement: Epidural catheter placed in the patient's midline to treat bilateral rib fractures. Note the blue depth markings along the catheter. Each single marking represents 1 cm, two single markings in succession represent 10 cm, three single markings represent 15 cm, four single markings represent 20 cm. The thick marking represents 12 cm. This catheter was placed at a depth of 10 cm at the skin (two single markings in succession are noticeable at the catheter/skin interface)

– *Erector spinae plane or serratus anterior*:

  • Fascial plane block or catheter, unilateral coverage (bilateral if two catheters/injections), minimal concern if patient on anticoagulants, minimal risk of hypotension (Figs. 29.3 and 29.4)

– *Intercostal blocks*: rapid relief but limited duration of action with additive risk of pneumothorax at each level attempted
– *Intrapleural local anesthetics*: not routinely used, higher risk of rapid systemic absorption of local anesthetic

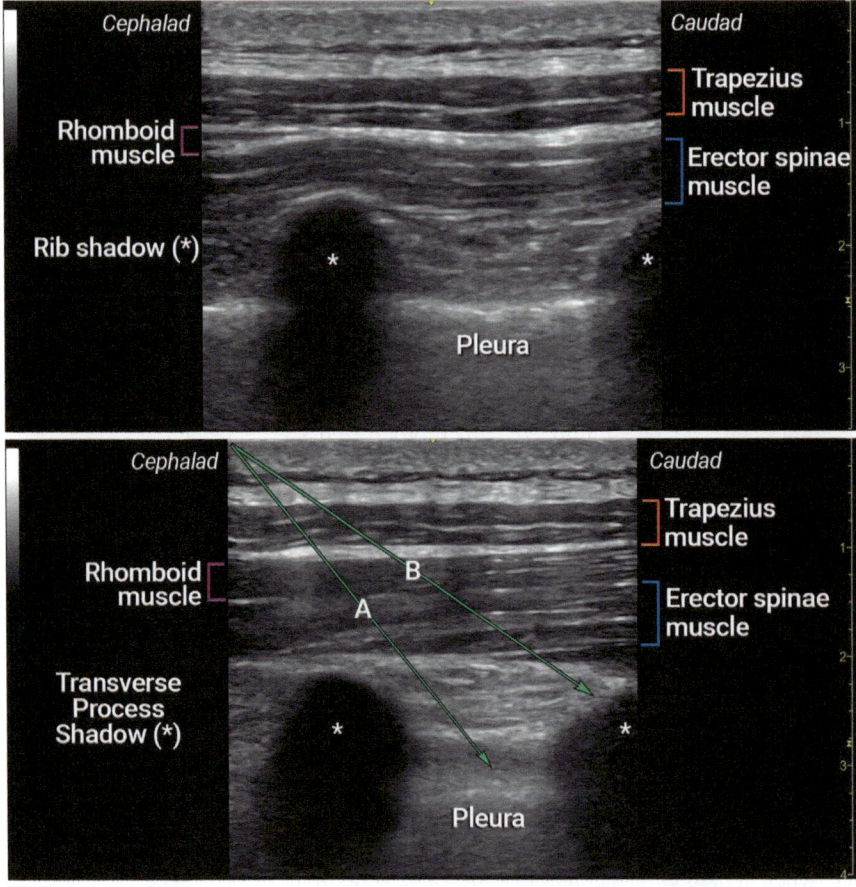

Figs. 29.3 and 29.4 ESP3 and ESP2: A linear ultrasound probe is placed in the sagittal plane on the patient's back. The probe is translated from lateral, where ribs are visualized more superficially and more rounded in shape (Fig. 29.3), toward midline. Transverse processes are viewed deeper and more rectangular in shape than ribs (Fig. 29.4). The needle trajectory and target for local anesthetic injection and catheter placement is depicted by the green arrows for **a** paravertebral and **b** erector spinae plane blockade

Falls

- Leading cause of death in adults >64 years of age
- Hip fracture is most serious and costly injury resulting from fall

    - >95% hip fractures are fall-related
    - Anatomy lends to peripheral nerve blockade, i.e., femoral nerve or fascia iliaca blockade for analgesia
    - Employ regional anesthetic techniques early to avoid opioid-related adverse effects in elderly

- Moderate to severe pain and use of opioids increases risk of delirium in elderly

Burns

- Burn Specific Pain Anxiety Scale (BSPAS): one of the pain assessments for a patient with an acute burn hospitalization [13]
- Multimodal analgesia is important, avoiding medications if indicated based on patient's history and lab trends, such as creatinine or kidney function
- Medications for neuropathic pain: adjunct to opioids, but together cause synergistic central nervous system depression (i.e., gabapentin, pregabalin)
- Ketamine: option for procedural sedation, i.e., dressing changes. Alternatively, sub-anesthetic infusions may be helpful to reduce opioid consumption
- Patients may need repeated procedures in or out of the operating room

Out-of-Operating Room Procedures

- Dressing changes, chest tubes, drain placements are anxiety- and pain-inducing
- Anxiolysis and analgesia options

    - Benzodiazepines, opioids, ketamine, dexmedetomidine
    - Existing CPNB catheters can be bolused with denser local anesthetic
    - Some procedures may lend to peripheral nerve blockade, i.e., shoulder reduction

Transition from Acute to Chronic Pain

- The development of chronic pain post-injury is a burden for the patient and the healthcare system. The most predictive risk factor for chronic pain development is the intensity of acute pain at the time of injury. It is crucial to treat traumatic pain early and aggressively.

- Chronic pain: Pain lasting >12 weeks
- Multiple risk factors:
  - Age, comorbidities, depression, anxiety, alcohol, and tobacco use

Take-Home Points

- Primary principle of pain management in trauma is to optimize the patient for recovery, including adequate respiration and early mobilization.
- Opioids are the most commonly administered analgesic in trauma patients; however, alternatives should be considered.
- Multimodal analgesia seeks to minimize adverse effects of opioids to promote recovery.
- Pain in the trauma patient is often undertreated, which may contribute to the development of chronic post-traumatic pain and impaired quality of life.
- Studies have highlighted disparities in analgesia for different genders and minority patients; therefore, physicians and clinicians should aim to provide effective and early analgesia.

References

1. Ali J. Chapter 92 Priorities in multisystem trauma. In: Hall JB, Schmidt GA, Wood LDH, editors. Principles of critical care. McGraw-Hill Education; 2015.
2. Berben SAA, Meijs THJM, van Dongen RTM, van Vugt AB, Vloet LCM, Mintjes-de Groot JJ, van Achterberg T. Pain prevalence and pain relief in trauma patients in the Accident & Emergency Department. Injury. 2008;39(5):578–85.
3. Banerjee M, Bouillon B, Shafizadeh S, Paffrath T, Lefering R, Wafaisade A, German Trauma Registry Group. Epidemiology of extremity injuries in multiple trauma patients. Injury. 2013;44(8):1015–21.
4. Saranteas T, Koliantzaki I, Savvidou O, Tsoumpa M, Eustathiou G, Kontogeorgakos V, Souvatzoglou R. Acute pain management in trauma: anatomy, ultrasound-guided peripheral nerve blocks and special considerations. Minerva Anestesiol. 2019;85(7):763–73.
5. Lauwens Y, Rafaatpoor F, Corbeel K, Broekmans S, Toelen J, Allegaert K. Immersive virtual reality as analgesia during dressing changes of hospitalized children and adolescents with burns: a systematic review with meta-analysis. Children (Basel). 2020;7(11):194.
6. Wong MS, Spiegel BMR, Gregory KD. Virtual reality reduces pain in laboring women: a randomized controlled trial. Am J Perinatol. 2021;38(S01):e167–72.
7. Eijlers R, Dierckx B, Staals LM, Berghmans JM, Van der Schroeff MP, Strabbin EM, Wijnen RMH, Hillegers MHJ, Legerstee JS, Utens EMWJ. Virtual reality exposure before elective day care surgery to reduce anxiety and pain in children: a randomised controlled trial. Eur J Anaesthesiol. 2019;36(10):728–37.
8. Sharma OP, Oswanski MF, Jolly S, Lauer SK, Dressel R, Stombaugh HA. Perils of rib fractures. Am Surg. 2008;74(4):310–4. PMID: 18453294.
9. Flagel BT, Luchette FA, Reed L, Esposito TJ, Davis KA, Santaniello JM, Gamelli RL. Half-a-dozen ribs: the breakpoint for mortality. Surgery. 2005;138:717–25.

10. Simon BJ, Cushman J, Barraco R, Lane V, Luchette FA, Miglietta M, Roccaforte DJ, Spector R, EAST Practice Management Guidelines Work Group. Pain management guidelines for blunt thoracic trauma. J Trauma. 2005;59(5):1256–67. PMID: 16385313.
11. Ho AMH, Karmakar MK, Critchley LAH. Acute pain management of patients with multiple fractured ribs: a focus on regional techniques. Curr Opin Crit Care. 2011;17:323–7.
12. Karmakar MK, Critchley LAH, Ho AMH, Gin T, Lee TW, Yim APC. Continuous thoracic paravertebral infusion of bupivacaine for pain management in patients with multiple fractured ribs. Chest. 2003;123:424–31.
13. Romanowski KS, Carson J, Pape K, Bernal E, Sharar S, Wiechman S, Carter D, Liu YM, Nitzschke S, Bhalla P, Litt J, Przkora R, Friedman B, Popiak S, Jeng J, Ryan CM, Joe V. American Burn Association guidelines on the management of acute pain in the adult burn patient: a review of the literature, a compilation of expert opinion, and next steps. J Burn Care Res. 2020;41(6):1129–51. https://doi.org/10.1093/jbcr/iraa119. PMID: 32885244.

Chapter 30
Traumatic Brain Injury

Holly B. Weis and Jose L. Pascual ⓘ

Introduction

Traumatic brain injury (TBI) occurs when a sudden forceful impact causes damage to the brain. TBI severity is variable, mirrored by a spectrum of management options that can be both emergent and complex.

Presentation

- TBI results from a sudden impact which damages the brain parenchyma. Common injury mechanisms include motor vehicle collisions (MVC), falls, pedestrian injuries, and assaults [1, 2].
- Symptoms of TBI can range from mild to moderate to severe depending on extent of damage to brain tissue [3].
- Bradycardia with hypertension and respiratory irregularities is representative of Cushing's triad which is indicative of intracranial hypertension, impending or progressing cerebral herniation and requires emergent intervention and management.
- Careful examination of the TBI patient is of paramount importance as early diagnosis and treatment can profoundly alter outcomes. All trauma patients should be evaluated in a systematic way, first prioritizing airway, breathing, and circulation

H. B. Weis
Baylor University Medical Center, Dallas, TX, USA

J. L. Pascual (✉)
University of Pennsylvania Perelman School of Medicine, Philadelphia, PA, USA
e-mail: Jose.Pascual@pennmedicine.upenn.edu

© The Author(s), under exclusive license to Springer Nature Switzerland AG 2025
T. S. Brahmbhatt, D. R. Scantling (eds.), *Trauma Surgery Clerkship*, Contemporary Surgical Clerkships,
https://doi.org/10.1007/978-3-032-01412-2_30

in accordance with the workup of all trauma patients (ATLS®). The neurologic exam is the next step in examination and is critical in assessment of the TBI patient. The well-validated Glasgow Coma Scale (GCS) is the instrument of choice and helps guide the next steps of evaluation. A pupillary exam should also be performed and documented.

Anatomy

Cranium

- TBI may be present with or without injury to the skull.
- In adults, the skull is rigid and non-expansile. This is the key concept behind the Monro-Kellie Doctrine which states that the sum of volumes of brain, CSF, and intracranial blood is constant; therefore, an increase in one will require a decrease in another or both remaining two. This principle is important when assessing or considering a patient's risk for cerebral herniation in the setting of cerebral edema or expanding hemorrhage.

Meninges

- The brain and spinal cord are covered and protected by three membranous layers (pia, arachnoid, and dura) termed "meninges."
- The dura mater is the outermost and most rigid layer. It divides the cranial cavity into compartments by folding on itself and creating dural reflections.

Brain

- The brain is composed of the cerebrum, cerebellum, and brainstem.
- The cerebrum contains gray matter in the form of the cerebral cortex and white matter at its center where initiation and coordination of movement, speech, judgment, problem solving, vision, hearing, and other sensory functions occur.
- The cerebellum primarily coordinates voluntary muscle movements and is responsible for posture, balance, and equilibrium.
- The brainstem serves to connect the cerebrum with the spinal cord. Its functions include regulation of heart rhythm and breathing, the brainstem is essential to survival.

Vascular

- The brain's blood supply is derived from two sets of large, paired vessels, the carotid, and vertebral arteries.
- The right and left vertebral arteries ultimately join to form the singular basilar artery.
- These vessels form a complex at the base of the brain called the "Circle of Willis." This structure then directs blood flow to different areas of the brain via the paired anterior cerebral arteries (ACA), middle cerebral arteries (MCA), and the posterior cerebral arteries (PCA) [4].

Imaging

Computed Tomography

- Non-contrast computed tomography (CT) is the current gold standard for TBI imaging. Acute hemorrhage will appear bright white in a non-contrast CT of the head.
- Indications for head CT include GCS ≤14, symptoms of nausea, vomiting, severe headache, or any neurologic deficit. More liberal triggers for head CT scanning should be used in patients taking anticoagulation or antiplatelet therapy.
- Repeat imaging is essential with any change in clinical status [5].

Magnetic Resonance Imaging

- Magnetic resonance imaging (MRI) has the highest sensitivity when assessing TBI; however, due to the lengthy timing of the exam, its use in the acute setting is limited [5].
- MRI is used primarily in the evaluation for diffuse axonal injury (DAI), characterization of non-hemorrhagic lesions, and assistance with neuro-prognostication.

Classification of TBI

Blunt Mechanisms

- *Concussion*

- Defined as a trauma-induced change in mental status with or without an associated loss of consciousness [6].
- Diagnosis is based on clinical assessment (headache, photophobia, memory
  difficulties, nausea). CT and MRI scans generally are normal [6].

- *Intracranial Bleed/Hemorrhage*

  - Epidural hematomas (EDH) occur when arterial blood accumulates between
    the dura mater and the skull (Fig. 30.1). These are rare and generally associ-
    ated with fracture of the skull and tear of the middle meningeal artery.
    Classically, patients are described as presenting with "lucid interval," which is
    followed by rapid decline in neurological status.
  - Subdural hematomas (SDH) occur when blood accumulates between the dura
    mater and the arachnoid mater. They are associated with tears of bridging
    veins (Fig. 30.2).
  - Subarachnoid hemorrhages (SAH) are seen after bleeding between the arach-
    noid and the pia mater. Resultant complications of SAH include seizures,
    vasospasm, and confusion (Fig. 30.3).
  - Intraparenchymal hemorrhages (IPH) or contusions are defined as bleeding
    into the brain parenchyma (Fig. 30.4). These can be complicated by evolution
    over the course of the first hours and days often referred to as "blossoming"
    and may be associated with progressive edema, mass effect, and ultimately
    ischemia [7].

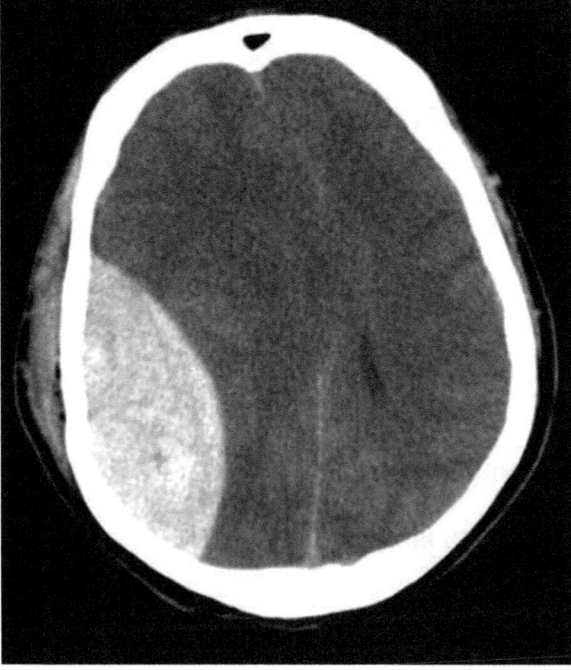

Fig. 30.1 Epidural hematoma in axial view demonstrating the characteristic lenticular shape

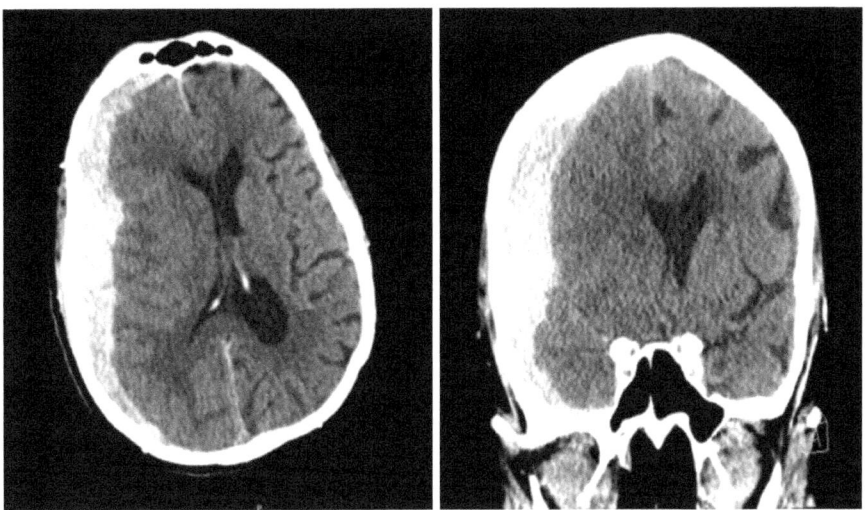

Fig. 30.2 Subdural hematoma in axial and coronal views demonstrating the crescent shape of SDH

- – Intraventricular hemorrhage (IVH) is bleeding into the brain's ventricular system which produces and manages cerebrospinal fluid. Following IVH, acute obstructive hydrocephalus, brain parenchymal damage related to breakdown of clot, and chronic hydrocephalus may occur.
- *Diffuse Axonal Injury (DAI)*

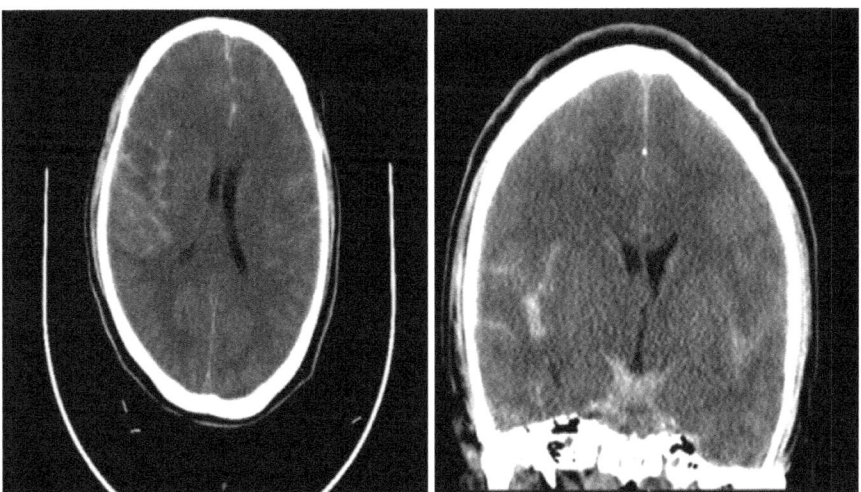

Fig. 30.3 Subarachnoid hemorrhage depicted in axial and coronal views with amorphous lesions apparent bilaterally

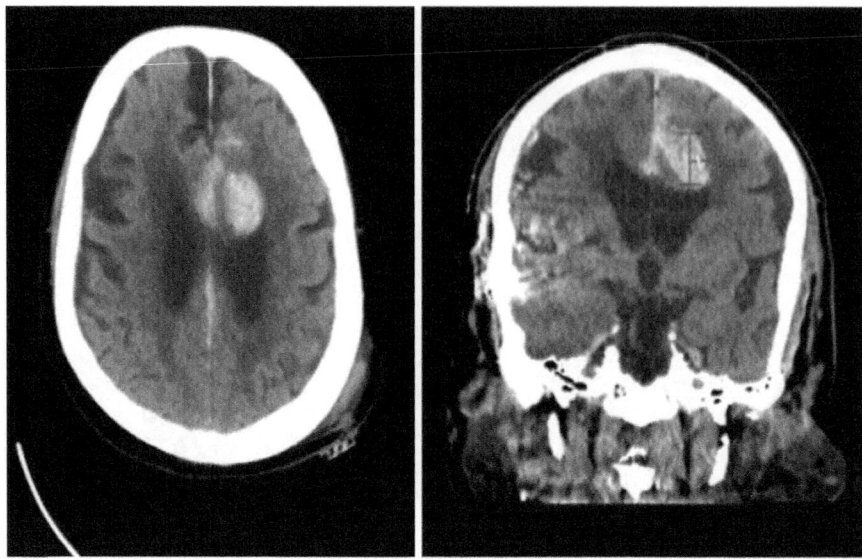

Fig. 30.4 Axial and coronal CT images of intraparenchymal hemorrhages with an associated sub-arachnoid hemorrhage

- Shear injury between white and gray matter sustained during acceleration/
  deceleration injuries can result in DAI and depressed mental status or coma in
  the setting of normal or near-normal head CT imaging. MRI is the imaging of
  choice. DAI carries a particularly poor prognosis.

Penetrating Mechanisms

Penetrating traumatic brain injuries (pTBI) are particularly lethal and result from
stab or gunshot wounds or any impalement of the head. Firearm injuries are the
leading cause of mortality in this group [8]. There are five categories of pTBI
wounds, including tangential, careening, penetrating, perforating, and ricochet [9].

Treatment

Non-surgical

- *Advanced Trauma Life Support® (ATLS®)*
  - Rapid and efficient assessment of ABCDEs.

– Loosening the cervical collar, reverse Trendelenburg bed positioning, avoidance or treatment of hypotension/hypoxia, and appropriate sedation management are strategies to decrease intracranial pressure.
– Early neurosurgical consultation is essential.

• *Observation and Medical Management*

– Mild TBI patients with normal neurologic exam and head imaging, few comorbidities, and/or concomitant traumatic injuries under the age of 65 may be discharged without significant observation as they have a low risk for deterioration [10, 11].
– Those patients at increased risk for interval development of intracranial hemorrhage (e.g., on therapeutic anticoagulation, history of renal disease) or those stable patients with abnormal head CT should be observed with repeat interval imaging at or before 24 h.
– Patients with moderate to severe TBI mandate admission to an intensive care unit (ICU) for close monitoring of vitals and management of intracranial pressure. ICP monitoring and interventions are typically aimed at achieving an optimal cerebral perfusion pressure (CPP).
– The American College of Surgeons (ACS) Trauma Quality Improvement Program (TQIP) has published three tiers of care for best practices in the management of TBI [12] with management goals summarized in Fig. 30.5.
– The most common noninvasive forms of decreasing ICP include elevation of the head, osmotherapy (hypertonic saline and mannitol), sedatives/analgesics/paralytics, avoiding hyperthermia, avoiding seizures and short-lived hyperventilation.

Fig. 30.5 Goals of treatment in the management of traumatic brain injury

	ICP 20–25 mmHg	Serum Sodium 135 –145
PaO2 100 mmHg		INR 1.4
PaCO2 35-45 mmHg	CPP 60 mmHg	Hemoglobin 7 g/dL
SBP 100 mmHg	Temperature 36 – 38 C	
	Glucose 80 –180 mg/dL	

PaO2: partial pressure of oxygen; PaCO2:partial pressure of carbon dioxide; SBP: systolic blood pressure; ICP: intracranial pressure; CPP: cerebral perfusion pressure; INR: international normalized ratio

Surgical

- *Intracranial pressure monitoring devices*
  - Are placed by neurosurgeons and can be intraventricular (allows CSF drainage, lower cost) or intraparenchymal (can measure temperature, and brain parenchymal oxygen, higher cost).
  - The most important reason for placing an ICP monitor is to measure ICP in a comatose patient (GCS <8) particularly when a mass lesion (hematoma) or cerebral edema is seen on head CT.

- *Craniotomy/Craniectomy*
  - Surgical evacuation (evacuative craniectomy) of large hematoma. Preferably performed prior to neurological deterioration, regardless of GCS.
  - Early (within 72 h of admission) decompressive craniectomy for severe diffuse TBI and refractory intracranial hypertension does not improve outcomes [13].
  - Decompressive craniectomy to treat refractory intracranial hypertension (late) may offer a mortality benefit [14].

Prognosis/Long-Term Outcomes

- Isolated TBI, or as part of other traumatic injuries, can lead to complications such as seizures, neuro-storming, wound infections, cerebrovascular accidents (stroke), and coma.
- Prognosis after TBI is extremely variable and dependent on the type and severity of injury as well as any complications incurred during the recovery process. There can be a wide range of cognitive outcomes from temporary amnesia to coma and permanent vegetative state. Neuro-prognostication can be an important part of patient care, particularly when families take on the role of decision-maker for their loved-one. A multi-disciplinary approach to these discussions, including the critical care team, neurosurgery, palliative care, and neurology or neurocritical care teams, can ensure that patients and families have the information they need to participate fully in goals of care conversations.

References

1. Baker CC, Oppenheimer L, Stephens B, Lewis FR, Trunkey DD. Epidemiology of trauma deaths. Am J Surg. 1980;140(1):144–50.
2. Asfaw S, Martin N. Traumatic brain injury. In: Martin N, Kaplan L, editors. Principles of adult surgical critical care. Switzerland: Springer International Publishing; 2016. p. 35–44.

3. Traumatic Brain Injury. National Institute of Neurological Disorders and Stroke; 2022 [cited 30 Aug 2022].
4. Kim DY, Biffl W, Bokhari F, Brakenridge S, Chao E, Claridge JA, et al. Evaluation and management of blunt cerebrovascular injury: a practice management guideline from the Eastern Association for the Surgery of Trauma. J Trauma Acute Care Surg. 2020;88(6):875–87.
5. Bodanapally UK, Sours C, Zhuo J, Shanmuganathan K. Imaging of traumatic brain injury. Radiol Clin North Am. 2015;53(4):695–715. viii.
6. Mullally WJ. Concussion. Am J Med. 2017;130(8):885–92.
7. Kurland D, Hong C, Aarabi B, Gerzanich V, Simard JM. Hemorrhagic progression of a contusion after traumatic brain injury: a review. J Neurotrauma. 2012;29(1):19–31.
8. Sosin DM, Sniezek JE, Waxweiler RJ. Trends in death associated with traumatic brain injury, 1979 through 1992: success and failure. JAMA. 1995;273(22):1778–80.
9. Van Wyck DW, Grant GA, Laskowitz DT. Penetrating traumatic brain injury: a review of current evaluation and management concepts. J Neurol Neurophysiol. 2015;6(6):336–43.
10. Leitner L, El-Shabrawi JH, Bratschitsch G, Eibinger N, Klim S, Leithner A, et al. Risk adapted diagnostics and hospitalization following mild traumatic brain injury. Arch Orthop Trauma Surg. 2021;141(4):619–27.
11. Barbosa RR, Jawa R, Watters JM, Knight JC, Kerwin AJ, Winston ES, et al. Evaluation and management of mild traumatic brain injury: an Eastern Association for the Surgery of Trauma practice management guideline. J Trauma Acute Care Surg. 2012;73(5 Suppl 4):S307–14.
12. Cryer H, Manley G, Adelson PD, Alali A, Calland J, Cipolle M, et al. American college of surgeons trauma quality improvement program guidelines, traumatic brain injury. Committee on Trauma Expert Panel 1/2015, American College of Surgeons; 2015.
13. Cooper DJ, Rosenfeld JV, Murray L, Arabi YM, Davies AR, D'Urso P, et al. Decompressive craniectomy in diffuse traumatic brain injury. N Engl J Med. 2011;364(16):1493–502.
14. Hutchinson PJ, Kolias AG, Timofeev IS, Corteen EA, Czosnyka M, Timothy J, et al. Trial of decompressive craniectomy for traumatic intracranial hypertension. N Engl J Med. 2016;375(12):1119–30.

Chapter 31
Ocular Trauma

Kelly Mayo and Andrew Mittelman

Overview

- Ocular trauma is a common and serious cause of ocular injuries worldwide.
- Ocular injuries are associated with blunt and penetrating trauma such as from motor vehicle collisions (MVCs), assault, sports-related trauma, and labor-related trauma.
- Blunt or penetrating ocular trauma can lead to both intraocular and extraocular injury.
- It is important to complete a comprehensive ocular exam to evaluate for associated and potentially more severe ocular injuries.
- Emergent or urgent ophthalmologic consultation is often required.

Epidemiology: It is thought that there are around 55 million ocular traumas worldwide annually, with about 19 million resulting in blindness or major vision loss. About two million of these injuries occur in the United States. These injuries happen more frequently in males than females, and most commonly affect patients in their third and fourth decade of life. Examples of possible trauma include gunshot wounds (GSWs), explosive devices, blunt trauma, and unintentional injuries from metalworking. These injuries are associated with lower socioeconomic status, poor education, and those people participating in labor-intensive occupations.

Pathophysiology: Different types of ocular injury exhibit different pathophysiology. Because of this, providers must thoroughly assess the mechanism of injury and

K. Mayo (✉) · A. Mittelman
Department of Emergency Medicine, Boston University Chobanian & Avedisian School of Medicine, Boston Medical Center, Boston, MA, USA
e-mail: Kelly.Mayo@bmc.org; Andrew.Mittelman@bmc.org

T. S. Brahmbhatt, D. R. Scantling (eds.), *Trauma Surgery Clerkship*, Contemporary Surgical Clerkships, https://doi.org/10.1007/978-3-032-01412-2_31

perform a comprehensive ocular exam that reflects a working knowledge of the ocular anatomy.

Anatomy: The sclera and cornea form the outer wall of the eye. The anterior structures (iris, cornea, anterior chamber) are separated from the posterior structures (retina, choroid, vitreous fluid, optic nerve) by the lens. Tears are drained from the medial eye into the nasopharynx through the canalicular system. There are seven bones within the bony orbit and together form the orbital floor, roof, medial and lateral walls. The orbital compartment also contains the extraocular muscles, retro-orbital fat, the ophthalmic artery, orbital veins, and optic nerve. Figure 31.1 [1].

Ocular Exam: VVEEPP (Visual acuity, Visual fields, External exam, Extraocular movements, Pupil exam, Pressure; OD = Oculus Dexter = Right Eye/OS = Oculus Sinister = Left Eye)

- Visual acuity (VA)

  - Patients who use corrective lenses should wear them if available; if not, use a pinhole to correct
- Visual fields
- External exam

  - Check for bony tenderness of the orbital rim and zygoma, crepitus, proptosis
  - Check for external abnormalities to the sclera, cornea, pupil, lid, lacrimal duct
  - As indicated, use fluorescein to evaluate for abrasion

- Extraocular movements (EOM)

Fig. 31.1 Horizontal cross section of eyeball [1]

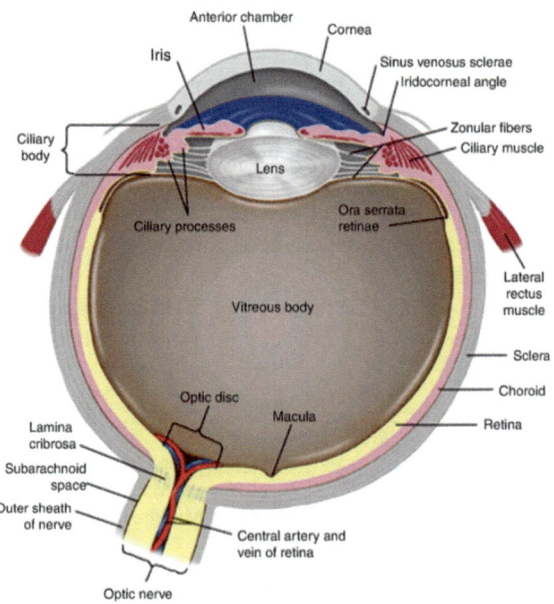

- Pupillary Evaluation

  - PERRL, check for afferent pupillary defect
- Intraocular Pressure (IOP)
- Slit lamp exam and/or dilated eye exam by ophthalmology

Types of Injuries

Corneal Abrasion/Laceration

- Pathophysiology:

  - Corneal epithelium is traumatically removed
  - Most commonly from fingernails, airbags, sports- or work-related injuries
  - Presents with eye pain, increased tearing, blurred vision, photophobia, foreign body sensation
- Exam:

  - VVEEPP
  - Topical anesthetic prior to fluorescein exam. Figure 31.2 [2].
- Diagnostics:

  - No imaging universally necessary unless additional ocular injury is suspected
- Treatment:

  - Topical anesthetics for exam only (not recommended for longitudinal use due to possibility of impaired healing)
  - Artificial tears QID
  - Erythromycin ointment

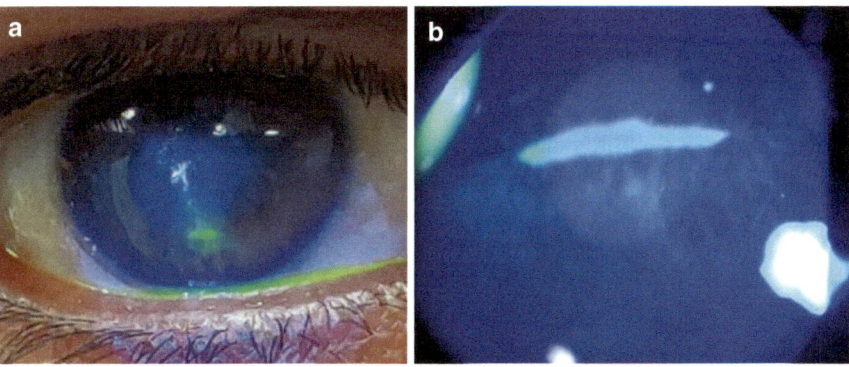

Fig. 31.2 Slit lamp photos showing (**a**) peripheral and (**b**) central linear corneal abrasions following trauma [2]

- Antibiotics with pseudomonas coverage in contact-lens wearers
- Outpatient Ophthalmologic referral within 48–72 h [3, 4]

Ruptured Globe/Penetrating Ocular Trauma

- Pathophysiology:

  - Full thickness disruption of the sclera or cornea
  - Suspect globe rupture based on mechanism (blunt trauma, projectile injury, eyelid or periorbital laceration)

- Exam:

  - VVEEP
  - Do not check ocular pressure if globe rupture is suspected
  - May see "teardrop pupil", decreased visual acuity, visible foreign body or vitreous extruding from eye, afferent pupillary defect, external prolapse of iris or ciliary body. Figure 31.3 [5]

- Seidel Test

  - Used to reveal leaks from the cornea, sclera, or conjunctiva following injury
  - Contraindicated if there is strong concern for globe rupture. Figure 31.4

- Diagnostics:

  - CT may be useful to identify an ocular foreign body and/or associated injuries (i.e., orbital fractures), but is not sensitive or specific enough to evaluate for globe rupture

- Treatment:

  - Emergent Ophthalmology consultation
  - Prevent IOP elevation (elevate head of bed to 30 degrees, avoid eye manipulation, give prophylactic antiemetics, cover eye with an eyeshield)
  - Broad spectrum antibiotics, Tdap, control pain
  - NPO for emergent surgical repair [7, 8]

Retrobulbar Hemorrhage

- Pathophysiology:

  - Rapidly progressive, vision-threatening emergency due to accumulation of blood behind the globe
  - Can lead to rapid increase in IOP and orbital compartment syndrome

- Exam:

Fig. 31.3 (Top) Teardrop pupil signifying full thickness globe injury. (Bottom) The Seidel Test: Fluorescein pattern enlarging from the corneal defect indicating a full thickness globe laceration [5]

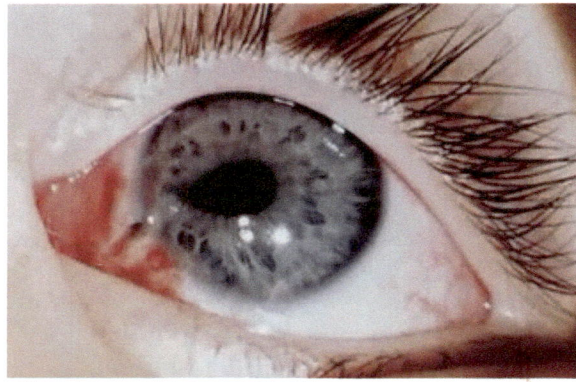

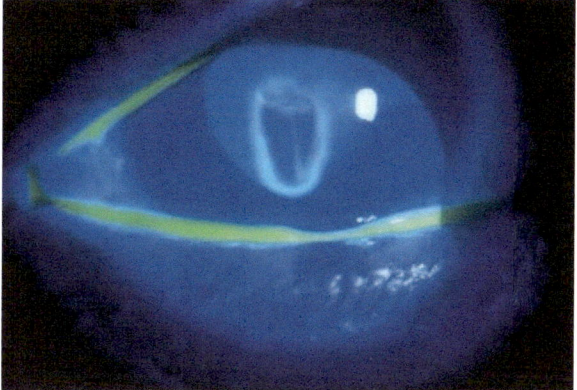

- – VVEEPP
- – May see proptosis, decreased visual acuity, afferent pupillary defect, decreased EOM, pain with EOM, increased IOP. Figure 31.4 [6].
- • Diagnostics:
  - – CT can identify a retrobulbar hematoma; however, do not delay management of orbital compartment syndrome if highly suspected based on exam
- • Treatment:
  - – Emergent Ophthalmology consult
  - – Lateral canthotomy if IOP >40 mmHg Fig. 31.5 [9]
  - – Nonsurgical interventions including IV acetazolamide, IV mannitol, and/or IM/IV steroids [10]

Fig. 31.4 Retrobulbar
hematoma with
proptosis [6]

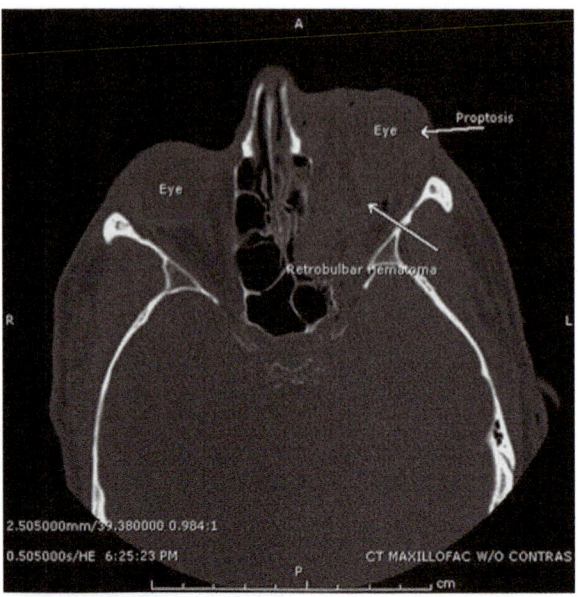

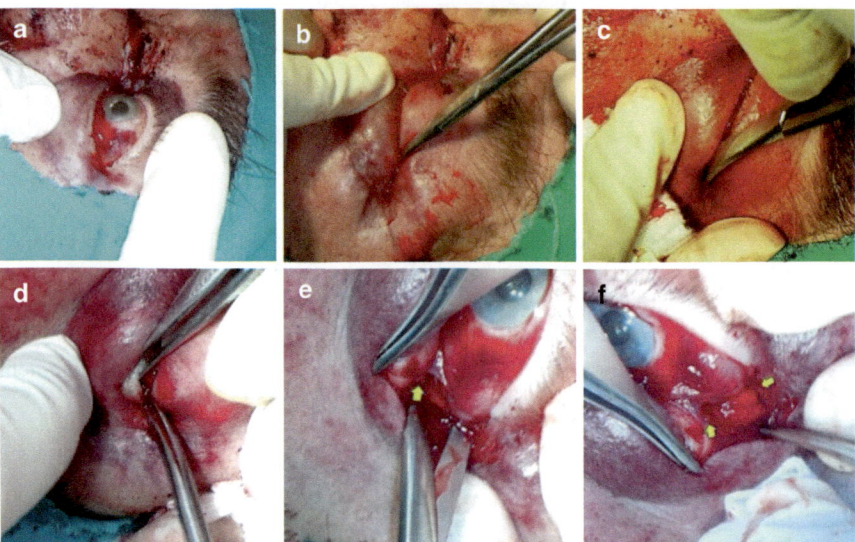

Fig. 31.5 (**a**) Patient with orbital compartment syndrome. (**b**) Hemostat to lateral canthus ~1 min.
(**c**) Incision of lateral canthus ~1 cm. (**d**) Exposure and incision of inferior crus. (**e**) Yellow arrow
showing cut edge of inferior crus. (**f**) Fat prolapse after successful septolysis. Recheck IOP, if still
>40mgHg cut superior crus [9]

Lacrimal Duct Laceration

- Pathophysiology:
    - Traumatic injury to the canalicular system of the eye leading to disruption of the duct. Figure 31.6 [11]
    - Often associated with penetrating trauma, MVCs, dog bites, and assaults
- Exam:
    - VVEEPP
    - Ophthalmology may need to perform more invasive exam
- Diagnostics:
    - Often need CT to evaluate for additional intra- or extraocular injury
- Treatment:
    - Ophthalmology consultation for urgent surgical repair
    - Tdap, consider rabies prophylaxis for animal bites, amoxicillin/clavulanate 3–5 days

Traumatic Iritis

- Pathophysiology:
    - Anterior chamber inflammation typically caused by blunt trauma
    - Presents with photophobia, blurry vision
- Exam:

Fig. 31.6 Upper and lower lacrimal canalicular lacerations after being bitten by a dog [11]

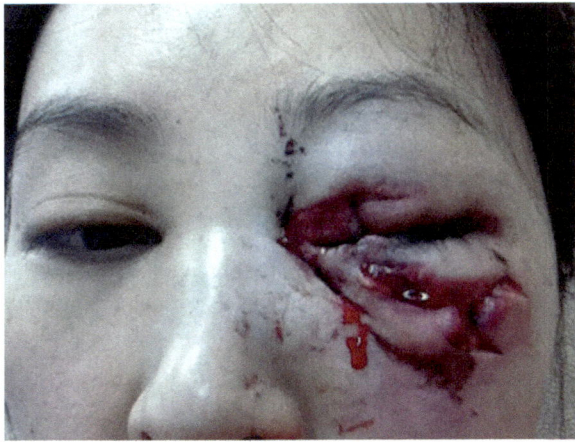

- – VVEEPP
- – May see sustained miosis, poorly reactive pupil, pain with pupillary constriction
- – Slit lamp will show cell and flare in anterior chamber
- Diagnostics:
  - – No imaging unless suspecting more concerning intra- or extraocular injury
- Treatment:
  - – Topical corticosteroids and cycloplegics
  - – Urgent Ophthalmology consult versus follow-up

Hyphema

- Pathophysiology:
  - – Blood in the anterior chamber typically from blunt trauma leading to tear of iris tissue and/or ciliary body
  - – Presents with decreased visual acuity, ocular pain, and photophobia
- Exam:
  - – VVEEPP
  - – Layered blood in anterior chamber, ~1/3 patients have elevated IOP. Figure 31.7 [12]
- Diagnostics:
  - – May need imaging if additional intra- or extraocular injury is suspected
- Treatment:
  - – Urgent Ophthalmology consult
  - – If elevated IOP, may need topical steroids, cycloplegics
  - – Anterior chamber washout or surgical evaluation if elevated IOP persists

Lens Dislocation

- Pathophysiology:
  - – Due to blunt compression force to the eye
  - – Presents with vision changes, eye pain, and monocular diplopia
- Exam:
  - – VVEEPP. Figure 31.8 [13].
  - – Dilated exam with Ophthalmology

Fig. 31.7 Slit lamp
showing blood fully filling
the anterior chamber [12]

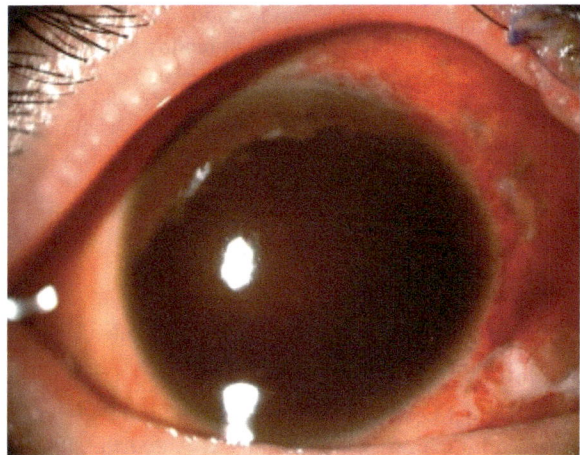

Fig. 31.8 Incomplete
dislocation of the lens [13]

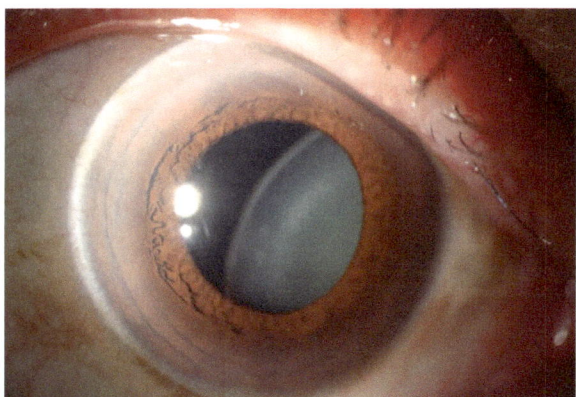

- Diagnostics:
  - CT scan to evaluate for associated intra- and extraocular injuries; ultrasound
    has high sensitivity
- Treatment:
  - Urgent Ophthalmology consult
  - IOP lowering meds as needed
  - Surgery versus conservative management [14]

Vitreous Hemorrhage

- Pathophysiology:

- Most cases due to ocular trauma such as blunt force, globe rupture, shaken baby syndrome that result in hemorrhage into the vitreous body
- Presents as painless vision disturbance with floaters or visual field deficits
- Exam:
  - VVEEPP
  - May have decreased VA or visual field defects
  - Slit lamp may show RBCs in vitreous fluid. Figure 31.9 [15].
- Diagnostics:
  - CT if suspect additional intra- or extraocular injury
- Treatment:
  - Urgent Ophthalmology consult within 24–48 h
  - Minimize strenuous activity, elevate head of bed, eye patch
  - Surgery with Ophthalmology versus observation

Retinal Detachment

- Pathophysiology:
  - May be secondary to closed or open globe injury
  - Presents as painless vision disturbance with floaters or visual field deficits
- Exam:
  - VVEEPP

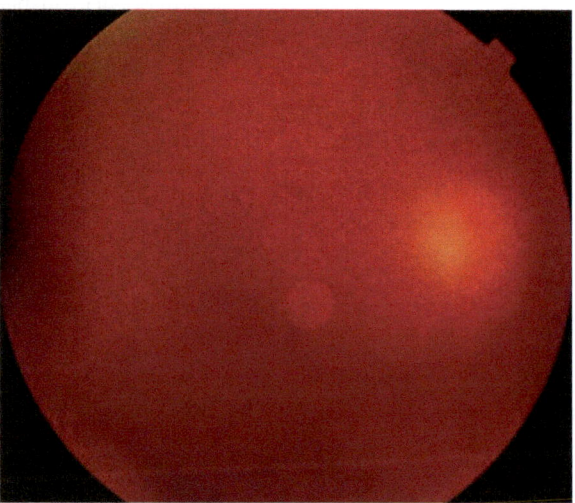

Fig. 31.9 Diffuse vitreous hemorrhage on ophthalmoscopic exam [15]

– Slit lamp and dilated eye exam with Ophthalmology, detachment will appear hazy and out of focus

- Diagnostics:

  – May need CT if additional intra- or extraocular injury is suspected; ultrasound has high sensitivity. Figure 31.10 [16]

- Treatment:

  – Urgent Ophthalmology consult
  – Minimize strenuous activity, elevate head of bed, eye patch
  – Surgery with Ophthalmology versus observation [17]

Take-Home Points for Patient Care

- Ocular injuries from trauma are extremely common and can go unnoticed
- Identified ocular injuries are often associated with additional intraocular and extraocular injuries
- Perform a complete eye exam on all ocular trauma patients
- Do not check IOP, perform bedside ocular ultrasound, or look for Seidel sign if there is high suspicion for globe rupture
- Ocular trauma often requires emergent or urgent Ophthalmologic evaluation and/or referral
- Timely evaluation and management of certain ocular traumatic ocular injuries will give the patient the best chance at regaining vision and salvaging the eye

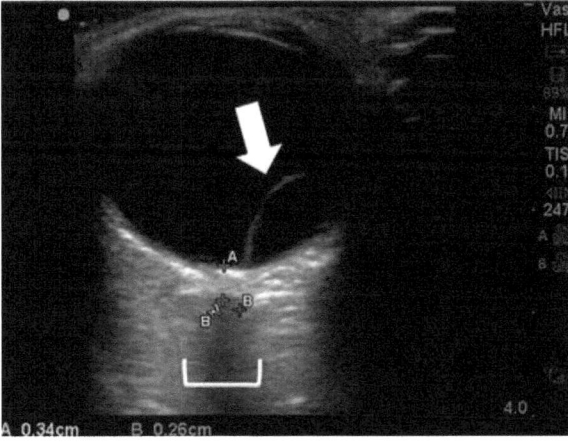

Fig. 31.10 Ultrasound image of retinal detachment, which appears as a hyperechoic linear structure (*white arrow*) attached posteriorly to the optic nerve [16]

References

1. Ng PC, Oliver JJ. Anatomy of the eye. In: Long B, Koyfman A, editors. Handbook of emergency ophthalmology. Cham: Springer; 2018. https://doi-org.ezproxy.bu.edu/10.1007/978-3-319-78945-3_1.
2. Raj N, Tandon R, Vanathi M, Lomi N, Gupta N. Minor corneal emergencies. In: Sharma B, Titiyal JS, editors. Corneal emergencies. Singapore: Springer; 2022. https://doi-org.ezproxy.bu.edu/10.1007/978-981-16-5876-1_5.
3. Kaufman SC, Rolain MA, Murchison A, Syed ZA, Stelzner SK. Anterior segment trauma: evaluation, considerations and initial management. In: EyeWiki. American Academy of Ophthalmology; 2022. https://eyewiki.org/Anterior_Segment_Trauma:_Evaluation,_Considerations_and_Initial_Management#Corneal_Abrasion.
4. Shi W, Wang T. Corneal injury. In: Yan H, editor. Atlas of ocular trauma. Ocular trauma. Singapore: Springer; 2019. https://doi-org.ezproxy.bu.edu/10.1007/978-981-13-1450-6_3.
5. Clark JD, Harold Lee HB. Ophthalmologic injuries as a complication of maxillofacial surgery. In: Ferneini E, Bennett J, editors. Perioperative assessment of the maxillofacial surgery patient. Cham: Springer; 2018. https://doi-org.ezproxy.bu.edu/10.1007/978-3-319-58868-1_49.
6. Kloss BT, Patel R. Orbital compartment syndrome from retrobulbar hemorrhage. Int J Emerg Med. 2010;3:521–2. https://doi-org.ezproxy.bu.edu/10.1007/s12245-010-0245-1.
7. Lam BC, Foster AA, Murchison A, Syed ZA, Gurnani B. Ruptured Globe. In: EyeWiki. American Academy of Ophthalmology; 2021. https://eyewiki.aao.org/Ruptured_Globe.
8. Patil B, Vanathi M, Raj N. Corneal laceration and penetrating injuries. In: Sharma B, Titiyal JS, editors. Corneal emergencies. Singapore: Springer; 2022. https://doi-org.ezproxy.bu.edu/10.1007/978-981-16-5876-1_6.
9. Papadiochos I, Petsinis V, Sarivalasis SE, Strantzias P, Bourazani M, Goutzanis L, Tampouris A. Acute orbital compartment syndrome due to traumatic hemorrhage: 4-year case series and relevant literature review with emphasis on its management. Oral Maxillofac Surg. 2022. https://doi-org.ezproxy.bu.edu/10.1007/s10006-021-01036-9.
10. Hasan A, Hwang FS, Feldman BH, Patel AS, Akkara JD, Murchison A, Stewart K, Yen MT, Burkat CN. Retrobulbar hemorrhage. In: EyeWiki. American Academy of Ophthalmology; 2022. https://eyewiki.org/Retrobulbar_Hemorrhage#cite_note-:5-9.
11. Tao H, Zhou X, Li Y. Lacrimal apparatus injury. In: Yan H, editor. Atlas of ocular trauma. Ocular trauma. Singapore: Springer; 2019. https://doi-org.ezproxy.bu.edu/10.1007/978-981-13-1450-6_9.
12. Wu N, Tao Z, Ji H. Iris and ciliary body injury. In: Yan H, editor. Atlas of ocular trauma. Ocular trauma. Singapore: Springer; 2019. https://doi-org.ezproxy.bu.edu/10.1007/978-981-13-1450-6_4.
13. Yan H, Guo C, Song H. Traumatic dislocation of the lens. In: Yan H, editor. Management on complicated ocular trauma. Ocular trauma. Singapore: Springer; 2022. https://doi-org.ezproxy.bu.edu/10.1007/978-981-16-5340-7_4.
14. Li H. Lens injury. In: Yan H, editor. Atlas of ocular trauma. Ocular trauma. Singapore: Springer; 2019. https://doi-org.ezproxy.bu.edu/10.1007/978-981-13-1450-6_5.
15. Williamson TH. Vitreous haemorrhage. In: Vitreoretinal surgery. Berlin, Heidelberg: Springer; 2013. https://doi-org.ezproxy.bu.edu/10.1007/978-3-642-31872-6_5.
16. Patel SS, Nickels LC, Patel RP. Ultrasound evaluation of retinal detachment. In: Ganti L, editor. Atlas of emergency medicine procedures. New York: Springer; 2016. https://doi-org.ezproxy.bu.edu/10.1007/978-1-4939-2507-0_49.
17. Patel SJ, Feldman BH, Phelps PO, Miller AM, Barash A, Murchison A, Justin GA, Bhagat N, Lim JL, Lai KE, Karth PA, Gullapalli V. Retinal detachment. In: EyeWiki. American Academy of Ophthalmology; 2022. https://eyewiki.org/Retinal_Detachment.

Chapter 32
Spinal Cord and Spine Injury

Shayan Rakhit, Amelia W. Maiga, and Mayur B. Patel

Introduction

Spinal injury is common in those with multiple and/or major traumatic injuries. The most concerning aspect of spinal injury is injury to the spinal cord and subsequent neurologic effects. Because of these resultant neurologic effects, spine injuries remain a major source of death and disability in the injured patient. The approach to

S. Rakhit · A. W. Maiga
Critical Illness, Brain Dysfunction, & Survivorship Center, Vanderbilt Center for Health Services Research, Vanderbilt Institute for Medicine and Public Health, Vanderbilt University Medical Center, Nashville, TN, USA

Division of Acute Care Surgery, Department of Surgery, Section of Surgical Sciences, Vanderbilt University Medical Center, Nashville, TN, USA
e-mail: shayan.rakhit.1@vumc.org; amelia.w.maiga@vumc.org

M. B. Patel (✉)
Critical Illness, Brain Dysfunction, & Survivorship Center, Vanderbilt Center for Health Services Research, Vanderbilt Institute for Medicine and Public Health, Vanderbilt University Medical Center, Nashville, TN, USA

Division of Acute Care Surgery, Department of Surgery, Section of Surgical Sciences, Vanderbilt University Medical Center, Nashville, TN, USA

Department of Neurosurgery and Hearing and Speech Sciences, Vanderbilt Brain Institute, Vanderbilt University Medical Center, Nashville, TN, USA

Surgical Service, Nashville VA Medical Center, Tennessee Valley Healthcare System, US Department of Veterans Affairs, Nashville, TN, USA

Geriatric Research, Education, and Clinical Center Service, Nashville VA Medical Center, Tennessee Valley Healthcare System, US Department of Veterans Affairs, Nashville, TN, USA
e-mail: mayur.b.patel@vumc.org

T. S. Brahmbhatt, D. R. Scantling (eds.), *Trauma Surgery Clerkship*, Contemporary Surgical Clerkships, https://doi.org/10.1007/978-3-032-01412-2_32

spinal injury described below is consistent with the principles of Advanced Trauma Life Support (ATLS), to which we adhere to at our center [1].

Epidemiology [2, 3]

- Spinal injuries (injuries to the bony, ligamentous, or neurologic components of the spinal column)

    - 10.5 injuries per 100,000 people worldwide
    - 226,000 people suffer specifically from spinal cord injury worldwide
    - Motor vehicle collisions most common cause, followed by falls
    - Decrease in incidence and mortality in the USA in the past few decades
    - Increasing proportion of spinal injuries are in older patients

- Burden of disease varies worldwide

    - ~5% of trauma patients have spinal injuries in the USA
    - High-income countries: 20%–25% of all spinal injuries have spinal cord injury
    - Middle-income countries: 30%–40% of all spinal injuries with spinal cord injury
    - Low-income countries: 70% of all spinal injuries with spinal cord injury

Anatomy

- Bones

    - 7 cervical, 12 thoracic, 5 lumbar vertebrae, plus sacrum and coccyx (Fig. 32.1)
    - Parts of vertebrae: body, pedicle, superior/inferior articular facets, lamina, transverse/spinal processes (Fig. 32.2)
    - In center: vertebral foramina form spinal canal
    - Canal widest from skull foramen magnum to C2
    - Below C2, bony injuries much more likely to cause cord injury
    - Low cervical spine and thoracolumbar junction: fulcrums connecting immobile thoracic spine and more mobile cervical and lumbar spines, thus injury prone

- Ligaments, cartilage, and discs

    - Anterior longitudinal ligament, posterior longitudinal ligament, ligamenta flava, interspinous ligaments, supraspinal ligament
    - Endplates (bone and cartilage): between discs and vertebrae
    - Intervertebral discs: outer (annulus fibrosus), inner (nucleus pulposus)

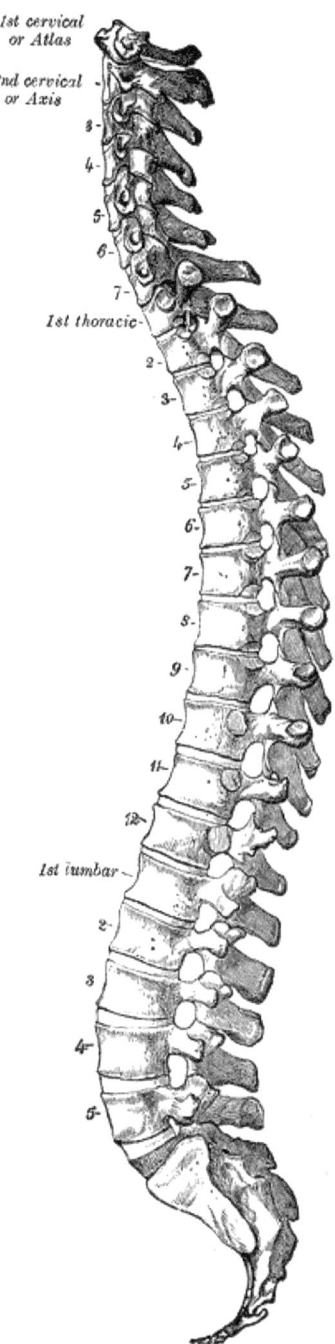

Fig. 32.1 Sagittal view of spinal column with cervical (C), thoracic (Th), lumbar (L), sacrum, and coccyx regions labeled. (Source: "Vertebral Column" by Henry Vandyke Carter, *Anatomy of the Human Body*, 20th Edition, in the Public Domain (CC0 1.0))

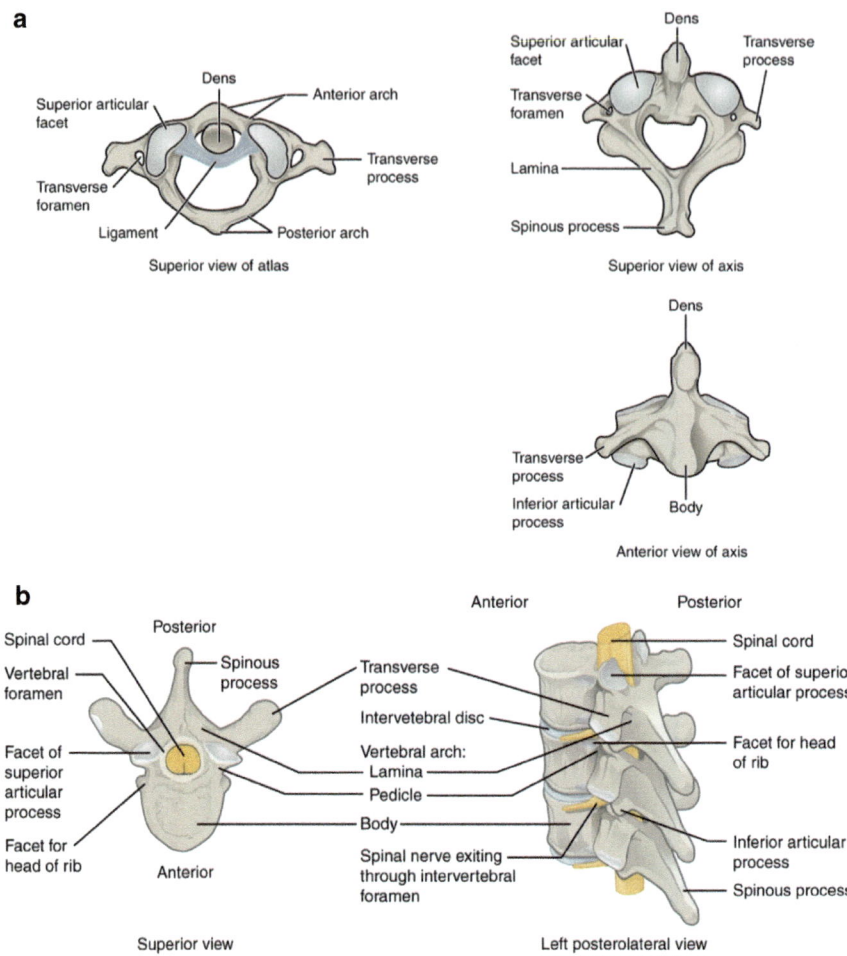

Fig. 32.2 (a) Transverse bony anatomy of the atlantoaxial joint, comprising vertebrae C1 (atlas) and C2 (axis); (b) Transverse bony anatomy of a generic vertebra with spinal cord (Source: OpenStax Anatomy and Physiology; Rice University; Houston, TX; under CC BY 4.0. Access for free at https://openstax.org/books/anatomy-and-physiology/pages/1-introduction)

- Spinal cord
  - Runs from medulla oblongata at the foramen magnum of skull to L1 vertebral level, the conus medullaris; below L1 is cauda equina
  - Three tracts amenable to clinical examination
    - Corticospinal tract: anterolateral part of cord, ipsilateral motor function
    - Spinothalamic tract: anterolateral part of cord, contralateral pain and temperature sensation

- • Dorsal tract: posteromedial part of cord, ipsilateral vibration and proprioception
- Segmental nerve roots (correspond with spinal level)

  - – Dorsal root exits posteriorly, contains sensory nerves
  - – Ventral root exits anteriorly, contains motor nerves
  - – Roots combine into spinal nerve, sensory and motor nerves combine
  - – Dorsal and ventral rami containing sensory/motor nerves spilt off spinal nerve to innervate posterior/anterior, respectively

- Sympathetic trunk

  - – Runs parallel to spinal cord
  - – Connects to spinal nerve via rami communicantes
  - – Houses most of sympathetic nervous system

Physiology

- Dermatomes: area of skin innervated by specific segmental nerve root (Fig. 32.3)

  - – For clinical examination, common nerve roots with corresponding skin areas

    - • C1–C2: variable distribution, not used for localization
    - • C2–C4: overlies pectoralis (cervical cape)
    - • C5: shoulder/deltoid
    - • C6: thumb
    - • C7: middle finger
    - • C8: little finger
    - • T4: nipple
    - • T8: xiphoid
    - • T10: umbilicus
    - • T12: pubic symphysis
    - • L4: medial calf
    - • L5: first/second toe web space
    - • S1: lateral foot
    - • S3: ischial tuberosity
    - • S4/S5: perianal

- Myotomes: muscles supplied by specific segmental nerve root

  - – Most muscles are supplied by more than one nerve root
  - – To simplify the clinical examination, common nerve roots with corresponding single muscles

    - • C5: elbow flexors (biceps, brachialis, brachioradialis)
    - • C6: wrist extensors (extensor carpi ulnaris/radialis brevis/longus)

Fig. 32.3 Dermatome map, anterior and posterior. (Source: "Dermatomes and major cutaneous nerves in a ventral view" by Mikael Häggström, MD, in the Public Domain (CC0 1.0))

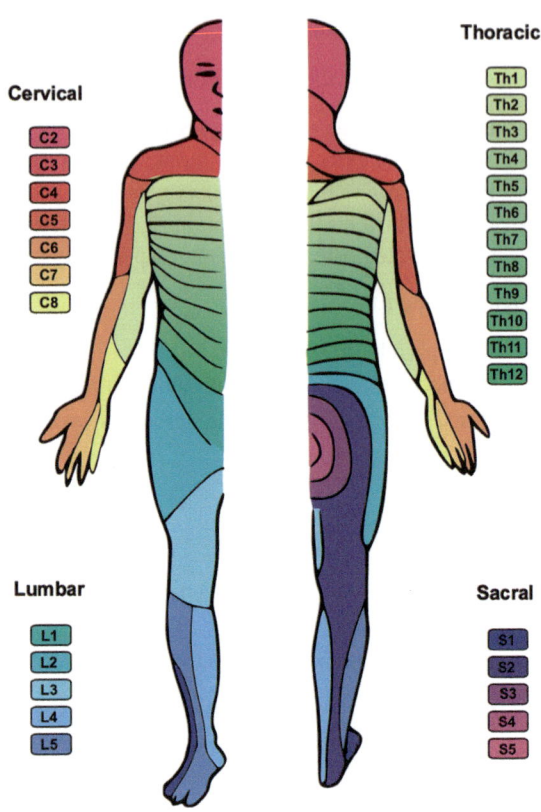

- C7: elbow extensors (triceps)
- C8: finger flexors (flexor carpi ulnaris/radialis, flexor digitorum profundus/superficialis, flexor pollicis longus, palmaris longus)
- T1: finger abductors (dorsal interossei)
- L2: hip flexors (iliopsoas, pectineus, sartorius)
- L3: knee extensors (quadriceps group)
- L4: ankle dorsiflexors (tibialis anterior)
- L5: toe extensors (extensor hallucis longus/digitorum longus)
- S1: ankle plantar flexors (gastrocnemius, soleus, plantaris)

- Pulmonary effects

    - Any spinal cord injury at risk for respiratory failure, especially cervical injuries
    - Central innervation at C2 or higher
    - Phrenic nerve innervated C3–5
    - Intercostals innervated lower cervical/upper thoracic
    - Respiratory failure can occur from any of these

- Cardiac effects

  - Neurogenic shock can result from spinal cord injury
  - Neurogenic shock: distributive shock subtype with the other subtype being septic (there are four main shock types: hypovolemic, cardiogenic, obstructive, and distributive)
  - Injury to sympathetic trunk above T6 and loss of vasomotor tone, resulting in:

    - Vasodilation and hypotension
    - Bradycardia (absolute or relative inability to mount tachycardiac response to hypovolemia)

  - *Neurogenic shock* is different from *spinal shock*

    - Neurogenic shock: type of shock as described above
    - Spinal shock: initial flaccidity and loss of reflexes after spinal cord injury, which develop into spasticity long term

- Effects on other organ systems

  - Inability to feel pain can mask injuries (e.g., abdominal or pelvic)
  - Bladder dysfunction
  - Bowel dysfunction: constipation or incontinence depending on level of injury

Common Injury Patterns [1]

- Mechanisms of injury to spine: axial loading, flexion, extension, rotation, lateral bending, distraction
- Noncontiguous spinal injury common: if injury found in one region (e.g., cervical), remainder of spine (thoracolumbar) should be evaluated
- Classification

  - Level

    - Bony: spinal level corresponding to vertebral (bone) level of injury
    - Sensory: spinal level corresponding to lowest dermatome with normal sensory function
    - Motor: spinal level corresponding to lowest muscle with at least three of six muscle strength

  - Complete versus incomplete

    - Incomplete: any motor or sensory function below injury other than local reflexes (e.g., sacral reflexes like bulbocavernosus or anal wink)
    - Complete: no motor or sensory function below injury
    - Incomplete with markedly better prognosis than complete

- Paraplegia versus quadriplegia

  - Paraplegia: motor level spares upper extremities, thoracic injury
  - Quadriplegia: motor level includes upper extremities, cervical injury

- American Spinal Injury Association (ASIA) Impairment Scale [4]

  - Standardized, detailed classification of spinal cord injury for research
  - May guide further assessment and treatment
  - Helps with prognostication, especially in predicting recovery of function

- Spinal cord syndromes

  - Posterior cord syndrome: not commonly caused by trauma
  - Anterior cord syndrome: paraplegia and bilateral loss of pain/temperature; from anterior ischemia; poorest prognosis
  - Central cord syndrome: motor strength loss in upper extremities > lower extremities, variable sensory loss; risk factor is preexisting cervical canal stenosis; better prognosis
  - Brown-Séquard syndrome: ipsilateral motor and position sense loss with contralateral loss of pain/temperature; cord hemisection from penetrating trauma; better prognosis
  - Conus medullaris syndrome: saddle anesthesia with bladder and rectal dysfunction; injury at L2
  - Cauda equina syndrome: often asymmetric weakness and anesthesia of lower extremities with bladder and rectal dysfunction; injury to cauda equina nerve roots

- Common injuries and terminology [5]

  - Atlanto-occipital dislocation: severe flexion/distraction; brainstem injury resulting in death or severe neurologic impairment such as ventilator dependence; unstable
  - Atlas (C1) fracture: axial loading (e.g., diving injury); often associated with C2 fractures; special type: burst (Jefferson) fracture with disruption of anterior and posterior rings with lateral displacement of lateral masses; usually cord sparing but unstable
  - Axis (C2) fracture: largest vertebrae and unusually shaped

    - Odontoid (dens) fracture: type I include just tip, uncommon; type II through base of dens, most common; type III through base of dens into body of axis
    - Posterior element (hangman's) fracture: severe extension; bilateral fractures of pars interarticularis (part of lamina); unstable

  - Facet subluxation and dislocation: extreme flexion/extension, more common in cervical spine; associated with ligamentous disruption; often causes spinal cord injury; often unstable

- Teardrop fracture: fracture of anterior corner of vertebral body, from flexion (anterosuperior corner) or extension (anteroinferior corner); highly unstable
- Anterior wedge compression: axial loading, anterior rarely >25% shorter than posterior, stable
- Burst fracture: axial loading; fracture of vertebral body endplates pushing body outward; ligaments often intact; spinal cord injury can result from fracture fragments moving outward
- Chance fracture: flexion (associated with incorrectly placed lap belt); transverse fracture through vertebral body; spinal cord injury rare; often associated with abdominal or retroperitoneal injuries
- Three column fracture: injuries to anterior column (anterior longitudinal ligament, anterior vertebral body), middle column (posterior longitudinal ligament, posterior vertebral body), and posterior column (supra- and interspinous ligaments, facet joint); stability based on two of three columns being intact

- Associated Injuries

  - Blunt cerebrovascular injury: blunt injuries to neck causing cervical fractures also associated with injuries to carotid or vertebral arteries; any cervical spine fracture should prompt diagnostic evaluation for blunt cerebrovascular injury (CT angiography of neck)
  - Abdominal injury: Chance fractures associated with retroperitoneal injuries (pancreatic, renal) and intraabdominal (mesenteric bucket handle injuries, small bowel and colonic perforation); may be associated with external seatbelt sign

Evaluation [1]

- Physical examination (as part of secondary survey *after* primary survey)

  - Sensory examination

    - Pinprick (pain and temperature)
    - Toe position sense (proprioception)
    - Tuning fork (vibration)

  - Muscle strength grading (0–5 scale) [6]

    - 0: no contraction
    - 1: trace or flicker
    - 2: movement with gravity eliminated
    - 3: movement against gravity but not resistance
    - 4: movement against some resistance
    - 5: movement against full resistance

- When imaging is not required to discontinue empirically placed cervical collar

  – Two decision rules (both sensitive, unclear which are more specific), both used in practice/protocols (CITE)
  – National Emergency X-Radiography Utilization Study (NEXUS): if all the following true, collar may be discontinued without imaging

    • No direct blows or penetrating injury to neck
    • Age 60 and younger
    • No posterior midline cervical spine tenderness
    • No evidence of intoxication
    • Normal level of alertness
    • No focal neurologic deficits
    • No painful distracting injuries

  – Canadian C-spine Rule: if all the following true, collar may be discontinued without imaging

    • Age 65 or younger
    • No dangerous mechanism (fall >1 m/5 stairs, axial load to head, motor vehicle collision greater than 62 mph, all-terrain vehicle accident, vehicle ejection, bicycle collision with larger object)
    • No extremity paresthesias
    • Able to rotate neck actively AND has a low-risk factor (simple rear-end MVC, sitting position in the emergency department, ambulatory at any time, delayed onset of neck pain, no midline cervical spine tenderness)

  – No similar decision rule exists for thoracic and lumbar spine imaging

- Radiologic evaluation

  – Plain radiography: should be used for primary evaluation when CT not available

    • Films from occiput to T1: lateral, anteroposterior (AP), and open-mouth odontoid views
    • Lateral: if unable to visualize all seven cervical and first thoracic vertebrae on lateral view, obtain swimmer's view of lower cervical and upper thoracic spine
    • AP: detects unilateral facet dislocation not seen laterally
    • Open-mouth odontoid: should include entire odontoid and lateral aspects of C1 and C2
    • Films from T1 to L5: lateral and AP views

  – Computerized tomography (CT): sensitive and specific, can be used for primary evaluation

    • Should include sagittal and coronal reconstruction
    • Posterior column fractures better visualized
    • Useful for determining spinal canal compromise

- Does not assess for ligamentous injury or epidural hematoma
  - Magnetic Resonance Imaging (MRI): most sensitive, but costly and time-consuming
    - Can assess soft-tissue injury, including cord contusion or disruption
    - Not appropriate for hemodynamically compromised patient
    - Indication: neurologic deficit without evidence of injury on CT
    - Otherwise performed at spine consultant discretion
  - Upright films: films performed after any stabilization modality (operative or nonoperative) to assess for effectiveness of stability therapy

Management [1]

- Spinal immobilization
  - Cervical collar: often placed in field empirically by EMS based on mechanism and local protocol; if patients present without collar, use decision rules above to determine if collar should be placed prior to imaging
  - Spine board: used for extrication and rapid patient movement in field or early in emergency department course; do not allow to lie on spine board >2 h or during surgery (high risk of pressure injury)
  - Supine on firm surface: spinal immobilization achieved when patient lying supine with cervical collar
  - Logroll: to evaluate spine/posterior, remove spine board, facilitate transfer, etc.; requires four team members
    - Team member 1: controls head and c-spine, responsible for directing other members of logroll team
    - Team member 2: controls torso, prevents undue motion to spine other than logroll movement
    - Team member 3: controls legs, providing stability for upper torso
    - Team member 4: responsible for examination, removal of spine board, placement of transfer device, changing sheets, any other activity, etc.
- Pulmonary management [7]
  - Intubation and mechanical ventilation:
    - Pulmonary issues most common complication of spinal cord injury: respiratory failure, pneumonia, pulmonary embolism, pulmonary edema
    - Primary mechanism: hypoventilation causing hypoxic and/or hypercarbic respiratory failure
    - In spinal cord injury: diaphragm or accessory muscle paralysis or weakness
    - Additional cause: supine position prior to spinal injury assessment or stabilization, especially in obese patients

- Tracheostomy

  - Performed for prolonged mechanical ventilation, 7–10 days
  - High cervical cord injuries particularly likely to need tracheostomy, in some cases permanent ventilator dependency

- Cardiac management [8]

  - Neurogenic shock:

    - Must rule out hemorrhagic shock first in trauma patients!
    - IV fluid resuscitation important, but shock often resistant to volume; judicious fluid management essential to prevent spinal cord and pulmonary edema
    - Bradycardia also common: may require atropine or pacing, especially in high cervical lesions; vasopressors may assist
    - Vasopressors often required: norepinephrine preferred (mixed alpha and beta for both hypotension and bradycardia); phenylephrine (pure alpha-1 agonist: peripheral vasoconstriction but reflex bradycardia)

  - MAP goals: maintaining higher mean arterial pressure (MAP) to promote perfusion of spinal cord (mixed empiric data); often between 80 and 90 mmHg; requires hemodynamic monitoring (arterial line for MAP measurement) and often vasopressor support; often continued for 2–3 days following operative stabilization for spinal cord injury

- Prophylaxis and other medical care

  - Venous thromboembolism (VTE): all trauma patients at risk for VTE but spinal cord injury highest risk for VTE; most common in first 2 weeks after injury; all spinal cord injury patients should receive VTE chemoprophylaxis when feasible [7]
  - Pain control: multimodal regimens best; balance need for pain control with opiates with opiate side effects (respiratory depression, ileus)
  - Pressure sores: most common on buttocks and heels after spinal cord injury; can develop quickly (within hours); removal of spine board and regular turning to prevent
  - Urinary catheterization: initial placement of Foley catheter when immobilized; if long-term immobilization (spinal cord injury), transition to intermittent catheterization (q4-6h)
  - Stress ulcer prophylaxis: stress ulcers more common in high cervical injuries; prophylaxis as in other critically ill patients
  - Bowel regimens: on top of normal risk (from opiates), spinal cord injury patients at high risk for paralytic ileus/Ogilvie's and resultant complications (aspiration, bowel perforation); bowel regimens should be instituted early
  - Nutrition: early nutrition to promote healing in injury and critical illness; if unable to eat, should initiate enteral nutrition via tube feeding, and if that is not possible, consider parenteral nutrition

- Nonoperative stabilization and reduction: indications for nonoperative management of spinal injuries are beyond the scope of this chapter; spine consultant drives decision-making; nonoperative modalities reviewed for familiarity

  - Mobilization without brace: certain fractures can be treated without brace and mobilization if pain control adequate
  - Collars (cervical injury): hard Aspen or Miami-J collars
  - Braces (thoracolumbar injury): thoracolumbar sacral orthosis (TLSO) including Jewett brace; soft brace (often for comfort)
  - Closed reduction (cervical injury): halo brace holds head in place in relation to thoracolumbar spine

- Indications for surgical decompression and stabilization; indications for operative management of spinal injuries beyond the scope of this chapter; below are *common* indications; spine consultant drives decision-making

  - Neurologic deficit: presumed unstable as spinal canal impinged or bony fragments have damaged spinal cord
  - Unstable fractures: fracture patterns described above as unstable often require surgical fixation
  - Penetrating injury: may require debridement and washout for removal of foreign bodies/reduce contamination burden to prevent infection

Prognosis [9]

- Without spinal cord injury: primary long-term complication is chronic pain
- With spinal cord injury: predictors of survival and functional (motor) recovery include age, level of injury, and completeness of neurologic injury
- Concomitant injuries (especially traumatic brain injury), medical comorbidities, and medical complications (especially infection) decrease survival and functional recovery
- Chronic complications of spinal cord injury include the following:

  - Orthostatic hypotension
  - Autonomic dysreflexia: severe/life-threatening hypertension after stimuli (most common: bladder catheterization)
  - Bladder dysfunction
  - Bowel dysfunction
  - Chronic pain syndromes
  - Spasticity
  - Pressure ulcers
  - Osteoporosis

References

1. Committee on Trauma, American College of Surgeons. Advanced Trauma Life Support: Student Course Manual. 10th ed. Chicago, IL: American College of Surgeons; 2018.
2. Kumar R, Lim J, Mekary RA, et al. Traumatic spinal injury: global epidemiology and worldwide volume. World Neurosurg. 2018;113:e345–63. https://doi.org/10.1016/j.wneu.2018.02.033.
3. Oliver M, Inaba K, Tang A, et al. The changing epidemiology of spinal trauma: a 13-year review from a Level I trauma centre. Injury. 2012;43(8):1296–300. https://doi.org/10.1016/j.injury.2012.04.021.
4. Roberts TT, Leonard GR, Cepela DJ. Classifications in brief: American Spinal Injury Association (ASIA) impairment scale. Clin Orthop Relat Res. 2017;475(5):1499–504. https://doi.org/10.1007/s11999-016-5133-4.
5. Preston-Suni K, Kaji AH. Spinal trauma. In: Walls RM, editor. Rosen's emergency medicine: concepts and clinical practice. 10th ed. Philadelphia: Elsevier; 2023:chap Spinal Trauma.
6. O'Brien M. Aids to the Examination of the Peripheral Nervous System. 5th ed. Edinburgh, Scotland: Saunders-Elsevier; 2010.
7. Brown R, DiMarco AF, Hoit JD, Garshick E. Respiratory dysfunction and management in spinal cord injury. Respir Care. 2006;51(8):853–70.
8. Yue JK, Tsolinas RE, Burke JF, et al. Vasopressor support in managing acute spinal cord injury: current knowledge. J Neurosurg Sci. 2019;63(3):308–17. https://doi.org/10.23736/s0390-5616.17.04003-6.
9. Sezer N, Akkuş S, Uğurlu FG. Chronic complications of spinal cord injury. World J Orthop. 2015;6(1):24–33. https://doi.org/10.5312/wjo.v6.i1.24.

Chapter 33
Maxillofacial Trauma

Kevin Kiang, Ali Khodadad-Hossaini, and Armando Uribe-Rivera

Assessment of Maxillofacial Trauma

Categories of Maxillofacial Trauma

- Emergent: life threatening injuries (airway obstructions, severe hemorrhage), eyesight threatening injuries
- Treatment within hours: extremely contaminated injuries in hemodynamically stable patient
- Treatment within 24 h: some facial injuries
- Treatment after 24 h: most facial fractures

Initial Assessment of Maxillofacial Trauma Within the Initial Trauma Assessment

1. Airway/Breathing:

   - Protect airway with endotracheal intubation versus surgical airway if appropriate.
   - Unfavorable bilateral mandible fractures may cause airway obstruction. Stabilize the fracture by bridle wire.

K. Kiang · A. Khodadad-Hossaini · A. Uribe-Rivera (✉)
Department of Oral and Maxillofacial Surgery, Boston University Henry M. Goldman School of Dentistry, Boston, MA, USA
e-mail: Kkiang@bu.edu; alikh@bu.edu; aur@bu.edu

T. S. Brahmbhatt, D. R. Scantling (eds.), *Trauma Surgery Clerkship*, Contemporary Surgical Clerkships,
https://doi.org/10.1007/978-3-032-01412-2_33

2. Circulation:

- Bleeding from highly vascularized head and neck (e.g., scalp lacerations control with Raney clips, sutures, staples).
- Epistaxis: due to midface fracture, bleeding through oropharynx presents with risk for airway obstruction, aspiration, and shock.
- Packing of nasal cavities: control posterior bleed with a 16-Fr Foley catheter to tamponade bleeding. Control anterior bleed with half-inch gauze with bacitracin (start by placing at nasal floor and extend upward) or use commercially available nasal packing.
- Rule out coagulopathy.
- Oral cavity: managed bleeding with packing and pressure. Reduce fractures with bridle wire.
- Other control measures: reduce facial fractures, angiography, and embolization.

3. Disability:

- Ocular examination: pupil size, reactivity to light, symmetry, and relative afferent pupillary defect.

Taking a History

- Mechanism of injury (object, direction and magnitude, location of injury)
- Time elapsed since injury
- Head and neck review of systems should include at minimum:

  Headache, (2) nausea and/or vomiting, (3) loss of consciousness, (4) dizziness, (5) numbness, (6) weakness, (7) change in vision, (8) pain on eye movement, (9) change in hearing, (10) bleeding or discharge from the nose, (11) changes in occlusion, (12) pain on opening/closing the jaw, (13) missing teeth, (14) facial weakness, (15) cervical spine tenderness, (16) throat pain, (17) voice change, and (18) pain on swallowing.

Clinical Exam

- Visually inspect for changes to facial contour, asymmetry, ecchymosis, bleeding, lacerations, abrasions.
- Observe for abnormal mandibular movements (deviation, trismus), maximal interincisal opening (40 mm is normal), changes in globe position (exophthalmos, proptosis, enophthalmos).
- Palpate the skeletal framework and entirely around the orbital rims in 360°, check for altered sensation, crepitus, mobility, step-offs, palpable fracture lines.

- Examine the cranial nerves.
- Ophthalmologic exam: visual disturbances, blindness, restricted ocular movement, pupillary response, globe position. Consult ophthalmology as appropriate.
- Internal nasal exam: check intranasal lacerations, septal deviation, septal hematoma, and nasal discharge.
- Intraoral exam: inspect for malocclusion, lacerations, bleeding, gaps in dentition, and ecchymosis.

Imaging in Maxillofacial Trauma

- Panoramic X-ray
- Computed tomography: axial, coronal, sagittal, and 3D-reconstruction

Exam Pearls

- Consultation to the oral and maxillofacial surgeon is appropriate. Consult ophthalmology when orbital or ocular involvement is suspected.
- Cranial nerve evaluation and ophthalmologic exam should always be performed (altered sensation of the face suggests further evaluation to rule out bony facial fractures). Anosmia suggests involvement of cribriform plate.
- Avulsed or fragmented teeth may be lodged into surrounding tissues.
- Assessment for open wound of the nose, epistaxis, and septal hematoma in any setting with trauma to the midface. Open wound of the nose is the strongest predictor for nasal fractures.
- Assessment for fracture can be done by palpation of the orbital, nasal and zygomatic region and bimanual manipulation of the maxillary and mandibular region for mobility, deformities, or step-offs.
- Enophthalmos typically associated with fracture to the medial orbital wall.
- Increased inter-canthal width suggests injury to the naso-orbitoethmoid complex. Normal measurements: Women: 28.6–33.0 mm, Men 28.9–34.5 mm.
- Ocular muscle entrapment can be tested with a "forced duction test."
- Difficulty opening or closing the jaw suggests traumatic bony injury as a possible cause.
- Avoid any packing if there is suspicion for a cerebrospinal fluid (CSF) leak to avoid meningitis.

  - Confirmatory test for CSF: beta-2 transferrin test
  - Bedside test (CSF will also form concentric rings when poured on line or soft filter paper)

Dentoalveolar (DA) and Mandibular Fractures

Epidemiology

- Incidence of DA fractures, highest between the ages of 8 and 12 years in children and between the ages of 18 and 23 years in adults.
- The number of mandibular fractures per patient ranges from 1.5 to 1.8. An estimated 50% of patients with mandibular fractures have more than one fracture.
- Incidence of Injury by Anatomical Site

Condyle	29.1%	Dentoalveolar	3.1%
Angle	24.5%	Ramus	1.7%
Symphysis	22%	Coronoid process	1.3%
Body of mandible	16%		

Mandible Fracture Classification [1]

- Favorable: the pull of muscles minimizes displacement of the fracture
- Unfavorable: the pull of muscles further destabilizes the segments

Additional Imaging

- *DA fractures.* Head, neck, chest, and or abdominal imaging as necessary to rule out aspiration, swallowed, or displaced teeth and/or prosthetic appliances [2].
- *Mandible fractures.* PA or reverse Towne's view is adequate if CT is not available in addition to a panoramic radiograph.

Treatment [3]

- Stabilize the DA fractured segment using orthodontic wire and dental bonding
- For avulsed teeth, tooth reimplantation is highly advised.
- Critical factors for avulsed teeth prior to reimplantation: storage media and time in solution.

  - Hanks Balanced Salt Solution (HBSS) (24 h) > Pasteurized milk (2 h) > Saline solution (2 h) > Saliva (30 min)

Table 33.1 Indications for closed and open surgical approach for mandibular fractures

Closed reduction approach	Open surgical approach
Minimally or non-displaced favorable fractures	Displaced unfavorable fractures
Grossly comminuted fractures with an undisturbed periosteum	Multiple fractures of the facial bones
Pediatric mandibular fractures with developing dentition	Midface fracture with bilateral condylar fractures
Coronoid process fractures	Delayed treatment of mandible fracture
Intracapsular condylar fractures	Systemic conditions contraindicating intermaxillary fixation (seizures, pulmonary disease, GI disorders, psychiatric conditions)
Significant loss of overlying soft tissue	Edentulous maxilla

Note: wire-cutting scissors should always be present at bedside

- Mandible fracture treatment goal is to restore function by reestablishing occlusion. See Table 33.1 for indications for closed and open surgical approaches.

Midface and Frontal Sinus Fracture

Epidemiology

Maxillary fracture. High risk of life-threatening hemorrhage in Le Fort II and III fractures (5.5%).

- ⅓ of Le Fort fracture patients require intubation to protect airway
- Associated with cervical spine injuries (1.5%–2%) and traumatic brain injury (51%)

Isolated nasal fracture. Most common presenting type of facial fracture, owing to its prominence and exposure on the face [4].

- 58% of all facial fractures in trauma patients, 93% of nasal fractures are closed

Naso-orbitoethmoid fracture. Presents with increased inter-canthal width [4].

- Rare—2%–15% of patients with facial fractures, often part of Le Fort II and III fractures.

Frontal sinus fracture.

- Reported from 5% to 15% of all facial fractures in major trauma centers.

Classification

Maxillary fracture.

- LeFort I: horizontal maxillary fracture above the apices of maxillary teeth
- Lefort II: Pyramidal fracture pattern due to trauma infraorbital rim and nasofrontal junction
- Lefort III: separation of the facial skeleton from skull base (craniofacial disjunction) due to trauma to nasofrontal junction and upper lateral orbital rim

Naso-orbitoethmoid (NOE) fracture [4].

- Type I: A single fractured segment, which maintains the attachment site of the medial canthal tendon (MCT)
- Type II: Comminution present and the MCT remains attached to non-comminuted bony segment
- Type III: Comminution extending into the attachment site of the MCT

Frontal sinus (FS) fracture.

- Type 1: Fractures of the anterior wall (1/3 of fractures).
- Type 2: Anterior and posterior table fractures (2/3 of fractures)
- Type 3: Posterior table fracture (rare <1%)
- Type 4: Very severe comminuted fractures of the whole frontal area, involving the orbit, nasal base, and the ethmoid bones

Treatment

- ATLS stabilization.
- Options for treatment:
  - Observation: no mobility or displacement of fractures, no change in occlusion (maxillary fractures)
  - Indications for Closed Reduction: minor change in occlusion (maxillary fractures). Absence of nasal deformity.
  - Indications for Open Surgery: malocclusion (maxillary fracture), loss of normal midface and/or nasal form, abnormal orbital volume, eyelid function and lacrimal drainage, increased inter-canthal width with or without canthal and nasal deformity (NOE fracture). Presence of cerebrospinal fluid (CSF) (FS fracture)

Zygomaticomaxillary Complex (ZMC) and Orbital Fracture

Epidemiology

ZMC fracture. Second in frequency after nasal fractures

- Diplopia in orbital fractures is common and often spontaneously resolves
- Incidence of ocular injury is higher in patients without orbital fractures, suggesting the fracture of the orbit plays a protective role in ocular trauma
- Most common orbital fractures involve the anterior medial orbital floor and medial wall

Classification

- *Linear "Greenstick"*: do not typically result in defect with orbital content herniation. Can result in increased orbital volume (enophthalmos).
- *Blow-out*: limited to one wall; typically, 2 cm or less in diameter.
- *Blow-in*: Orbital roof fracture resulting in herniation of the brain into the orbit. Characteristic: "pulsatile globe" due to cerebrovascular pulsation.
- *Complex*: Extensive fracture affecting two or more orbital walls. Often extend to the posterior orbit and may involve the optic canal.

Additional Imaging

- Water's and Submentovertex view for ZMC fracture if CT reconstruction is not available

Treatment [5]

- Goals include restoration of function and cosmesis.
- Observation
  - Stable, minimally displaced fractures without any significant clinical findings. Absence of orbital deformity
- ZMC: Indication for closed reduction
  - For minimal to moderately displaced isolated zygomatic arch fractures with trismus or aesthetic concerns

- ZMC: Indications for reduction and internal fixation

  - Significant comminution of anterior portion of ZMC
  - Posterior segmentation
  - Reconstruction of orbit
  - When exposure is required for adequate reduction and fixation

- ZMC: Indication for Open Surgery

  - When exposure is required for adequate reduction and fixation

- Orbital Fractures: Indications for Surgical Repair

  - Enophthalmos >2 mm or hypoglobus
  - Floor defect greater than 50% of the surface area
  - Ocular muscle entrapment
  - Diplopia within 30° of primary gaze or persistent diplopia

- Contraindications to Surgical Repair for Orbital Fracture

  - Hyphema, globe rupture, retinal tears, recent ophthalmologic injury
  - Obtain ophthalmology consult and clearance prior to surgery

References

1. Morris C, Bebeau NP, Brockhoff H, Tandon R, Tiwana P. Mandibular fractures: an analysis of the epidemiology and patterns of injury in 4,143 fractures. J Oral Maxillofac Surg. 2015;73:951.e1–951.e12.
2. Khinda VI, Brar GS, Kallar S, Khurana H. Clinical and practical implications of storage media used for tooth avulsion. Int J Clin Pediatr Dent. 2017;10:158–65.
3. Fonseca RJ, Eberts A. Oral & maxillofacial trauma. 4th ed. St. Louis: Elsevier; 2013.
4. Li L, Zang H, Han D, Yang B, Desai SC, London NR. Nasal bone fractures: analysis of 1193 cases with an emphasis on coincident adjacent fractures. Facial Plast Surg Aesthet Med. 2020;22:249–54.
5. Miloro M, McKeon M, Ackerman MB. Peterson's principles of oral and maxillofacial surgery. 3rd ed. Shelton: People's Medical Publishing House; 2011.

Chapter 34
Cardiac and Major Vascular Injury of the Chest

Patrick McGillen and Kenji Inaba

Abbreviations

ATLS	Advanced trauma life support
BCI	Blunt cardiac injury
CTA	Computed tomography angiography
FAST	Focused assessment with sonography in trauma
IV	Innominate vein
IVC	Inferior vena cava
LAD	Left anterior descending artery
LCx	Left circumflex artery
LMCA	Left main coronary artery
MTP	Massive transfusion protocol
NGT	Nasogastric tube
OGT	Orogastric tube
PCI	Penetrating cardiac injury
PW	Pericardial window
RA	Right atrium
RT	Resuscitative ED thoracotomy
SP	Subxiphoid pericardiotomy
SVC	Superior vena cava
TTE	Transthoracic echocardiogram

P. McGillen (✉) · K. Inaba
Division of Trauma, Emergency Surgery and Surgical Critical Care, Los Angeles General Medical Center, Los Angeles, CA, USA

Department of Surgery, University of Southern California Keck School of Medicine, Los Angeles, CA, USA
e-mail: Patrick.Mcgillen@med.usc.edu; Kenji.Inaba@med.usc.edu

© The Author(s), under exclusive license to Springer Nature Switzerland AG 2025
T. S. Brahmbhatt, D. R. Scantling (eds.), *Trauma Surgery Clerkship*, Contemporary Surgical Clerkships,
https://doi.org/10.1007/978-3-032-01412-2_34

Cardiac Injury

Surgical Anatomy

The Thoracic Cage, Thoracic Outlet, and Cardiac Box

- The heart, lungs, thoracic aorta, and great vessels are enclosed by the thoracic skeleton made up of the manubrium, sternum, clavicle, rib cage, and vertebral bodies [1]. The cage protects the thoracic cavity but in cases of penetrating injuries, it can deflect missiles and knives leading to unique and nonlinear injury vectors or create secondary fragments [1].
- Historically, the cardiac box or "box" is the area of the anterior thorax with the highest risk of cardiac injury in trauma. The box is bordered superiorly by the clavicles, laterally by a vertical line intersecting the medial third of the right clavicle and the left midclavicular line, and inferiorly by the costal margins, projecting posteriorly to the spine. Because all penetrating injuries to the thorax including those outside the "box" can cause a cardiac injury, the clinical utility of this anatomic construction is questionable [2].
- The thoracic outlet refers to the confined space between clavicle and manubrium anteriorly, the first rib and costal cartilage laterally, and T1 vertebrae posteriorly. It is the space through which the subclavian vein, subclavian artery, and brachial plexus travel from their central origins to the upper extremities.

Surface Anatomy of the Heart

- The pericardium envelops the heart and attaches to the roots of the ascending aorta, pulmonary artery, pulmonary veins, the last 2–4 cm of superior vena cava, and inferior vena cava [3].
- The atria are significantly thinner (2–3 mm) than the right (4 mm) and left (12 mm) ventricles
- Left main coronary artery (LMCA) supplies blood to the left side of the heart. The LMCA arises from the left coronary cusp of the ascending aorta and runs branches into the left anterior descending coronary artery (LAD), which perfuses the anterior ventricular septum and the anterior portion of the left ventricle as well as the left circumflex artery that supplies the lateral wall of the left ventricle and occasionally the posteroinferior heart in individuals with left heart dominance. The right coronary artery arises from the anterior ascending aorta and supplies blood to the right atrium, right ventricle, sinoatrial nodal artery, AV node, and posterior third of the interventricular septum via the posterior descending artery branch.
- Left and right phrenic nerves originate from C3 to C5 spinal nerves and descend along the anterior scalene muscle before running anterior to the brachiocephalic artery (right phrenic) and subclavian artery (left phrenic) and posterior to the subclavian veins (Fig. 34.1).

Fig. 34.1 Surface anatomy of the heart and great vessels. (Reprinted from Demetriades et al. [3, pp. 104–117]. Copyright 2020 by Cambridge University Press. Reprinted with permission)

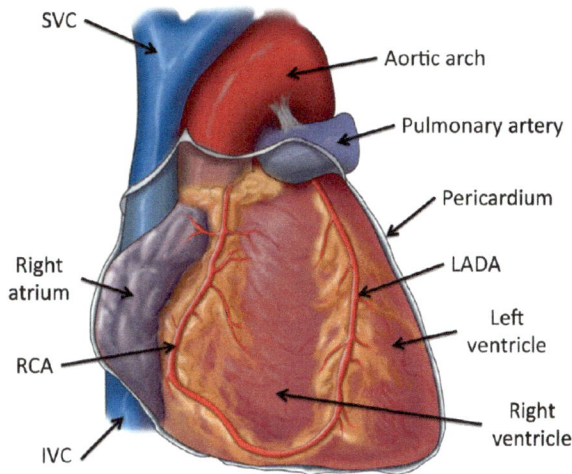

Blunt Cardiac Injury (BCI)

Background and Epidemiology

- There is no agreed upon definition of BCI and there is no universally accepted diagnostic workup or management algorithm. Diagnostic criteria include elevated troponins [4], novel ECG abnormalities, or structural cardiac defects seen on echocardiography [5]. In general, BCI can be defined as either new dysrhythmia on ECG or structural abnormalities of the myocardial wall, valve, or coronary arteries [4].
- Electrical disturbances are more commonly seen than structural injury in patients with BCI. Sudden cardiac death is exceedingly rare and can occur after a direct impact to the heart that alters the electrical stability of the myocardium causing ventricular fibrillation [4].
- Blunt cardiac rupture is the most severe form of BCI and has a poor prognosis [1]. The exact incidence is unknown and over 75% of patients with cardiac rupture after blunt chest trauma die at the scene [5].

Mechanism

- Any blunt force to the chest can cause BCI. Blunt forces can lead to crush, traction, or torsion injuries to the heart and great vessels. During rapid deceleration the heart is compressed between the sternum and spine.

Presentation

- Patients with BCI can be asymptomatic, though, if not immediately recognized, some can quickly develop complications such as pulmonary edema, pericardial effusion, hemorrhagic shock, tamponade, and cardiogenic shock.
- Signs and symptoms of BCI include hypotension, chest pain, dyspnea, chest bruising, and distended neck veins. Auscultation to detect signs of structural injuries is usually not practical in the noisy trauma bay [4]. Patients may also be asymptomatic.
- BCI is associated with additional thoracic injuries such as aortic or great vessel injury, rib and sternal fractures, flail chest, pulmonary contusion, and hemothorax or pneumothorax [4].
- Nonspecific ECG changes are the most common electrical disturbances in patients with BCI. Possibilities include sinus tachycardia, atrial fibrillation, ventricular tachycardia, etc., or new conduction abnormalities (heart blocks). With the exception of sinus tachycardia, the estimated incidence dysrhythmia after blunt chest trauma is approximately 6% [6, 7].
- Most structural injuries with the exception of wall contusion will cause rapid clinical deterioration from either tamponade or frank rupture if the pericardium is lacerated. Because of its anterior location, the right ventricle is the most commonly injured chamber [4]. Two or more chambers are injured in more than 50% of cases [9].
- While rare, pericardial tear and cardiac herniation with displacement of the heart into pleural or abdominal cavities most often occurs secondary to a sudden increased intra-abdominal pressure or lateral deceleration force. Right-sided herniation can result in twisting of heart and reduced venous return whereas left-sided herniation can result in trapped apex ("strangulated heart") and is highly lethal. Loss of pulse or hypotension when repositioning patient with BCI is the hallmark of cardiac herniation [12].

Screening for BCI

- The goal in screening for BCI is to identify those that will develop clinically significant cardiac injury. Any patient with significant blunt force trauma to the chest should be screened for BCI with 12 lead ECG and troponins [4].
- Basic screening modalities include ECG, serum troponin and Transthoracic echocardiogram (TTE); transesophageal echocardiography (TEE), Magnetic Resonance Imaging (MRI), ventriculography, Positron Emission Tomography (PET), and myocardial perfusion scintigraphy can be utilized to further characterize injuries [8].
- ECG is highly sensitive but not specific for BCI. If performed serially it has a negative predictive value >95% [4].
- Elevated troponin levels are very sensitive for detecting cardiomyocyte necrosis. However, simple elevations of troponin do not necessarily indicate clinically sig-

nificant BCI. The extent of troponin release and duration of release can be useful in judging the severity of cardiac contusion. Serial troponins obtained every 4–8 h have a high negative predictive value for BCI [10].
- When used in combination, serial EGC and serial troponin measurements have a negative predictive value for clinically significant BCI that approaches 100% [11].
- TTE is an ideal modality for definitive diagnosis in patients with suspected structural injuries. TTE is noninvasive and easily performed in a stable patient but due to length of exam time it is not an ideal screening test in the acute setting and should only be performed once hemorrhage and other life-threatening injuries have been ruled out or addressed [12].
- A practical approach for any patient with significant chest trauma is to perform 24 h of inpatient cardiac monitoring along with screening serial ECG and troponin levels every 8–12 h. Any hemodynamic or lab abnormalities should trigger a TTE.

Penetrating Cardiac Injury (PCI)

Background

- Unlike BCI, PCI is a well-defined and understood pathology. PCI includes any penetrating injury resulting in injury or violation of the pericardium or deeper cardiac structures. PCI can lead to rapid tamponade or exsanguination and death. PCI should be suspected in any patient presenting with any signs of penetrating injury to the thorax or missile trajectories in proximity to the mediastinum.
- Rapid transport to a trauma center, successful endotracheal intubation, and expeditious access to the heart is paramount in the survival of PCI. With improvements in rapid transport prehospital management and well-defined treatment algorithms, patients with PCI arriving signs of life have an overall survival of 30%–85%.
- Hemodynamic status is the best way to approach evaluation and management of patients with suspected PCI. Patients should be grouped into those in extremis with ongoing cardiac arrest requiring immediate resuscitative thoracotomy in the trauma bay and all other patients including those with or without hemodynamic stability. Survival rates for patients who are not in extremis and undergo operative repair in the OR ranges from 74% to 86% compared with an overall survival of <8% for those requiring emergency department thoracotomy [1, 13].
- Young males are disproportionately affected by PCI and constitute greater than 85% of victims with a penetrating injury to the thorax [2, 14, 15].

Mechanism

- Penetrating wounds anywhere to the thorax or missile trajectory entering the thorax can cause PCI.
- Low energy mechanisms include stab wounds. Historically, stab wounds are more common than GSW to the thorax. SW represent approximately 70% of all isolated thoracic penetrating injuries and 54%–60% of all PCI [2, 14, 15].
- High energy mechanisms include gunshot wounds and blast injuries. Gunshot wounds constitute an estimated 24%–42% of all PCI [2, 14, 15].
- The right ventricle is at greatest risk of injury due to its anterior location [15, 16]. Isolated injuries to the right ventricle also carry the best prognosis [17]. Due to its posterior location the left atrium is the least common cardiac chamber injured [14, 16].
- Compared with stab wounds (SW), patients with Gunshot wounds (GSWs) to the thorax result in more severe injuries to other thoracic structures and lead to a higher burden of injury and overall increase of mortality [2]. Survival after PCI due a SW is approximately fivefold higher than with GSW [16].

Presentation

- Spectrum of clinic presentation is variable from asymptomatic stable patient to a patient in extremis with full cardiac arrest.
- The majority of PCI involve a single cardiac chamber and only one-fifth of PCI involve multiple cardiac structures [5]. Multichamber PCI is more likely to result from GSW than SW [15].
- Up to 80% of SW that result in PCI will cause pericardial tamponade [1]. Only 60–100 mL of hemopericardium can produce clinically significant tamponade [18].
- Tamponade pathophysiology: Accumulation of pericardial blood → decreased ventricular filling → decreased stroke volume → decreased cardiac output → compensatory increase in catecholamines → tachycardia and increased right heart filling pressures → right-sided distensibility decreases and shift of ventricular septum to left → further decrease in stroke volume and cardiac output → cardiovascular collapse.
- Classic finding of Beck's Triad (muffled heart sounds, hypotension, distended neck veins) pulsus paradoxus (significant decrease in systolic pressure during inspiration) and Kussmaul's sign (increased jugular vein distension with inspiration) are only present in the minority of patients (<10%) and are not reliable with PCI and associated tamponade [1, 19, 20].
- Narrowed pulse pressure is a more valuable and reproducible sign of tamponade even with volume resuscitation.

Evaluation of Suspected Cardiac Injury

Initial Evaluation

- Initial evaluation should include a primary survey of the airway, breathing and circulation to identify life-threatening injuries per advanced trauma life support (ATLS) protocol. The trauma team should perform a rapid survey of the entire body to identify all penetrating wounds.
- Immediate life-threatening injuries to identify include tension pneumothorax, massive hemothorax, open pneumothorax, and cardiac tamponade.
- A well-choreographed multidisciplinary trauma team approach is essential for the successful management of traumatic injuries to the heart or great vessels.
- Simultaneous endotracheal intubation, placement of large bore IV access, resuscitation with blood products via massive transfusion protocol activation, NGT or OGT placement, cardiac FAST, chest tube placement and, if needed, resuscitative thoracotomy should occur in concert for patients arriving with life-threatening cardiac or great vessel injuries.
- There is a high incidence of concomitant intra-abdominal injuries in this population, which should be identified and treated in coordination with cardiothoracic injuries.
- In general, foreign bodies retained in the chest such as a knife with signs of PCI should be left in place until the patient is in the operating room, intubated, and the surgical team is ready for operative exploration. Foreign bodies in the thorax can be removed in the emergency department (ED) if there is no immediate indication for operation, the patient is hemodynamically normal, has a negative FAST, and there is immediate access to the operating room.

Imaging and Investigations

- Time to diagnosis and treatment is critical for survival in patients with cardiac injury. Imaging should not delay ED thoracotomy or transport to the operating in patients arriving in extremis or significant hemodynamic instability.
- Cardiac FAST is a highly accurate, noninvasive and widely available point of care test performed as part of the primary survey during the evaluation of a trauma patient at risk of PCI and should be the first test performed as soon as feasible [23].
- The sensitivity, specificity, and accuracy of FAST are all near perfect for identifying PCI in the hands of an experienced surgeon [21]. A caveat to this is the case of a false negative from a large concurrent laceration of the pericardial sac where hemopericardium can be missed due to blood decompression into the ipsilateral thoracic cavity [22].
- Presence of pericardial fluid on FAST in a patient with suspected acute cardiac injury warrants immediate transfer to the operating room for sternotomy [23].

Great Vessel Injuries

Surgical Anatomy

- The thoracic great vessels include the aorta, innominate (brachiocephalic) artery, pulmonary arteries, pulmonary veins, superior vena cava (SVC), intrathoracic inferior vena cava (IVC), innominate and azygos veins.
- The thymus and surrounding mediastinal fat are the first tissues encountered when entering the upper mediastinum and lie over the left innominate vein and the aortic arch.
- Left innominate vein is approximately 6 cm long and traverses the upper mediastinum anterior to the superior border of the aortic arch and its branches [3]. The right innominate vein is approximately 3 cm long and joins the left innominate vein at a 90° angle just lateral of the sternum at the level of the first intercostal space to form the SVC [24].
- The ascending aorta is contained within the pericardium while the aortic arch begins at the superior attachment of the pericardium [24]. The descending aorta typically begins at the fourth thoracic vertebra.
- The innominate artery (zone 0) is the first branch of the aortic arch and branches into the right subclavian and right common carotid arteries. The second branch of the arch is the left common carotid artery (zone 1), followed by the left subclavian artery (zone 2).
- Common thoracic aorta anatomic variants include bovine arch (common origin of innominate and left common carotid arteries), right subclavian takeoff from the descending thoracic aorta, origin of left vertebral artery off the aortic arch and persistent left ductus arteriosus.
- The right trunk of the pulmonary artery is posterior to the aortic arch and SVC. The left trunk is superior to the left mainstem bronchus and left pulmonary veins.
- The ligamentum arteriosum is a small ligament attaching the left pulmonary artery and aortic arch distal to the left subclavian artery take off (zone 3). It is the remnant of the ductus arteriosus. This anchoring point is often the site of blunt aortic injury.
- The phrenic nerve runs anterior along the anterior scalene muscles and posterior to the subclavian veins.
- The brachial plexus is posterior to the subclavian artery and anterior to the middle scalene.
- Esophagus lies on the right side of the aorta in the upper mediastinum before moving anterior to the thoracic aorta and crossing over as it enters the abdomen at the level of T10 via the esophageal hiatus of the diaphragm.
- The ligamentum arteriosum is an important landmark for identifying the left recurrent laryngeal nerve, which loops around the aortic arch behind the ligamentum arteriosum before ascending to the larynx (Fig. 34.2, 34.3, 34.4, and 34.5).

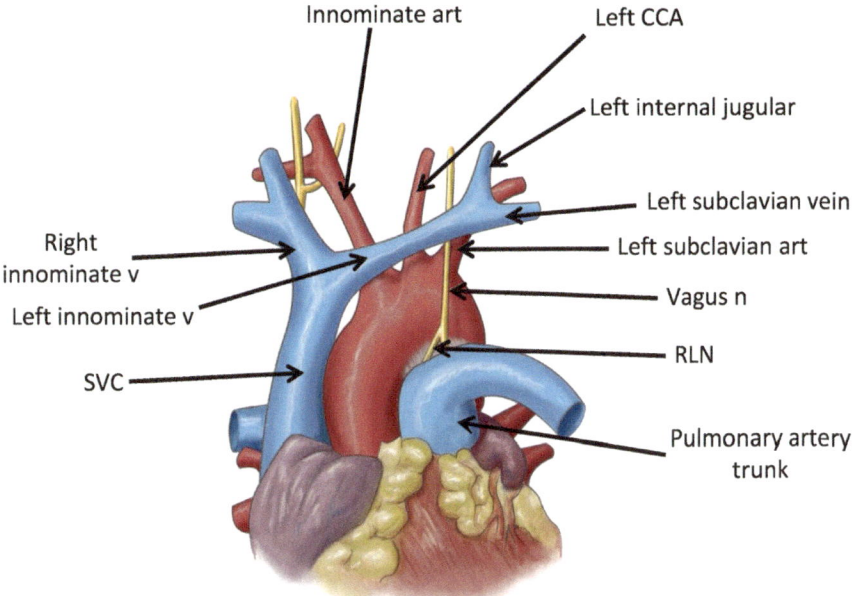

Fig. 34.2 Anatomy of the vessels of the superior mediastinum. (Reprinted from Demetriades et al. [3, pp. 118–129]. Copyright 2020 by Cambridge University Press. Reprinted with permission)

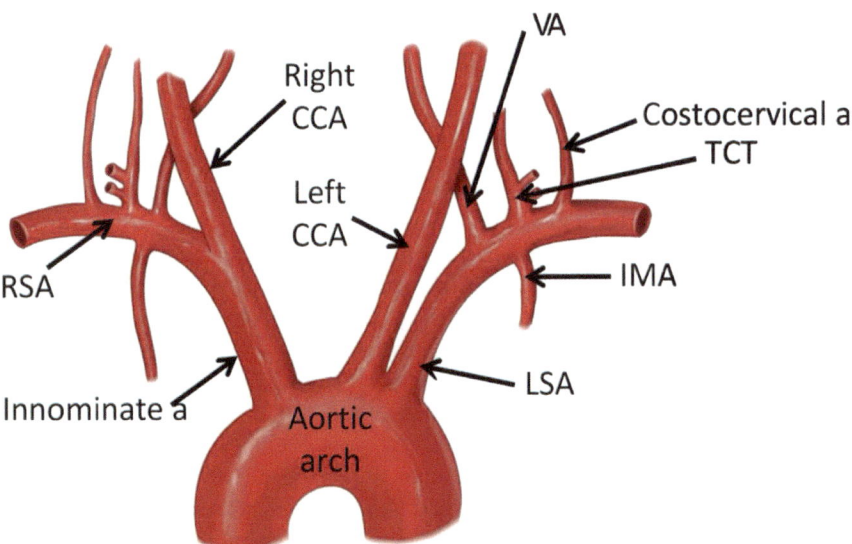

Fig. 34.3 The major vessels of the aortic arch. (Reprinted from Demetriades et al. [3, pp. 118–129]. Copyright 2020 by Cambridge University Press. Reprinted with permission)

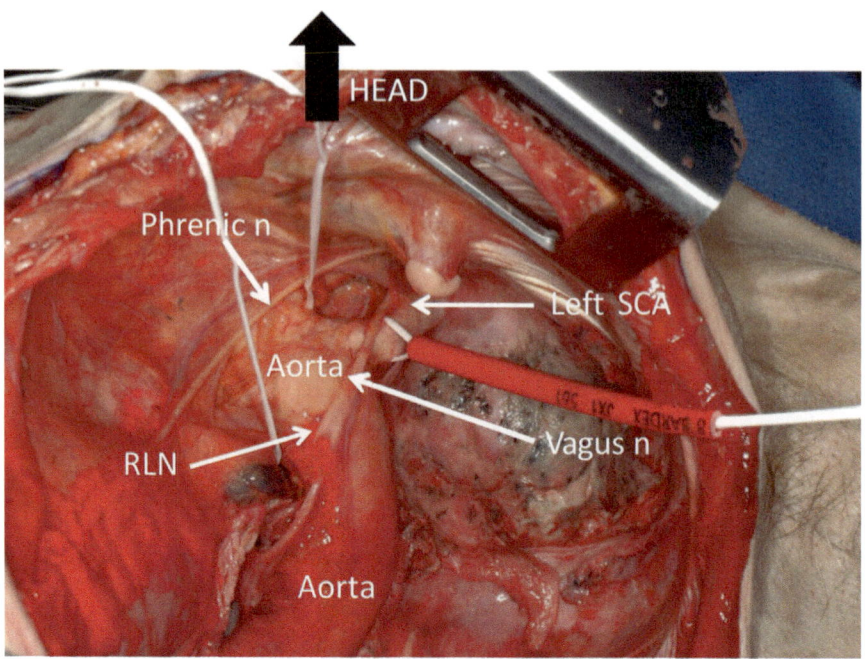

Fig. 34.4 Left thoracic cavity demonstrating left vagus nerve crossing over the proximal left sub-clavian artery and the aortic arch. (Reprinted from Demetriades et al. [3, pp. 118–129]. Copyright 2020 by Cambridge University Press. Reprinted with permission)

Workup and Initial Management of Suspected Great Vessel Injury

- A well-coordinated multidisciplinary approach is imperative to have along with an immediate primary survey and FAST to identify and treat life-threatening injuries. A rapid and thorough secondary survey follows, with a focus on identifying immediately life-threatening injuries.
- Clinical findings that should raise suspicion for thoracic vessel injury include hard signs of vascular injury in the thoracic outlet or upper extremities (expanding hematoma, pulsatile bleeding, signs of distal ischemia, palpable thrill, audible bruit), hypotension, isolated upper extremity hypertension, pulse exam and blood pressure differences between upper extremities, signs of major chest trauma, sternal deformities, massive hemothorax, flail chest, or thoracic spine fractures [30].
- Patients with suspected great vessel injury should be initially managed in a similar fashion to suspected cardiac injuries. Unstable patients with dwindling physiologic reserve or already in extremis require ED thoracotomy with extension to the right if required, with the goal of rapidly obtaining hemorrhage control. Simple temporizing measures such as vessel ligation, vessel cross clamping, or

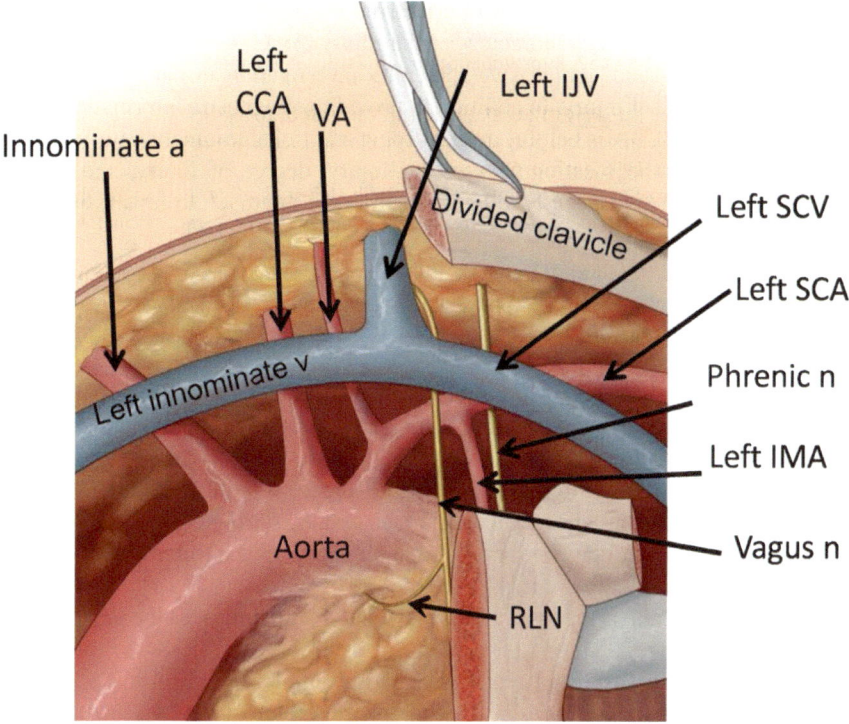

Fig. 34.5 Anatomy of the aortic arch and its major trunks. (Reprinted from Demetriades et al. [3, pp. 118–129]. Copyright 2020 by Cambridge University Press. Reprinted with permission)

intrapleural packing can provide time for transfer to the operating room for definitive repair.
- Like PCI and BCI, expedient diagnosis, repair or ligation of the injured great vessel in order to control hemorrhage is the key to preventing poor outcomes.

Imaging for Suspected Great Vessel Injury

- Initial screening radiograph with a supine anteroposterior chest X-ray should be obtained in the stable patient with thoracic trauma to assess for pneumothorax, hemothorax, and the presence of retained fragments.
- Radiographic findings associated with blunt and penetrating great vessel injury include large hemothorax, intrathoracic bullets, or other intrathoracic foreign bodies with trajectories that traverse the mediastinum, widening of the superior mediastinum >8 cm, multiple rib fractures, sternal fracture, tracheal deviation, downward displacement of the bronchus, loss of normal aortic knob contour, and presence of a left apical cap.

- CT angiography (CTA) is the most effective imaging modality in hemodynamically stable patients with thoracic vascular injury [3]. CTA is a readily available, quick, accurate, and noninvasive screening investigation in patients with suspected great vessel injury. In addition to providing diagnostic information about vascular injury, CTA is helpful in identifying additional traumatic injuries [31].
- CTA identifies the location of vascular injury, degree of injury, and vessels involved, which significantly aids in selecting the approach to repair, timing of repair, and, if needed, access.

Blunt Thoracic Vessel Injury

- Motor vehicle crashes are a common mechanism of blunt thoracic vessel injury. Other sources of injury include blast injuries, auto-pedestrian and auto-bicyclist crashes, and falls from heights greater than 30 feet.
- Blunt injury is thought to result from shear forces on mobile portion of a great vessel adjacent to an adjacent fixed portion created during abrupt deceleration, vessel compression between bony structures, and rapid intraluminal hypertension during a traumatic event [1].
- With the exception of the thoracic aorta, isolated blunt injury to the great vessels of the chest is rare.
- All patients with suspected blunt great vessel injury should go to the OR for exploration and or endovascular stenting unless stable.
- Although rarely encountered, isolated great vessel injury after blunt trauma identified by CTA in hemodynamically stable patients should be immediately repaired by open operative techniques or by endovascular stenting. Blunt thoracic aortic injury in a stable patient is an exception to immediate repair and can be addressed in a delayed fashion.

Blunt Thoracic Aortic Injury

- The fixed attachments of the descending aortic arch at the ligamentum arteriosum and diaphragm as well as the pulmonary veins and vena cavae to the pericardium make these structures particularly vulnerable to blunt injury.
- The medial aspect proximal descending aorta just distal to the left subclavian artery takeoff is by far the most commonly involved site of injury [1]. This portion of the descending aorta has a naturally weaker tensile strength compared to the proximal aorta. The aorta is fixed at this position due to the ligamentum arteriosum. As a result, the proximal descending aorta is more prone to injury from sudden increases in intra-aortic pressure combined with rotational forces [25].
- This medial aspect of this portion of the aorta is particularly prone to injury as tensile strength of the aorta is naturally weaker compared to the more proximal

aorta and sudden increases in intra-thoracic pressure combined with a site of aortic fixation from the ligamentum arteriosus.

- Blunt injury can result in partial thickness injury to the intima or media. Full thickness injuries result in a traumatic false aneurysm (pseudoaneurysm), acute arteriovenous fistula, or free rupture much like a contained ruptured aortic aneurysm.
- In cases of full thickness injury, an intact parietal pleura may help contain the hematoma and prevent exsanguination.
- Blunt thoracic aortic injuries are classified according to the anatomical layers of the aortic wall involved to guide management: intimal tear (grade I), intramural hematoma (grade II), pseudoaneurysm (grade III), rupture (grade IV) [26].
- Hemodynamically stable patients with blunt thoracic aortic injury should be managed expectantly with permissive hypotension and arterial pressure impulse reduction ("anti-impulse control") similar to the management of aortic dissection or aortic aneurysm rupture. The goal of anti-impulse therapy is to reduce vessel wall sheer stress by preventing tachycardia (HR < 80 BPM) and hypertension (SBP < 120 mm Hg). Beta-blockers such as esmolol and calcium channel blockers such as clevidipine and nicardipine are commonly used medications to achieve anti-impulse control goals.
- Initial nonoperative management with purposeful delay of surgical repair >24 h allows time resuscitation and workup in stable patients with blunt thoracic aortic. Delayed aortic repair is associated with improved survival, regardless of presence or not of major associated injuries [7]. Patients undergoing nonoperative or delayed operative management should receive anti-impulse control therapy.
- Serial CTA should be obtained in patients undergoing initial nonoperative management in order to assess interval progression of injury or pseudoaneurysm formation that would warrant delayed operative or endovascular repair.

Endovascular Repair of Blunt Thoracic Aortic Injury

- Endovascular techniques and devices have made significant advances since their initial FDA approval in 2005 [32].
- Thoracic endovascular aortic repair (TEVAR) is the most common repair approach for blunt thoracic aortic injuries and now considered first-line approach for acute management of blunt aortic injury in patients with small intimal tears, pseudoaneurysm and rupture due to its lower rates of mortality, paraplegia, and stroke [27, 28].
- Preoperative CTA is important in preoperative evaluation prior to endovascular as it helps define: (1) size and extent of vessel injury, (2) angulation of the aortic arch, (3) relationship between the arch aorta, the descending aorta, and origin of the great vessel branches to determine graft placement, (4) diameter of aorta, and (5) diameter of potential access vessels (common superficial femoral and brachial arteries) [32].

- Endovascular approach to great vessel injury includes diagnostic angiography, which is advantageous in identifying occult injuries not seen on preoperative imaging.

Penetrating Thoracic Vessel Injury

- Great vessel injury can occur by blunt or penetrating mechanisms resulting in partial or complete vessel wall injury. Greater than 90% of thoracic vessel injury are due to penetrating or iatrogenic injury [24, 29].
- Due to the significant portion of blood volume within the great vessels, injury can result in rapid life-threatening exsanguination. Most patients with penetrating trauma to the major mediastinal vessels die at the scene [24].
- The majority of patients surviving to the hospital will present with hemodynamic instability and require emergent transfer to the operating room without any diagnostic studies [24].
- Injury to the great vessels can result in external or internal hemorrhage, vascular thrombosis from intimal flaps, acute arteriovenous fistula, or pseudoaneurysms. Therefore, the absence of visible large volume hemorrhage does not rule out a thoracic vessel injury [24].
- A chest tube should be placed in the emergency room if chest X-ray demonstrates the presence of a large hemothorax. Chest tube output greater than 1500 mL of blood over the initial 15 min or sustained bloody output greater than 200 mL per hour for 3–4 consecutive hours are indications for emergent exploratory thoracotomy.

Management of Mediastinal Venous Injuries

- Venous injuries should be immediately occluded with direct compression or vascular clamps to reduce the risk of a potentially lethal intraoperative air embolism.
- Ligation of the innominate vein can be performed for destructive vessel injuries or to improve exposure. Ligation is well tolerated, and transient arm edema is the most common complication [24]. In general, reconstruction of mediastinal veins should be avoided. Repair with lateral venorrhaphy should only be attempted if it can be performed without vessel narrowing in hemodynamically stable patients.
- Repair or reconstruction of the SVC should always be attempted as ligation leads to development of massive brain edema and death.

Sources

1. Mattox KL, Moore EE, Feliciano DV. Trauma. 9th ed. New York: McGraw-Hill; 2020.
2. Kim JS, Inaba K, de Leon LA, et al. Penetrating injury to the cardiac box. J Trauma Acute Care Surg. 2020;89(3):482–7.
3. Demetriades D, Inaba K, Velmahos G. Atlas of surgical techniques in trauma. Cambridge University Press; 2019. https://doi.org/10.1017/9781108698665.
4. Joos E, Tadloc MD, Inaba K. Diagnosis, work-up and management of blunt cardiac injuries. Trauma (London, England). 2014;16(2):93–8. (15).
5. Teixeira PG, Georgiou C, Inaba K, Dubose J, Plurad D, Chan LS, Toms C, Noguchi TT, Demetriades D. Blunt cardiac trauma: lessons learned from the medical examiner. J Trauma. 2009;67(6):1259–64. https://doi.org/10.1097/TA.0b013e318187a2d2. PMID: 20009675..
6. Ismailov RM, Ness RB, Redmond CK, et al. Trauma associated with cardiac dysrhythmias: results from a large matched case-control study. J Trauma. 2007;62:1186–91. (20).
7. Hadjizacharia P, O'Keeffe T, Brown CVR, et al. Incidence, risk factors, and outcomes for atrial arrhythmias in trauma patients. Am Surg. 2011;77:634–9. (21).
8. Bock JS, Benitez MR. Blunt cardiac injury. Cardiol Clin. 2012;30:545–55.
9. Schultz JM, Trunkey DD. Blunt cardiac injury. Crit Care Clin. 2004;20:57–70. (23).
10. Rajan GP, Zellweger R. Cardiac troponin I as a predictor of arrhythmia and ventricular dysfunction in trauma patients with myocardial contusion. J Trauma. 2004;57:801–8. (27).
11. Velmahos GC, Karaiskakis M, Salim A, et al. Normal electrocardiography and serum troponin I levels preclude the presence of clinically significant blunt cardiac injury. J Trauma. 2003;54:45–1. (28).
12. Co SJ, Yong-Hing CJ, Galea-Soler S, et al. Role of imaging in penetrating and blunt traumatic injury to the heart. Radiographics. 2011;31:101–15. (29).
13. Rhee PM, Acosta J, Bridgeman A, Wang D, Jordan M, Rich N. Survival after emergency department thoracotomy: review of published data from the past 25 years. J Am Coll Surg. 2000;190(3):288–98.
14. Wall MJ Jr, Mattox KL, Chen CD, Baldwin JC. Acute management of complex cardiac injuries. J Trauma. 1997;42(5):905–12. (6).
15. Morse BC, Mina MJ, Carr JS, et al. Penetrating cardiac injuries: a 36-year perspective at an urban, Level I trauma center. J Trauma Acute Care Surg. 2016;81(4):623–31. (7).
16. Tang AL, Inaba K, Branco BC, et al. Postdischarge complications after penetrating cardiac injury: a survivable injury with a high postdischarge complication rate. Arch Surg (Chicago 1960). 2011;146(9):1061–6. (45).
17. Demetriades D, van der Veen BW. Penetrating injuries of the heart: experience over two years in South Africa. J Trauma. 1983;23(12):1034–41. (46).
18. Ivatury RR. The injured heart. In: Moore EE, Feliciano DV, Mattox KL, editors. Trauma. 5th ed. New York: McGraw-Hill; 2004. p. 555–68. (13).
19. Ameli S, Shah PK. Cardiac tamponade: pathophysiology, diagnosis, and management. Cardiol Clin. 1991;9:665–74. (11).
20. Hancock EW. Cardiac tamponade. Heart Dis Stroke. 1994;3:155–8. (12).
21. Rozycki GS, Feliciano DV, Ochsner MG, et al. The role of ultrasound in patients with possible penetrating cardiac wounds: a prospective multicenter study. J Trauma Injury Infect Crit Care. 1999;46(4):543–52. (43).
22. Ball CG, Williams BH, Wyrzykowski AD, Nicholas JM, Rozycki GS, Feliciano DV. A caveat to the performance of pericardial ultrasound in patients with penetrating cardiac wounds. J Trauma. 2009;67(5):1123–4. (44).
23. Inaba K, Chouliaras K, Zakaluzny S, Swadron S, Mailhot T, Seif D, Teixeira P, Sivrikoz E, Ives C, Barmparas G, Koronakis N, Demetriades D. FAST ultrasound examination as a predictor of outcomes after resuscitative thoracotomy: a prospective evaluation. Ann Surg. 2015;262(3):512–8; discussion 516–8. (41).
24. Symbas PN. Cardiothoracic trauma. Philadelphia: W. B. Saunders; 1989. (3).

25. Demetriades D, Velmahos GC, Scalea TM, Jurkovich GJ, Karmy-Jones R, Teixeira PG, Hemmila MR, O'Connor JV, McKenney MO, Moore FO, London J, Singh MJ, Spaniolas K, Keel M, Sugrue M, Wahl WL, Hill J, Wall MJ, Moore EE, Lineen E, Margulies D, Malka V, Chan LS. Blunt traumatic thoracic aortic injuries: early or delayed repair—results of an American Association for the Surgery of Trauma prospective study. J Trauma. 2009;66(4):967–73. (9).
26. Waller CJ, Cogbill TH, Kallies KJ, Ramirez LD, Cardenas JM, Todd SR, Chapman KJ, Beckman MA, Sperry JL, Anto VP, Eriksson EA, Leon SM, Anand RJ, Pearlstein M, Capano-Wehrle L, Cothren Burlew C, Fox CJ, Cullinane DC, Roberts JC, Harrison PB, Berg GM, Haan JM, Lightwine K. Contemporary management of subclavian and axillary artery injuries-a Western Trauma Association multicenter review. J Trauma Acute Care Surg. 2017;83(6):1023–31. (47).
27. Demetriades D. Blunt thoracic aortic injuries: crossing the Rubicon. J Am Coll Surg. 2012;214:247. (36).
28. Tang GL, Tehrani HY, Usman A, et al. Reduced mortality, paraplegia, and stroke with stent graft repair of blunt aortic transections: a modern meta-analysis. J Vasc Surg. 2008;47(3):671–5. https://doi.org/10.1016/j.jvs.2007.08.031. (37).
29. Mattox KL, Feliciano DV, Burch J, Beall AC Jr, Jordan GL Jr, De Bakey ME. Five thousand seven hundred sixty cardiovascular injuries in 4459 patients. Epidemiologic evolution 1958 to 1987. Ann Surg. 1989;209(6):698–705; discussion 706–7.
30. Villa M, Sarkaria IS. Great vessel injury in thoracic surgery. Thorac Surg Clin. 2015;25(3):261–78. (32).
31. Wall MJ Jr, Tsai PI, Gilani R, et al. Challenges in the diagnosis of unusual presentations of blunt injury to the ascending aorta and aortic sinuses. J Surg Res. 2010;163:176. (38).
32. Brown C, de Moya M, Brasel K, Hartwell J, Inaba K, Ley E, Moore E, Peck K, Rizzo A, Rosen N, Sperry J, Weinberg J, Moren A, DuBose J, Coimbra R, Martin M. Blunt thoracic aortic injury: a Western Trauma Association critical decisions algorithm. J Trauma Acute Care Surg. 2023;94(1):113–6.

Chapter 35
Lung and Noncardiac Thoracic Injury

Abraham E. Jaffe and Aliyah N. Gaines

Overview

- Traumatic thoracic injuries are widespread and occur in blunt and penetrating trauma
- Potential types of lung and noncardiac thoracic injuries include but are not limited to the following:

  - Rib fractures
  - Sternal fractures
  - Pneumothorax and hemothorax
  - Pulmonary contusion and laceration
  - Esophageal injury
  - Tracheal/airway injury

- Keys to management include early identification and determination of the need for surgical intervention

A. E. Jaffe (✉)
Boston University Chobanian & Avedisian School of Medicine, Division of Trauma & Acute Care Surgery, Boston Medical Center, Boston, MA, USA
e-mail: Abraham.Jaffe@bmc.org

A. N. Gaines
Boston University Chobanian & Avedisian School of Medicine, Boston Medical Center, Boston, MA, USA
e-mail: Aliyah.Gaines@bmc.org

© The Author(s), under exclusive license to Springer Nature Switzerland AG 2025
T. S. Brahmbhatt, D. R. Scantling (eds.), *Trauma Surgery Clerkship*, Contemporary Surgical Clerkships,
https://doi.org/10.1007/978-3-032-01412-2_35

Epidemiology

Thoracic injury following trauma is widespread, occurring in approximately 20% of all trauma patients and accounts for 25% of trauma-related deaths. Approximately 70% of thoracic injuries, especially chest wall trauma, are associated with blunt trauma [1]. The incidence of specific injuries will vary by anatomical location and mechanism of injury.

Two or more rib fractures can be identified in 10% of patients with multisystem trauma and 39% with blunt chest trauma. High morbidity is associated with these injuries, including the need for mechanical ventilation, pneumonia, prolonged length of stay, chronic pain, and disability [2].

Pulmonary contusion is the most identified lung injury, seen in 30%–75% of blunt chest traumas with a mortality rate of 10%–25%. Pulmonary contusion is particularly common in children, who tend to have more flexible chest bones that are less prone to fracture, resulting in large forces transmitted to the lung tissue and significantly more severe contusions [3].

Pneumothorax occurs in 40%–50% of patients with thoracic trauma and is the most common cause of hemothorax [4]. Approximately 16,000–30,000 deaths per year are due to trauma-associated hemothorax. The hemothorax can result from bleeding of the lung parenchyma, chest wall, or major vessels within the chest leading to hemorrhagic shock and death if untreated [5].

In contrast to other thoracic injuries, traumatic aerodigestive injury is rare. Among trauma patients, the incidence of esophageal injury is less than 10% and occurs more frequently in penetrating thoracic injuries. Furthermore, the most common injury site is the cervical esophagus, which is less protected than the thoracic esophagus [6]. Trauma to the intrathoracic trachea and airway tree occurs in approximately 2%–3% of cervical or thoracic trauma patients. These injuries carry a high level of mortality, with most patients dying at the scene. Only 0.5%–0.9% of these patients will arrive at the trauma bay for evaluation. Like the esophagus, there is intrinsic protection by rigid surrounding structures, including the sternum, rib cage, and thoracic spine. Nevertheless, penetrating trauma and significant blunt forces can disrupt these structures with potentially fatal clinical consequences [7].

Pathophysiology

Trauma patients with suspected thoracic injury should undergo a primary survey and initial stabilization and resuscitation as outlined via ATLS guidelines (discussed in a previous chapter). The secondary survey includes an assessment for external signs of injury, equal chest rise, and auscultation of bilateral breath sounds. Key findings suggesting chest wall trauma and the likely correlating diagnosis are listed in Table 35.1.

Table 35.1   Key secondary exam findings

Suspected diagnosis	Physical exam finding
Tension pneumothorax	Absent unilateral breath sounds + Jugular vein distension + tracheal deviation
Non-tension pneumothorax or hemothorax	Absent/decreased unilateral breath sounds WITHOUT Jugular vein distension + tracheal deviation
Flail chest	Paradoxical chest wall motion

The above findings are suggestive of significant chest wall injury. Adjunct to the secondary survey is rapid radiographic evaluation via chest X-ray (CXR). Initial CXR should be completed to rapidly assess for pneumothorax, hemothorax, rib fractures, or widening of the mediastinum. The addition of an Extended Focused Assessment with Sonography in Trauma (eFAST) exam with the absence of lung sliding can further indicate the presence of pneumothorax or hemothorax [2].

Rib Fracture and Flail Chest

Rib fractures are often secondary to blunt or penetrating trauma. As stated previously, most rib fractures can be identified on plain CXR. However, computed tomography (CT) scan carries superior sensitivity and specificity with precise identification and localization of rib fractures. As the number of rib fractures increases, so do morbidity and mortality. Simple, single, non-displaced fractures, even if multiple, are often tolerated well in the absence of underlying cardiopulmonary pathology. The most common site of rib fractures are ribs 4–10. Injuries to ribs 1–3 are associated with blunt cerebrovascular injury and indicative of significant trauma, given that they are the most difficult to break. Injury to ribs 9–12 is often associated with injuries to abdominal organs such as the spleen or liver. Significantly posterior rib fractures (within 3 cm of the transverse process) tend to have the least morbidity and mortality as the erector spinae muscles often stabilize the fractures [2, 8].

Flail chest can be defined clinically or anatomically. *Anatomic* flail chest is a *flail segment* consisting of one or more ribs fractured in two or more places and thus disconnected from the thoracic cage. *Clinical* flail chest is a paradoxical chest wall motion where the chest wall moves inward during inspiration. Clinical flail chest can present with or without a flail segment. It can present in severely displaced contiguous or bilateral rib fractures near the sternum. Both clinical and anatomical flail chest carry significant morbidity and mortality, between 10% and 15% [8]. Flail chest is often associated with pulmonary contusion, hemothorax, and/or pneumothorax.

Sternal Fracture

Sternal fractures are most often associated with motor vehicle crashes. One-fourth of sternal fractures are isolated, and the remaining three-fourth often coincide with other injuries (i.e., extremity fracture, head/neck injury, rib fracture, spine injury, pulmonary contusions). The most feared but least common (less than 2%) associated injuries are blunt cardiac injury (discussed in another chapter) and great vessel injuries. Given the significant mortality and morbidity associated with blunt cardiac and great vessel injury, a patient with concern for sternal fracture should be promptly evaluated with CT angiography, EKG, and echocardiogram [2].

Pneumothorax

Pneumothorax occurs when air enters the pleural space resulting in the separation of visceral and parietal pleura. Pneumothorax can be occult (seen on CT but not identified on CXR), small (lung line <2 cm from chest wall on CXR), or large (lung line >2 cm from the chest wall). Pneumothorax due to blunt trauma is secondary to alveolar rupture, acceleration and deceleration injury, or rib fractures damaging the pleura [1]. Penetrating trauma can cause pneumothorax due to violation of the pleura and introduce air into the pleural space. Traumatic, iatrogenic pneumothorax can occur during resuscitative procedures in the trauma bay (i.e., central line placement in the internal jugular or subclavian vein, positive pressure ventilation) [2]. At presentation, patients may present with chest pain, dyspnea, anxiety, tachypnea, tachycardia, and hyperresonance with decreased respiratory sounds on the affected side. If left without intervention, the presentation can progress to decreased consciousness, tracheal deviation, hypotension, distension of cervical veins, and cyanosis.

In tension pneumothorax, the creation of a one-way valve occurs, causing air to enter the pleural space with inspiration and be trapped in the pleural space. Continuous accumulation of air in the pleura collapses the lung resulting in severe hypoxia. Concurrent hypotension occurs secondary to heart compression as air accumulates within pleural space. Any pneumothorax, spontaneous, iatrogenic, or traumatic, can progress into a tension pneumothorax. Tension pneumothorax is always a clinical, not radiological, diagnosis. When identified, rapid intervention should ensue [2].

Clinical findings and physical examination are precious in the rapid identification of pneumothorax. However, as discussed earlier, imaging methods play an important role. CXR can often be sufficient for identifying pneumothorax. However, in occult pneumothorax, the air in the pleural cavity may not be visible on CXR. Occult pneumothorax occurs in 2%–20% of patients with blunt trauma [1]. In addition, occult pneumothorax can develop in 51% of trauma patients and may progress to clinically significant non-tension or tension pneumothorax. Therefore, there should be high suspicion of occult pneumothorax in patients with subcutaneous emphysema, rib fractures, and pulmonary contusion. These patients, if stable, should be thoroughly evaluated via CT scan [9]. For patients not appropriate for presentation to CT, ultrasound can be utilized with a sensitivity of 98.1% and specificity of 99.2% [1].

Hemothorax

Hemothorax is the accumulation of blood within the pleural space. This blood can be secondary to blunt or penetrating trauma of the chest wall and intercostal arteries, intraparenchymal pulmonary vessels, diaphragmatic or abdominal injury, and cardiac or mediastinal large vessel rupture. The presentation's severity depends on the location of the injury, patient functional reserve, blood volume, and accumulation rate. Hemothorax can develop in the presence or absence of rib fracture or with concurrent pneumothorax [1, 2, 10].

Blood in the pleural space will diminish the lung's functional vital capacity by creating alveolar hypoventilation, V/Q mismatch, and anatomic shunting. A large hemothorax can increase hydrostatic pressure and exert pressure in the vena cava and pulmonary parenchyma, resulting in reduced preload and increased pulmonary vascular resistance. Large hemothorax can thus create a physiologic presentation resembling tension hemothorax and cause hemodynamic instability, cardiovascular collapse, and death without intervention [10].

Clinical findings of hemothorax often overlap with signs and symptoms associated with pneumothorax, including respiratory distress, tachypnea, and decreased or absent breath sounds. Dullness to percussion is often present secondary to blood accumulation within the pleura. On CXR, opacification of the entire chest can be seen if the patient is supine. On eFAST, oblique views of both hemidiaphragm can evaluate for dependent fluid suggestive of hemothorax [10].

Retained or residual hemothorax can occur without tube thoracostomy within 48–72 h of injury or insufficient blood drainage. A retained clot in the pleural space can result in post-traumatic empyema or the accumulation of adhesions and impaired lung function [1, 2].

Pulmonary Parenchymal Injury

The two most common pulmonary parenchymal traumatic injuries are pulmonary contusion and laceration. A pulmonary contusion occurs because of the transmission of kinetic energy to the lung parenchyma, resulting in destruction of lung parenchyma and subsequent alveolar hemorrhage, inflammation, and edema of pulmonary tissue even without laceration or disruption of the parenchyma or pleura. This bleeding and edema can be severe and lead to disruption of oxygenation resulting in hypoxia. Parenchymal destruction will peak within the first 24 h of injury. In the instance of severe blunt thoracic trauma, the presence of a pulmonary contusion should always be suspected. These patients can experience chest pain, dyspnea, and tachypnea on presentation. Hypoxemia and hypercarbia may occur, especially in contusions associated with other injuries. For this reason, an argument can be made that early intubation in severe cases of pulmonary contusion is warranted to prevent clinically significant hypoxia, hypercarbia, and increased mortality. The overall mortality of pulmonary contusion varies between 10% and 25%. Concomitant injuries contribute significantly to this mortality. Pulmonary contusion is usually associated with concurrent rib fractures. However, pulmonary contusion can occur without rib fractures, especially in pediatric patients [1].

It can be challenging to diagnose pulmonary contusion based on clinical findings alone as the presentation is variable, and some patients may be initially asymptomatic. Historically, CXR was the initial modality for diagnostic imaging. However, in greater than one-third of patients, contusion may not be visualized on CXR. CT provides much higher sensitivity for the diagnosis of pulmonary contusion. Pulmonary contusion increases the risk of pneumonia or progression to Acute Respiratory Distress Syndrome (ARDS). Noncomplex pulmonary contusion recovery may be observed on CXR as early as 48–72 h post-injury. However, complete recovery can take up to 14 days [1].

Pulmonary laceration involves the disruption of the parenchymal tissue of the lung and is usually caused by penetrating injuries. Unlike pulmonary contusion, which is very common in blunt chest trauma, the incidence of pulmonary laceration in blunt chest trauma varies between 4% and 12% [1]. Pulmonary lacerations usually overlap with concomitant pulmonary contusions, making it challenging to identify lacerations on CXR. CT scan is thus the imaging modality with the highest sensitivity. Pulmonary lacerations can result in bleeding, respiratory distress, and air leakage. If the laceration extends into the pleural cavity, hemothorax or pneumothorax may develop. Pneumatocele may develop if air enters pulmonary cavities, and hemato-pneumatocele may occur if air and blood enter these spaces. Respiratory sounds can be decreased on the side of pulmonary laceration [1].

Tracheal/Airway Injury

Tracheal and airway injury can result from penetrating trauma, blunt trauma, or iatrogenic causes in the trauma patient. Injuries can be divided into cervical and thoracic. Thoracic injury includes the thoracic trachea, carina, and mainstem bronchi. Penetrating injury is more common than blunt injury in the cervical trachea as it is more exposed and accessible. Blunt tracheal and airway injury is less common but often occurs at the intrathoracic tracheal and airway tree levels, most common at the carina and mainstem bronchi levels. Injuries can include transverse or longitudinal tears (75% vs. 18% of cases, respectively), partial or complete tears, cartilage fractures, dislocations, or airway avulsion. Blunt intrathoracic tracheal and airway injury can be secondary to high energy or direct impact on the structure. Iatrogenic tracheal injuries can occur from endotracheal intubation or overinflation of the endotracheal tube balloon [7].

The clinical presentation of tracheal and airway injury can range from subtle to life-threatening airway obstruction or tension pneumothorax. Because penetrating injuries are generally more apparent, a high level of clinical suspicion for detection in the context of blunt trauma is required. Classic signs of tracheal or airway injury include stridor, air moving through the wound, subcutaneous emphysema, and hemoptysis. Unexplained persistent pneumothorax, pneumomediastinum, subcutaneous emphysema, or difficulty with ventilation or oxygenation should raise suspicion for tracheal and airway injury. In the setting of penetrating injury, the presence of hard signs (air or bubbling from the wound, stridor) may warrant operative exploration. However, in blunt injury, additional diagnostic testing is indicated most often. Definitive diagnosis requires a combination of clinical suspicion about the presence and likely location of the injury and imaging modalities to confirm the diagnosis and define the injury [7].

Initial CXR is abnormal in 80%–90% of patients, with common findings including pneumothorax, pneumomediastinum, and subcutaneous emphysema. Near-complete airway transection with intact adventitia may not show typical radiographic findings indicative of airway disruption, so a high level of suspicion, along with direct airway visualization, is imperative. On CT scan, bronchial step-offs, fluid within the bronchial tree, locules of air outside the airway, pneumomediastinum, pneumopericardium, or pneumothorax can be identified. The gold standard for diagnosing traumatic tracheal and airway injury is fiberoptic bronchoscopy with direct visualization of the airway and injury. Flexible bronchoscopy is highly accurate, sensitive, and specific in identifying tracheal and airway injury [7].

Existing or impending airway compromise, secondary to edema or from the injury, often make securing the airway of utmost importance early in evaluating patients with suspected tracheal and airway injury. Direct or video laryngoscopy to visualize the larynx and vocal cords can be utilized. Blind intubations should always be avoided, given the potential to disrupt the airway further and cause complete obstruction. Awake endotracheal or nasotracheal intubation over a bronchoscope is often preferred. Awake intubation allows for successful airway management and direct visualization of the injury. Awake intubation with fiberoptic bronchoscopy typically does not require head and neck extension, preventing further disruption of the injured airway and protecting the cervical spine [7].

Esophageal Injury

Blunt or penetrating traumatic injury of the thoracic esophagus is rare. The mediastinum and trachea protect the thoracic esophagus. However, the presence of esophageal perforation is uniformly fatal if left without appropriate management. Even with prompt diagnosis and management, mortality rates range from 15% and 20%

[5]. Adequate source control, sepsis eradication, and intensive care management are required to ensure and maximize survival. Esophageal perforation results in extravasation of oral and gastric secretions into the mediastinum and rapid and progressive subsequent inflammatory response. Symptoms depend on the anatomic location of the perforation, the time since inciting injury, and other patient comorbidities. Chest pain is often the most common complaint; however, patients may also have dysphagia or dysphonia. Tachycardia is present secondary to the significant mediastinal inflammatory response [11].

Diagnostic imaging is needed to confirm and localize esophageal perforation. CXR may show nonspecific findings like pleural effusion, subcutaneous emphysema, pneumomediastinum, or hydropneumothorax. However, in most individuals, CXR may appear normal. Thus, the gold standard of evaluation is barium esophagography; however, there are low risks of false-negative assessment. Endoscopy can be utilized to directly identify the anatomic location of the injury, associated pathologic changes of the esophagus, and assessment of the esophagus distal to the injury [11].

Current Management Practices

Rib and Sternal Fractures

- Mainstay of treatment is pain control (see Table 35.2) and pulmonary hygiene
- Isolated rib fractures: Conservative therapy is usually adequate (pain control, rest)
- Adequate pain control encourages good ventilation to help prevent:

Table 35.2 Example of standardized pain regimen in setting of multiple rib fractures, options for management of refractory pain from rib fractures, and indications for surgical rib fixation

Standardized pain regimen in setting of multiple rib fractures	Refractory pain (pain score >6 despite standardized pain regimen)
Acetaminophen 650 mg q6h Ibuprofen 600 mg q6h Gabapentin 300 mg q8h Oxycodone 5 mg q6h prn	Intercostal block or paracostal infusion catheter Ketamine drip IV narcotics (i.e., patient-controlled analgesia) Epidural catheter
Indications for surgical rib fixation [2, 5]	
Flail chest (anatomic or clinical) ≥3 displaced rib fractures Pain score >6 despite medical management Respiratory insufficiency requiring ICU transfer or intubation Concurrent thoracotomy for another indication Chronic nonunion or malunion of fracture Lung impalement Three or more rib fractures with displacement Pulmonary herniation	

- Splinting
- Pulmonary atelectasis
- Pneumonia
- Acute respiratory failure and need for intubation

- Important to minimize narcotic use and decrease risk of:

  - Sedation
  - Respiratory depression
  - Cough suppression
  - Hypotension
  - Constipation

- Surgical rib fixation can be considered in select patients (see Table 35.2)

Pneumothorax

- Gold standard treatment is tube thoracostomy
- ATLS recommends tube thoracostomy for all traumatic pneumothorax cases due to the risk of tension pneumothorax
- If mechanical ventilation support is required, the risk of tension pneumothorax increases
- Occult pneumothorax: If patient remains stable and asymptomatic continuous monitoring is recommended
- Tension pneumothorax is ALWAYS a clinical diagnosis

  - Emergent tube thoracostomy should be performed if identified
  - If delay in chest tube placement, consider angiocatheter decompression first

Hemothorax

- Gold standard of treatment is tube thoracostomy
- Irrigation of the pleural cavity with 1 L of warmed sterile saline within first 24 h of chest tube placement can reduce need for additional intervention and reduce risk of retained hemothorax
- Massive hemothorax (blood loss of 1.5 L or continuous blood loss of >200 mL/h for 2–4 h) may warrant urgent thoracotomy to control hemorrhage

Pulmonary Parenchymal Injury

- Pulmonary contusion

- – Mainstay of treatment is supportive therapy

  - Close monitoring of vital signs
  - Oxygen support
  - Pain control
  - Early mobilization
  - Chest physiotherapy

- – Euvolemia is imperative; fluid overload can worsen pulmonary edema and lead to respiratory distress and hypoxemia
- – Noninvasive respiratory support preferred over intubation given increased risk of barotrauma and pneumonia

- Pulmonary laceration

  - – Severity of laceration varies and will dictate treatment
  - – Tube thoracostomy recommended if associated pneumothorax or hemothorax
  - – Hemodynamic instability secondary to parenchymal bleeding is rare but may require surgical intervention or IR angioembolization

Tracheal/Airway Injury

- Key to initial management is securing the airway without expansion of injury
- Location and severity of injury will dictate management
- Intervention criteria:

  - – Presence of pneumothorax or hemothorax
  - – Air leaks that do not resolve with chest tube
  - – Injury >1/3 airway circumference or defect >2 cm

- Nonoperative management can be considered in select stable patients

  - – Humidified air, voice rest, antibiotics, PPI
  - – Repeat interval bronchoscopy

- Operative management criteria:

  - – Hemodynamically or respiratory unstable
  - – Failure of nonoperative management
  - – Large injuries or injuries with devitalized tissue require debridement, resection, and reconstruction

    - Endotracheal/endobronchial tube placement distal to injury post-repair if possible (avoids direct positive pressure ventilation and allows healing)

Esophageal Injury

- Basic principles of management:

  - Control of leak
  - Infection drainage
  - Sepsis eradication
  - Maintenance of gastrointestinal continuity and nutrition

- Operative intervention often required; approach and procedure depend on location and nature of injury, general principles include the following:

  - Debridement of devitalized tissue
  - Two-layer repair of esophagus
  - Wide drainage
  - Alternative means of nutrition

- Nonoperative management can be considered in patients with small, contained perforations who are hemodynamically stable with minimal symptoms
- Nonoperative therapy includes the following:

  - Nasogastric decompression
  - Broad-spectrum antibiotics
  - Percutaneous drainage
  - Nutritional support

Take-Home Points for Patient Care

- Traumatic thoracic injuries are widespread and occur in both blunt and penetrating trauma.
- Adequate multimodal pain control is imperative in the management of rib fractures.
- Surgical rib fixation can be considered in select patients with flail chest or multiple displaced rib fractures and associated respiratory failure.
- Tube thoracostomy is the mainstay of treatment for pneumothorax and hemothorax, except when very small.
- Tension pneumothorax is a clinical diagnosis and requires emergent decompression.
- Massive hemothorax (blood loss of 1.5 L or continuous blood loss of >200 mL/h for 2–4 h) may warrant urgent thoracotomy to control hemorrhage.
- Pulmonary contusion and laceration vary in severity, and management is based on clinical findings.

- Injuries to the trachea and airway are rare, can be difficult to identify, and require a high degree of suspicion and care not to disrupt the airway further.
- Traumatic injury of the thoracic esophagus is rare but often requires surgical intervention and carries a high mortality rate without appropriate management.

References

1. Dogrul BN, Kiliccalan I, Asci ES, Peker SC. Blunt trauma related chest wall and pulmonary injuries: an overview. Chin J Traumatol. 2020;23(03):125–38.
2. Semon G, McCarthy M. Chest wall, pneumothorax, and hemothorax. In: Cameron AM, Cameron JL, editors. Current surgical therapy. 13th ed. Philadelphia: Elsevier; 2020. p. 1146–50.
3. Choudhary S, Pasrija D, Mendez MD. Pulmonary contusion. [Updated 2022 Aug 22]. In: StatPearls [Internet]. Treasure Island (FL): StatPearls Publishing; 2022. Available from: https://www.ncbi.nlm.nih.gov/books/NBK558914/.
4. Tran J, Haussner W, Shah K. Traumatic pneumothorax: a review of current diagnostic practices and evolving management. J Emerg Med. 2021;61(5):517–28.
5. Zeiler J, Idell S, Norwood S, Cook A. Hemothorax: a review of the literature. Clin Pulm Med. 2020;27(1):1.
6. Schraufnagel DP, Mubashir M, Raymond DP. Non-iatrogenic esophageal trauma: a narrative review. Mediastinum. 2022;6:23.
7. Antonescu I, Mani VR, Agarwal S. Traumatic injuries to the trachea and bronchi: a narrative review. Mediastinum. 2022;6:22 https://doi.org/10.21037/med-21-21. PMID: 36164365; PMCID: PMC9385878.
8. Kuo K, Kim AM. Rib fracture. [Updated 2022 Aug 8]. In: StatPearls [Internet]. Treasure Island (FL): StatPearls Publishing; 2022. Available from: https://www.ncbi.nlm.nih.gov/books/NBK541020/.
9. McKnight CL, Burns B. Pneumothorax. [Updated 2022 Aug 8]. In: StatPearls [Internet]. Treasure Island (FL): StatPearls Publishing; 2022. Available from: https://www.ncbi.nlm.nih.gov/books/NBK441885/.
10. Pumarejo Gomez L, Tran VH. Hemothorax. [Updated 2022 Aug 8]. In: StatPearls [Internet]. Treasure Island (FL): StatPearls Publishing; 2022. Available from: https://www.ncbi.nlm.nih.gov/books/NBK538219/.
11. Lambright E. Management of esophageal perforation. In: Cameron AM, Cameron JL, editors. Current surgical therapy. 13th ed. Philadelphia: Elsevier; 2020. p. 78–80.

Chapter 36
Diaphragm Injury

Andrew W. Wang and Bradley M. Dennis

Overview

- The diaphragm is a large, fibromuscular, thoracoabdominal structure that separates the thoracic and peritoneal cavities.
- Injury to the diaphragm is uncommon in the traumatically injured patient and found more commonly in penetrating than blunt trauma.
- Diagnosis requires a high index of suspicion in the evaluation of a trauma to avoid future morbidity, which is very high in the setting of a delayed presentation of a missed injury.
- There is limited role for nonoperative management of diaphragm injuries; most will require operative repair.

Epidemiology

The diaphragm is uncommonly injured in the traumatically injured patient and is found in approximately 5% of blunt trauma patients and 10%–15% of patients with a penetrating mechanism of trauma.

- In patients found to have traumatic injury to the diaphragm, 2/3 of cases involve penetrating trauma in comparison to the 1/3 of cases with a blunt mechanism. Motor vehicle collisions, falls from height, and crush injuries particularly in the elderly are at high risk for blunt injury to the diaphragm.

A. W. Wang (✉) · B. M. Dennis
Vanderbilt University Medical Center, Nashville, TN, USA
e-mail: bradley.m.dennis@vumc.org

© The Author(s), under exclusive license to Springer Nature
Switzerland AG 2025
T. S. Brahmbhatt, D. R. Scantling (eds.), *Trauma Surgery Clerkship*,
Contemporary Surgical Clerkships,
https://doi.org/10.1007/978-3-032-01412-2_36

- Over 80% of cases are identified in male patients.
- Approximately 2/3 of injuries to the diaphragm are left sided. Injury to the right diaphragm in both blunt and penetrating trauma is associated with a higher degree of mortality due to the highly vascular structures (liver, inferior vena cava) intimately involved with the right side of the structure.
- Conventional imaging modalities including CT scan have limited sensitivity in the detection of diaphragmatic injury and many, up to 2/3 of injuries, may be missed during the index presentation.

Pathophysiology

Anatomy

The diaphragm is a unique anatomical structure in the human body. Understanding external landmarks that approximate diaphragm location is important for managing traumatic thoracoabdominal injuries.

- It is a dynamic organ with positional variation during the respiratory cycle.
- Externally, the diaphragm roughly extends from the nipples to the costal margins anteriorly and from the inferior tip of the bilateral scapulae to the costal margins bilaterally
- The diaphragm attaches to the xiphoid anteriorly, the underside of the 6th through 12th ribs laterally, and lumbar vertebra posteriorly.
- From the cartilage of the lumbar vertebrae extend two fibromuscular structures that wrap around the esophagus and insert on the central tendon. These structures are known as the left and right diaphragmatic crus. The left and right crus originate on either side of the aorta creating the aortic hiatus.
- The aorta passes posterior to the diaphragm at the level of L1 (Fig. 36.1). Proximal control of the supraceliac aorta can be achieved at this level, a hemorrhage control maneuver sometimes facilitated by the division of the right diaphragmatic crus.
- Centrally the diaphragm forms a dome arching into a fibromuscular central tendon underlying the pericardium. It receives innervation via the phrenic nerves bilaterally, which arise from the C3 to C5 cervical nerve roots and traverse the middle mediastinum along the lateral pericardium to divide into four main trunks bilaterally at or above the dome of the diaphragm.
- The inferior vena cava (IVC), esophagus, and aorta all traverse the diaphragm through separate portals, the IVC foramen, the esophageal foramen, and the aortic hiatus, respectively.

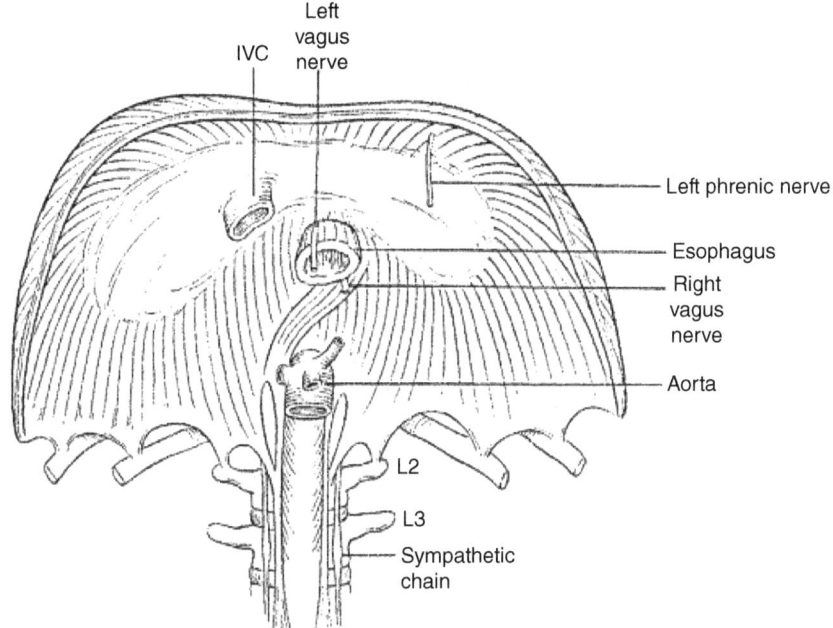

Fig. 36.1 Diaphragm anatomy demonstrating the IVC and esophageal foramen and aortic hiatus as well as posterior attachments to the inferior ribs and lumbar vertebrae. (Reproduced with permission from [1])

Penetrating Injury

Penetrating injuries to the thoracoabdominal region place the diaphragm at risk for injury. Penetrating wounds between the nipple and the umbilicus circumferentially place the diaphragm at risk. Trajectory of penetrating injuries should be evaluated to determine if they have potential to cross the diaphragm.

- Penetrating injuries to the diaphragm are typically focal and often small. They can easily be missed without a high index of suspicion. The left diaphragm is more commonly injured in cases of penetrating trauma thought to be related to the higher proportion assaults inflicted by the right hand of individuals.

Blunt Injury

- Blunt injury to the diaphragm occurs via massive acute pressure rise in the intraabdominal cavity transferred to the dome of the diaphragm, resulting in disruption.

- Injuries due to blunt trauma are typically large tears arranged in a radial orientation extending from centrally to peripherally. Lateral impacts place the diaphragm at risk for avulsion from the chest wall.
- A common pattern of injury occurs posterior-laterally between the aortic hiatus and the spleen due to developmental weakness. The left diaphragm is thought by some to be less developmentally robust than the right side thus contributing to the higher frequency of injury on the left in blunt trauma. The right diaphragm is reinforced and bolstered by the liver, which absorbs and dissipates an acute rise in intraperitoneal pressure over a greater surface area of the diaphragm in blunt trauma. Thus, significantly greater force is required for disruption of the right hemidiaphragm compared to the left, resulting is greater prehospital mortality in patients with right-sided injuries.
- This survival bias is likely the greatest contributor toward the observed predominance of left-sided injuries in patients who arrive to the hospital alive.

Associated Injuries

- Injuries associated with both penetrating and blunt diaphragmatic injury include those to the heart, lungs, aorta, IVC, ribs, stomach, spleen, liver, small bowel, colon, pancreas, and kidneys. Injury to the diaphragm implies multicavity injury to both the thoracic and peritoneal spaces and therefore should be considered a marker of significant trauma burden.
- Traumatic diaphragm injury carries a mortality rate up to 25% in the injured patient.
- The most common concomitant injury seen in blunt diaphragm trauma is pelvic fractures in approximately 40% of patients followed by solid organ injury (liver and spleen) in roughly 25% of patients.

Acute Presentation and Diagnosis

- Patients with acute traumatic injury to the diaphragm have a high degree of variation in their presentation owing to the differences in blunt versus penetrating mechanisms of injury and presence or absence of associated injuries.
- Rarely, patients can present in respiratory distress or with a picture of obstructive shock owing to the presence of herniated abdominal contents in the chest approximating a tension pneumothorax physiology.
- Exceedingly rare cases in blunt trauma include visceral herniation through the central tendon into the pericardium approximating the obstructive shock picture of pericardial tamponade. On physical exam, a pathognomonic finding is the auscultation of breath sounds in the chest.

- On plain films of the chest and/or abdomen, the sharp contour of the diaphragm may be lost or blunted (Fig. 36.2). Air-filled loops of bowel can occasionally be seen in the thoracic domain most commonly in the left hemithorax. An orogastric or nasogastric tube seen above the level of the diaphragm is a classic radiographic finding suggesting injury to the diaphragm.
- However, nearly half of all plain films in patients with traumatic diaphragm injury appear normal. Therefore, any abnormality on chest X-ray in the traumatically injured patient may suggest the presence of a diaphragm injury.
- CT scan is the best imaging modality for identifying diaphragm injuries. It is specific for diaphragm injury especially in the presence of intrabdominal contents visualized above the diaphragm in the thorax.
- A "collar sign" or narrowing of herniated structures can demonstrate the region of disruption in the diaphragm (Fig. 36.3). However, the sensitivity of this CT for diagnosis is limited to approximately 80%. Axial imaging should be thoroughly inspected for injury for associated structures, which may point to concomitant

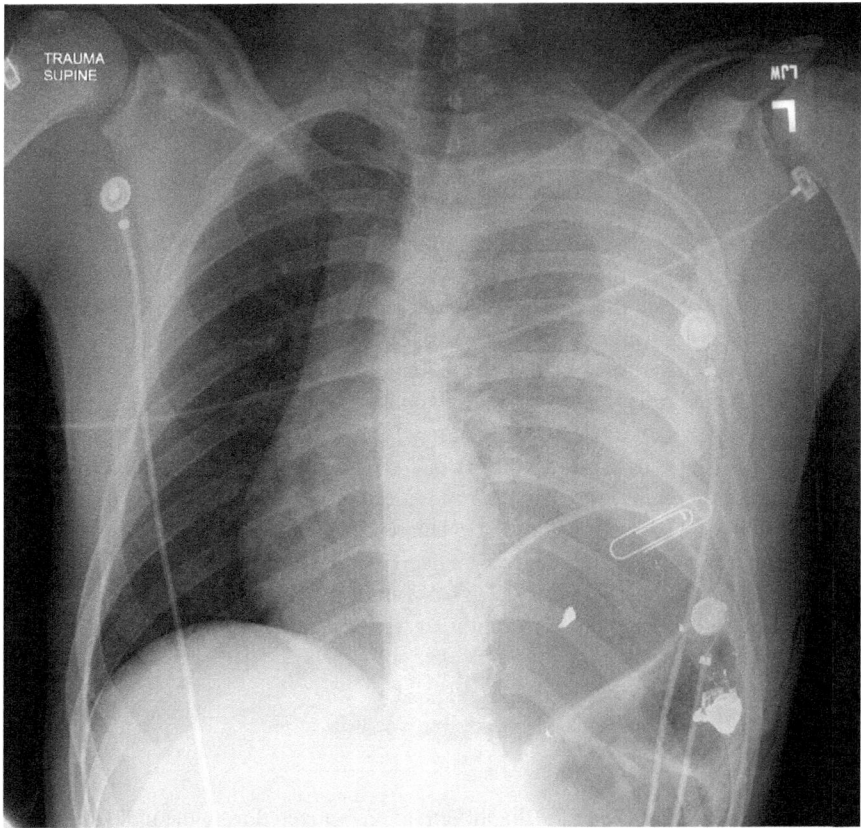

Fig. 36.2 Chest film demonstrating ballistic injury to the left upper quadrant with associated hemothorax, elevation of the left hemidiaphragm, and visceral structures in the left chest

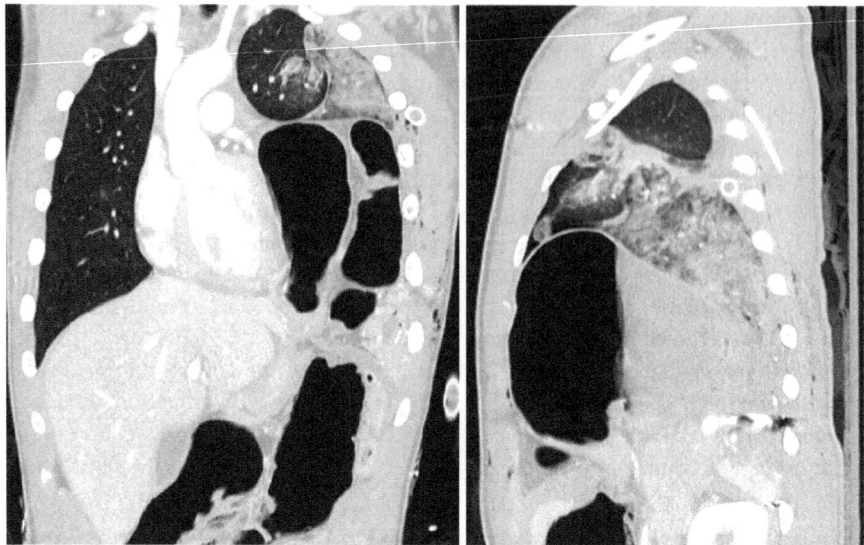

Fig. 36.3 Coronal and sagittal CT scan of the patient in Fig. 36.2 demonstrating traumatic rupture of the left hemidiaphragm with stomach, colon, and small bowel herniated into the chest

diaphragm injury in patients with suggestive mechanisms for thoracoabdominal injury. Sagittal and coronal reconstructions can demonstrate contour irregularity or interruption in the continuity of the diaphragm.

- Most injuries to the diaphragm are diagnosed intraoperatively in patients with associated injuries requiring operative intervention. The diaphragm should be carefully inspected both visually and via palpation during operative intervention when concern for injury exists.
- In patients with penetrating thoracoabdominal injuries concerning the possibility of diaphragm injury, laparoscopy is a valuable adjunct for further evaluation with a negative predictive value approaching 100%.
- Video-assisted thoracoscopic surgery (VATS) is another tool available for diagnosis of diaphragm injury and may provide superior views of the posterior sulci, particularly on the right compared to laparoscopy due to the presence of the liver.
- Detection requires a high degree of suspicion to avoid the potential high degree of morbidity associated with the risk of future herniation of intraabdominal viscera leading to ischemia, perforation, and even death.

Chronic/Missed Injuries

- Patients with an injury to the diaphragm unrecognized during the index presentation may present in a delayed fashion often months to years subsequent from the inciting traumatic event. This is thought to represent a gradual process as the

negative intrathoracic pressure during the respiratory cycle gradually draws visceral structures into the chest.
- In fact, acute injuries may initially be masked in patients requiring positive pressure ventilation during the acute phase of their trauma resuscitation.
- Similar to acute diaphragm injury, the presentation of chronic diaphragm injury is highly variable ranging from the asymptomatic, incidental finding on routine chest X-ray to the unstable patient in extremis resulting from the delayed herniation of visceral structures through the defect and resultant visceral ischemia.
- Mortality in these patients is high exceeding 1/3 of patients in some series and as high as 50% in patients with visceral ischemia at presentation.

Operative Repair

- The diaphragm does not spontaneously heal without defect following traumatic injury. Therefore, except for carefully selected penetrating injuries to the right diaphragm, which are at low risk for future visceral herniation due to the bolstering presence of the liver, traumatic diaphragm injuries should be surgically repaired. Principles of operative repair include the reduction of herniated contents back to their native domain along with restoration of the continuity of the fibromuscular septum between the chest and abdomen. This is most common achieved with a tension free, watertight, primary suture repair following the debridement of tissue edges back to viable tissue.
- To facilitate visualization and repair, the edges of the defect are grasped with allis clamps to bring the diaphragm into the operative field from below the costal margin and evert the tissue edges (Fig. 36.4). Care should be taken to ensure all layers of the diaphragm are included in the suture to prevent subsequent hernia formation later. In the absence of significant tissue loss or devitalization, mesh is not commonly required.
- However, higher grade injuries may require use of biologic mesh and/or tissue transfer techniques to secure the diaphragm to adjacent ribs. Controversy exists regarding the use of suture material and running or interrupted techniques. However, there is no objective evidence to support the use of one suture material and/or technique over another. It is commonly accepted that permanent suture should be used as recurrences are seen with the use of absorbable suture. Especially in the presence of significant contamination of the chest from injury to hollow viscus organs, the chest should be irrigated and thoracostomy tube(s) should be placed.
- The operative approach may be via open or minimally invasive (thoracoscopy or laparoscopy) techniques.
- In cases of isolated diaphragm injury, laparoscopic repair is the favored approach. However, the approach to individual cases is commonly dictated by a combination of surgeon preference along with the presence of concomitant injuries in the chest or abdomen.

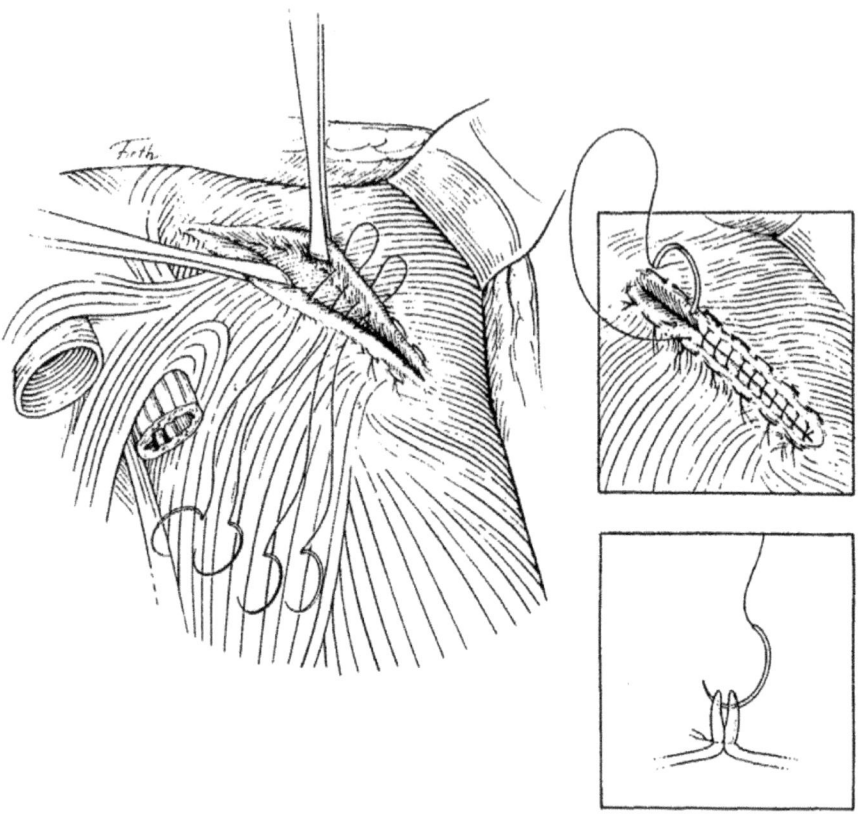

Fig. 36.4 Primary repair of diaphragm laceration incorporating full thickness of the diaphragm in a watertight closure using permanent suture. (Reproduced with permission from [1])

- The operative repair of missed or chronic diaphragm injuries is similar in principle to the techniques deployed in the acute setting. However, often more complex repairs requiring insertion of mesh prosthesis and/or tissue transfer techniques are required to achieve a tension-free, watertight closure due to tissue atrophy and retraction of the diaphragm over time.
- Similarly, visceral ischemia requiring concomitant bowel resection can also complicate repairs in this setting. Some surgeons suggest that a thoracic approach to the operative management of chronic diaphragm injuries is favored owing to the tenacious adhesions between visceral and thoracic structures that commonly form from the absence of a peritoneal lined hernia sac due to the traumatic mechanism of the inciting injury. A dual cavity approach may be required for these repairs.

Current Management Practice

- Left-sided, penetrating injuries to the diaphragm require operative repair.
- A minimally invasive approach to repair of isolated injuries is favored. Associated injuries are often present and may require an open approach.
- Diagnostic laparoscopy is superior to CT to evaluate for diaphragm injury in left-sided, penetrating thoracoabdominal injuries.
- Thoracoscopy may be superior to laparoscopy to evaluate the diaphragm in right-sided posterior, penetrating thoracoabdominal injuries.
- Nonoperative management is an acceptable approach to isolated traumatic diaphragm injury on the right in a stable patient. Delayed diaphragm hernia on the right is rare due to the presence of the liver.
- In hemodynamically stable patients with acute injury to the diaphragm, an abdominal approach may be favored over thoracic approach though concomitant injuries may factor into the operative approach.
- Patients presenting with delayed identification of a traumatic diaphragm hernia require careful consideration concerning operative approach, recognizing that a dual cavity approach may be required during operative repair.
- Repair of diaphragm injury should be coupled with irrigation and drainage of the associated hemithorax.

Take-Home Points for Patient Care

- Diaphragm injury is an uncommon entity encountered in the care of the traumatically injured patient. It is more commonly seen in penetrating versus blunt mechanisms.
- A high index of suspicion is required to diagnose injury to the diaphragm, and the cost of a missed injury for future patient morbidity and mortality is high.
- Patient clinical status and anatomic features (side, location, size, etc.) of the injury must be considered in management decisions regarding this injury. Most injuries to the diaphragm will require operative repair.

References

1. Petrone P, Asensio JA, Marini CP. Diaphragmatic injuries and post-traumatic diaphragmatic hernias. Curr Probl Surg. 2017;54:11–32.

Chapter 37
Liver and Biliary Trauma

Michael E. Huffner and Joshua A. Marks

Introduction

Liver and biliary trauma, from both blunt and penetrating mechanisms, are responsible for approximately 5% of all trauma admissions [1]. Injury to the liver, and particularly the biliary system, comes with significant morbidity and mortality. Management has evolved over the last few decades, with conservative management including admission and close monitoring becoming a more commonly accepted strategy, in certain circumstances, for treating these complex injuries.

Anatomy

- The liver is the largest solid abdominal organ fixed in the right upper quadrant.
- There are eight segments in total, including the caudate lobe (Segment 1), which lies behind the porta hepatis receiving blood supply from both the right and left hepatic arteries, the portal vein, and venous drainage directly into the inferior vena cava (IVC) via the hepatic veins.

M. E. Huffner
Sidney Kimmel Medical College at Thomas Jefferson University, Philadelphia, PA, USA
e-mail: Michael.Huffner@jefferson.edu

J. A. Marks (✉)
Division of Acute Care Surgery, Department of Surgery, Sidney Kimmel Medical College at Thomas Jefferson University, Philadelphia, PA, USA
e-mail: Joshua.Marks@jefferson.edu

© The Author(s), under exclusive license to Springer Nature Switzerland AG 2025
T. S. Brahmbhatt, D. R. Scantling (eds.), *Trauma Surgery Clerkship*, Contemporary Surgical Clerkships,
https://doi.org/10.1007/978-3-032-01412-2_37

353

- Cantlie's line divides the right lobe (segments 6–8) and left lobe (segments 2–4) traversing the gall bladder fossa posteriorly to the inferior vena cava (IVC). The falciform ligament is therefore located on the left lobe of the liver.
- Coronary ligaments: liver dome to the diaphragm. Triangular ligaments are the medial and lateral extensions of coronary ligaments forming the bare area.

Vascular Supply

- Hepatic artery: branch of the celiac axis, ultimately separating into the right and left hepatic arteries, providing 25% of the flow and is responsible for 50% of the oxygenation.
- Aberrant anatomy is common with the arterial supply with the most common being a replaced R hepatic artery originating off of the superior mesenteric artery (SMA) coursing behind the duodenum. A replaced left hepatic coming off of the left gastric artery running in the hepato-gastric ligament is the second most common.
- Portal vein: 75% of the flow, only 50% of the oxygenation.
- Hepatic veins: three veins total, middle hepatic joins the left hepatic in 90% of individuals prior to entering the IVC. Right hepatic vein drains directly to the IVC.

Classification

- American Association for the Surgery of Trauma (AAST) Liver Injury Scale (Table 37.1)

Table 37.1 American Association for the Surgery of Trauma (AAST) Liver Injury Scale [2]

Grade	Injury Type	Injury Description
I	Hematoma	Subcapsular <10%
	Laceration	Capsular tear, <1 cm depth
II	Hematoma	Subcapsular, 10%–50% area, intraparenchymal <10 cm
	Laceration	1–3 cm depth, <10 cm length
III	Hematoma	Subcapsular, >50% surface area or expanding; ruptured hematoma, intra-parenchymal hematoma >10 cm or enlarging
	Laceration	>3 cm depth
IV	Laceration	Parenchymal disruption 25%–75%
V	Laceration	Parenchymal disruption >75% of hepatic lobe
	Vascular	Juxtavenous hepatic injuries (IVC/Central hepatic veins)
VI	Vascular	Hepatic avulsion

Management of Liver Injury

- Same as any abdominal trauma: Patient stability dictates appropriate management both for blunt and penetrating injury and the standard trauma resuscitation workup and management are followed.
- Secondary survey may be suggestive of abdominal trauma, chest X-ray may have rib fractures on the right side.
- Fast exam sensitivity dependent on volume of blood in the abdomen, with >1 L approaching 97% sensitivity [3]
- Pain, tenderness, rebound, and guarding may be present in patients with intra-abdominal trauma; however many patients may have a completely benign exam.
- Blunt and penetrating liver injuries can both be conservatively managed depending on hemodynamic stability. Penetrating injuries are at higher risk for additional associated abdominal injuries so trajectory and injury pattern must be considered.
- Conservative management approaches a success rate of 88% for isolated blunt liver injury[4.]

Stable Patient

- Following advanced trauma life support (ATLS) protocols, in the hemodynamically stable patient, additional imaging may be considered to determine the extent of injury as well as the presence of additional injuries.
- CT scan: mainstay for diagnosis of liver and biliary injury. Evaluates grade, presence of hemoperitoneum, and evidence of pseudoaneurysm or active extravasation of contrast (active uncontained bleeding).
- All grades may be observed safely if the patient is stable. Higher grades (4/5) should be admitted to the ICU for close observation.

  - Conservative management of higher-grade injuries has become more common and has improved survival. Operative intervention should be reserved for unstable patients, those with suspected or proven concomitant injury or significant complications.
  - Failure of conservative management approaches 40% for severe liver injury (grade 4/5) [4].

- Active extravasation on CT scan

  - If stable, interventional radiology (IR) embolization is the mainstay of therapy.
  - In some situations, with low-grade injury and minimal risk factors, observation in the ICU with serial abdominal exams and hemoglobin (Hg) level checks is reasonable.

- If persistent transfusion requirement, patient may require IR evaluation even without evidence of active extravasation on CT scan or operative intervention to address or evaluate for other injury.

Unstable Patient

- Following ATLS with a patient who is persistently hypotensive despite resuscitation, abdominal exploration is often indicated.
- The operative decisions for the unstable patient and the steps involved in the trauma laparotomy are discussed elsewhere; however, if suspicion is high for abdominal trauma, exploratory laparotomy is indicated.

Operative Management of Liver Injury

- Trauma laparotomy: midline incision, possible extension with a right-sided Kocher incision (subcostal). Divide the falciform ligament. Pack the abdomen, with removal in a systematic approach identifying any additional injuries— focusing first on hemorrhage control, then on control of contamination.
- Pack the four quadrants of the abdomen with folded laparotomy pads. Quality is more important than quantity! Under-packing results in continued hemorrhage, while over-packing can compress the inferior vena cava (IVC), cause decrease in venous return, and result in hypotension.
- Regardless of the extent of the injury (and you likely will not know the full extent initially), the first step is to pack the liver. Hemorrhage not well controlled by packing will require further mobilization and exploration.
- Recreate the anatomy by packing above and below the liver (Fig. 37.1).

  - Anterior hepatic packing

    - Divide the falciform ligament as previously described.
    - Retract the liver inferiorly with one hand and place packs over the retracting hand between the anterior surface of the liver and the diaphragm.

  - Lateral hepatic packing

    - Retract the liver medially one hand and place packs over the retracting hand between the right lateral surface of the liver and the abdominal sidewall.

  - Posterior hepatic packing

    - Retract the liver superiorly with one hand and place packs under the retracting hand between the posterior surface of the liver and the infrahepatic structures.

Fig. 37.1 Liver injury
with packing in place
above and below the liver
to compress the injury and
restore native anatomy

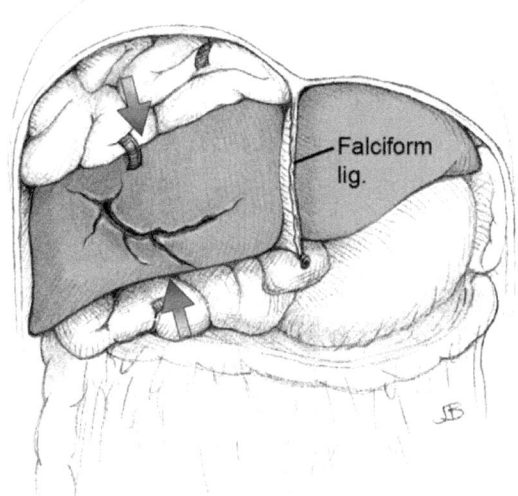

- If bleeding stops after packing, leave the packs in place! Premature removal of the packing may result in further bleeding from peeling the packs off the injured parenchyma.
- To remove the packing, slowly irrigate with water to loosen the packs.
- Localize and control any residual areas of bleeding.

Minor Liver Injury

- Electrocautery, argon laser, aquamantys bipolar or direct suture ligation for bleeding. Consider fibrin glue/floseal in tracts or directly on liver injury.
- Consider packing the liver to compress and bring the damaged edges together to return liver to its native anatomy. This maneuver will tamponade bleeding.
- If hemorrhage is controlled, may close the abdomen and monitor in ICU. If there is concern for rebleeding or if the patient is unstable (shows lethal triad), consider damage control procedure and leave the packing in place with plans to return to the OR in 24–48 h after resuscitation in the ICU.
- Upon closure, drain placement may be indicated depending on the size and risk for bile leak.

Significant Liver Injury

- May require manual compression with hands to decrease bleeding and restore native anatomy.
- As previously described, packing is the mainstay of therapy and can be used in large liver injuries.

  - If controlled, may perform damage control procedure with plans to return to the OR in 24–48 h.
  - Perihepatic sepsis risk increases as packs are left in place reaching 80% in 72 h.

- Uncontrolled hemorrhage despite compression/packing:

  - Full mobilization of the liver with takedown of the coronary and triangular ligaments, attempting to turn the liver into a midline organ to gain access to the retrohepatic IVC.

    - Mobilization of the right liver lobe may unroof the tamponade and cause severe hemorrhage if a retrohepatic caval injury is present.
  - Liver isolation: Pringle maneuver—clamp across the portal triad (inflow), release for 5 min every 20 min. Can safely clamp for 75 min without injury [3]. Also obtain infra- and suprahepatic IVC control (outflow).

    - Retract the anterior edge of the liver superiorly and to the right.
    - Insert the left index finger into the Foramen of Winslow.
    - Pinch the thumb on top of the index finger to control the portal triad (hepatic artery, portal vein, common bile duct).
    - A vascular clamp or a Rumel tourniquet can replace the fingers for long-term control.
    - Pringle is ineffective in patients with a replaced left hepatic artery or injuries to the hepatic veins and retrohepatic IVC. A replaced right hepatic artery commonly travels posterior to the portal vein. Feel for a pulsatile structure posterior to the portal vein to help identify this vessel.

- Direct Suture ligation: Large, blunt tip absorbable suture figure of eight or mattress ligation of bleeding vessels incorporating the uninjured liver parenchyma and capsule.

  - Taking too small of a bite of the liver parenchyma can cause the suture to tear through and result in more bleeding. When tying down the sutures, apply just enough tension to reapproximate the lacerated edges. Excessive tension during knot tying will further avulse the liver and exacerbate the injury.
  - Omental packing is useful in deep liver lacerations and needs to be secured with sutures.

- Tractotomy: Either with finger fracture or staple device, can open injuries further to gain access to large bleeding vessels.

- Through-and-through liver injuries can be controlled via balloon tamponade by using a Blakemore tube or a homemade balloon constructed from a Penrose drain over a hollow rubber catheter.
- Liver resection: Anatomic or wedge resection may be necessary in the setting of large injuries.
- Atrial-caval shunt (Schrock Shunt) and venovenous bypass are possible if injury is severe, however, are rarely used (and also rarely successful). Both the injury requiring it and the procedure itself have high associated morbidity and mortality with unclear benefit.
- Even more rare, but described—Auto-transplant: Complete removal of liver with reimplantation after ex vivo repair of liver/venous injury [5].
- Hepatic Transplant: Requires donor within 36 h. Very high mortality.

Complications of Liver Injury

- Nonoperatively and operatively managed liver injuries are both at risk for similar complications. There is increased risk for complications based on the severity of the injury.
- Increased risk of complications in patients with penetrating injury when compared to blunt injury (40.7% vs. 27.4%, respectively) [6].
- Presentation: Fever, worsening abdominal pain, nausea, vomiting, lab abnormalities including leukocytosis and elevated liver function tests.
- Imaging: CT scan (most common), ultrasound, consider HIDA (hepatobiliary iminodiacetic acid), MRCP (magnetic resonance cholangiopancreatography) and possible fistulagram via interventional radiology placed drain.
- Bile Leak: Leakage from the injured liver, which can lead to bilomas, abscesses and bile peritonitis (free bile throughout the abdomen).

  - Biloma: collection of bile, managed with IR drainage. ERCP (endoscopic retrograde cholangiopancreatography) must be considered if high output from the drain for possible direct stenting, or, more commonly, sphincterotomy. Sphincterotomy decreases the pressure in the biliary tree and increases the chances for successful nonoperative management.
  - Abscess: Management similar to biloma with IR drainage; however, antibiotics indicated and there is less likely a need for operative intervention.

- Hemorrhage—either delayed or rebleed: Management similar to initial injury. May require OR if unstable. If stable, recommended IR intervention for possible embolization.
- Hemobilia: Patient with recent liver injury presents with a brisk upper GI bleed. Likely from a hepatic pseudoaneurysm connecting to the biliary system leading to an upper GI bleed via the ductal system to the duodenum.

  - Management with IR intervention, unless unstable.

- Less common recently with increased conservative management of liver injury (thought to be due to previous direct suturing on the liver leading to iatrogenic connections between the arterial and biliary system).

- Hepatic Necrosis: Ischemic segment of liver (particularly after prior embolization). Observation is a viable option; however, some studies suggest early operative resection if large, symptomatic, or unstable.
- Budd-Chiari: Possible compression on the hepatic veins from hematoma compression leading to hepatic congestion. This is a rare complication and may require hematoma evacuation however high risk for rebleeding given loss of tamponade.

Follow-Up

- Routine imaging after liver injury is generally not necessary.
- Higher grade (3/4/5) often carry a recommendation of repeat CT scan.
- Okay to restart activity about 1 month after injury or 3 months after major injury (>grade 3) [3].

Biliary Tract Injuries

- 50% mortality due to vascular injury, mainly from portal vein and hepatic artery injury. 99% mortality if both artery and vein are injured.
- Gall bladder injury: Rarely an isolated injury, manage with cholecystectomy. Nonoperative management not indicated given increased risk of additional injuries and stasis/cholecystitis risk from blood in the biliary system.
- Bile Duct Injury: Management of hemorrhage, shock, and coagulopathy first. May just require wide drainage if instability continued.
- Duct laceration: Primarily repair small laceration <50% circumference, with consideration of T-tube placement, which acts as a drain for the duct.
- Extensive laceration/avulsion: Roux-en-y hepaticojejunostomy reconstruction.
- Ampullary/Intrapancreatic duct injury: Primary repair possible, however associated duodenal/pancreas injury likely and may require wide drainage, isolation, or rarely Whipple procedure.
- Wide drainage and closure is always an option with plans for takeback once acute injury is managed.

Summary

- ATLS protocol should be followed when assessing any trauma patient and the basic principles of resuscitation adhered to always.
- The liver is a highly vascular organ and associated with significant morbidity and mortality when severely injured.
- Overall management is based on stability of the patient and other concomitant injuries.

References

1. Mattox K, Moore E, Feliciano D. Trauma. 7th ed. McGraw Hill; 2015. p. 539. Elsevier.
2. Moore E, Cogbill T, Jurkovich G, et al. Organ injury scaling: spleen and liver (1994 revision). J Trauma. 1995;38:323–4.
3. Asensio J. Current therapy of trauma and surgical critical care. 2nd ed. Philadelphia; 2016.
4. Rouy M, Julien C, Birnbayum DJ, et al. Predictive factors of non-operative management failure in 494 blunt liver injuries: a multicenter retrospective study. Updat Surg. 2022. https://doi.org/10.1007/s13304-022-01367-6.
5. Bevilacqua L, Pace D, Aka A, Maley W, et al. Hepatic autotransplant for hepatic vein avulsion after blunt abdominal trauma. J Trauma Acute Care Surg. 2020;89:55–8.
6. Fu Y, Lewis M, Demtriades D, et al. Gunshot wound versus blunt liver injuries: different liver-related complications and outcomes. Eur J Trauma Emerg Surg. 2022. https://doi.org/10.1007/s00068-022-02096-6.

Chapter 38
Spleen Injury

Drew Farmer

Introduction

- The spleen is the most commonly injured solid abdominal organ following blunt trauma.
- The firm splenic capsule is susceptible to injury by direct compression and its ligamentous attachments make it vulnerable to avulsion during rapid deceleration. It is highly vascularized and possesses both closed and open circulation systems. Because of these features, injury to the spleen can result in profound hemorrhage.
- Although it is not an essential organ, the spleen performs immunologic and hematologic roles that make preservation preferable when feasible.
- With advances in imaging technology, injury grade stratification, and endovascular techniques, nonoperative methods for managing spleen trauma have become routine in the majority of cases.

Diagnosis and Evaluation

- Evaluation and diagnosis of splenic injury follows a standard pathway in the workup for abdominal trauma, which includes primary and secondary survey assessing hemodynamic stability, presence of peritonitis, evidence of blunt or penetrating injury to the abdomen.

D. Farmer (✉)
Texas Health Presbyterian Hospital, Dallas, TX, USA
e-mail: DrewFarmer@texashealth.org

© The Author(s), under exclusive license to Springer Nature Switzerland AG 2025
T. S. Brahmbhatt, D. R. Scantling (eds.), *Trauma Surgery Clerkship*, Contemporary Surgical Clerkships, https://doi.org/10.1007/978-3-032-01412-2_38

363

- Focused Assessment with Sonography for Trauma (FAST) exam may provide insight into the presence of hemoperitoneum, which should be performed on the hemodynamically unstable patient with blunt trauma.
- The standard imaging modality for diagnosis and assessment of severity of spleen injury is the abdominal CT scan with IV contrast. Arterial phase imaging has demonstrated increased detection rates of splenic vascular injuries resulting in more accurate injury grade classification, though its routine use to evaluate abdominal trauma is not standard practice in most institutions [5].

Approach to Initial Management, Part 1: Operative Intervention

- Patients with diffuse peritonitis or hemodynamic instability attributed to abdominal injury that is unresponsive or transiently responsive to blood product resuscitation should proceed directly to the operating room for emergency laparotomy [1].
- Options for surgical management include splenectomy and splenorrhaphy (or repair of the injured spleen). Of these, splenectomy is far and away the more common operation, and is the appropriate choice for the injured patient with hemodynamic instability.
- Splenectomy is performed quickly and effectively through a midline laparotomy incision. Packing laparotomy pads between the spleen and the diaphragm improves exposure of the organ, bringing it more anterior and thus nearer to the midline incision. The lateral attachments (splenorenal and splenophrenic ligaments) are then divided to allow for medialization of the spleen into the surgical incision. The gastrosplenic ligament is divided (commonly performed with a sealer/divider energy device), thus ligating the short gastric vessels taking care to avoid causing thermal injury to the greater curvature of the stomach. Then with the hilum isolated and avoiding injury to the pancreatic tail, the splenic vessels are ligated either with suture or a vascular stapler. The splenocolic ligament is then divided and the spleen is passed off the field. The short gastric vessels should be reexamined for hemostasis and oversewn as necessary to prevent postoperative bleeding (a common complication at this site).
- Splenorrhaphy should be reserved for low-grade injuries in patients who are otherwise stable and without other significant unresolved injuries who have proceeded to the operating room. The goal of splenorrhaphy is to reapproximate the capsule to achieve tamponade and hemostasis. This can be accomplished using absorbable monofilament suture on a blunt needle with or without felt pledgets, or it can be accomplished by encasing the spleen in an absorbable mesh to facilitate external compression and reapproximation of a multiple fracture capsule. This is uncommonly done.

Approach to Initial Management, Part 2: Nonoperative Management

- When hemodynamic stability and absence of peritonitis have been established in the initial evaluation, abdominal CT with IV contrast should be obtained and AAST grade of splenic injury should be established [2].
- Selective nonoperative management (NOM) of spleen injury has become progressively more common and successful over the last two decades with advances in imaging technology, endovascular interventions, and increasingly sophisticated injury severity stratification system with progressively more nuanced approaches to treatment.
- Advantages of NOM include less pain, easier recovery, shorter length of hospital stay, preserved spleen immunologic and hematologic functions, and avoidance of risks of surgical complications, which include wound infection, poor wound healing, injury to surrounding visceral structures including the pancreatic tail and stomach, and late complications including incisional hernia and peritoneal adhesions [12].
- NOM should only be considered in a setting capable of providing reliable monitoring (including serial lab work), frequent clinical reevaluation, and access to an operating room allowing for urgent surgical intervention should it become necessary due to delayed hemorrhage.
- The failure rate of NOM increases with increasing AAST injury grade. Splenic artery angiography and embolization (SAE) significantly mitigates failure rate in higher-grade injuries and should be considered in patients with AAST grade IV or V, presence of contrast blush on abdominal CT, moderate or large volume hemoperitoneum, or in patients with evidence of ongoing bleeding such as downtrending hemoglobin/hematocrit levels or transient hemodynamic response to volume expansion/transfusion [7].

Subsequent Management for Patients Undergoing NOM

- Vascular complications, such as development of a pseudoaneurysm may arise in patients with high-grade spleen injuries. Follow-up imaging with contrast-enhanced US or CT is often recommended in 48–72 h after admission for patients with AAST grade III injury or higher who have undergone NOM [13].
- Chemical VTE prophylaxis has not been shown to increase the risk of failure rate in NOM and may be initiated within 24 h for AAST Grade I–III injuries and 48–72 h for high-grade injuries if no other specific contraindications are present (i.e., persistently downtrending hemoglobin levels or concomitant intracranial hemorrhage precluding prophylactic anticoagulation).

- Early discharge should include education to the patient and caregiver on the signs, symptoms, and risks of delayed hemorrhage and need for immediate return to the hospital for reevaluation.
- Currently, there are no evidence-based guidelines for length of activity restriction following NOM of spleen injury, but surgeons generally agree that these patients should avoid contact sports, strenuous exercise, or other activities that place a patient at increased risk for secondary blunt abdominal trauma for some duration. A 2022 consensus document from the World Society of Emergency Surgery advised 3–5 weeks of restricted activity for adults with Grade I–II injuries and 2–4 months for adults with higher-grade injuries [9].

Vaccination Recommendations

- Patients who have had a splenectomy are at lifelong increased risk for bacterial infections and postsplenectomy septicemia. A small percentage of patients progress to overwhelming postsplenectomy infection (OPSI), which has a fatality rate approaching 50%. Organisms responsible for OPSI are most commonly the polysaccharide-encapsulated bacteria *Streptococcus pneumoniae*, *Neisseria meningitidis*, and *Haemophilus influenzae*. For this reason, pneumococcal, meningococcal, and Hib vaccines are recommended for patients following splenectomy [3, 6, 10, 11].
- Optimal timing of postsplenectomy vaccination is thought to be at about 14 days after surgery. Patients who were vaccinated earlier demonstrated inferior functional antibody response. Furthermore, waiting 28 days to vaccinate conferred no further immunologic benefit. It should be considered, however, that early vaccination is superior to no vaccination, and patients who are likely to be lost to follow-up should be considered for vaccination prior to discharge [4].
- Interestingly, patients who have undergone SAE do not demonstrate diminished splenic immune function when compared to control patients, and therefore the 2022 EAST Practice Management Guidelines conditionally recommend against routine vaccination in this group [8].

AAST Spleen Injury Scale (2018 Revision)	
Grade	CT Imaging findings
I	Subcapsular hematoma <10% surface area or Parenchymal laceration <1 cm depth or Capsular tear
II	Subcapsular hematoma 10%–50% surface area or Intraparenchymal hematoma <5 cm or Parenchymal laceration 1–3 cm depth
III	Subcapsular hematoma >50% surface area or Ruptured subcapsular or intraparenchymal hematoma ≥5 cm or Parenchymal laceration >3 cm depth

AAST Spleen Injury Scale (2018 Revision)	
Grade	CT Imaging findings
IV	Any injury in the presence of a splenic vascular injury or
	Active bleeding confined within the splenic capsule or
	Parenchymal laceration involving segmental or hilar vessels producing >25% devascularization
V	Any injury in the presence of splenic vascular injury with active bleeding extending beyond the spleen into the peritoneum or
	Shattered spleen

Bibliography

1. Chahine AH, Gilyard S, Hanna TN, Fan S, Risk B, Johnson JO, Duszak R Jr, Newsome J, Xing M, Kokabi N. Management of splenic trauma in contemporary clinical practice: a National Trauma Data Bank Study. Acad Radiol. 2021;28(Suppl 1):S138–47. https://doi.org/10.1016/j.acra.2020.11.010. Epub 2020 Dec 4. PMID: 33288400.

2. Crichton JCI, Naidoo K, Yet B, Brundage SI, Perkins Z. The role of splenic angioembolization as an adjunct to nonoperative management of blunt splenic injuries: a systematic review and meta-analysis. J Trauma Acute Care Surg. 2017;83(5):934–43. https://doi.org/10.1097/TA.0000000000001649. PMID: 29068875.

3. Cullingford GL, Watkins DN, Watts AD, Mallon DF. Severe late postsplenectomy infection. Br J Surg. 1991;78(6):716–21. https://doi.org/10.1002/bjs.1800780626. PMID: 2070242.

4. Freeman JJ, Yorkgitis BK, Haines K, Koganti D, Patel N, Maine R, Chiu W, Tran TL, Como JJ, Kasotakis G. Vaccination after spleen embolization: a practice management guideline from the Eastern Association for the Surgery of Trauma. Injury. 2022;53(11):3569–74. https://doi.org/10.1016/j.injury.2022.08.006. Epub 2022 Aug 4. PMID: 36038390.

5. Hemachandran N, Gamanagatti S, Sharma R, Shanmuganathan K, Kumar A, Gupta A, Kumar S. Revised AAST scale for splenic injury (2018): does addition of arterial phase on CT have an impact on the grade? Emerg Radiol. 2021;28(1):47–54. https://doi.org/10.1007/s10140-020-01823-z. Epub 2020 Jul 23. PMID: 32705369.

6. Howdieshell TR, Heffernan D, Dipiro JT, Therapeutic Agents Committee of the Surgical Infection Society. Surgical infection society guidelines for vaccination after traumatic injury. Surg Infect. 2006;7(3):275–303. https://doi.org/10.1089/sur.2006.7.275. PMID: 16875461.

7. Miller PR, Chang MC, Hoth JJ, Mowery NT, Hildreth AN, Martin RS, Holmes JH, Meredith JW, Requarth JA. Prospective trial of angiography and embolization for all grade III to V blunt splenic injuries: nonoperative management success rate is significantly improved. J Am Coll Surg. 2014;218(4):644–8. https://doi.org/10.1016/j.jamcollsurg.2014.01.040. Epub 2014 Jan 28. PMID: 24655852.

8. Peitzman AB, Heil B, Rivera L, Federle MB, Harbrecht BG, Clancy KD, Croce M, Enderson BL, Morris JA, Shatz D, Meredith JW, Ochoa JB, Fakhry SM, Cushman JG, Minei JP, McCarthy M, Luchette FA, Townsend R, Tinkoff G, Block EF, Ross S, Frykberg ER, Bell RM, Davis F 3rd, Weireter L, Shapiro MB. Blunt splenic injury in adults: multi-institutional study of the Eastern Association for the Surgery of Trauma. J Trauma. 2000;49(2):177–87. https://doi.org/10.1097/00005373-200008000-00002; discussion 187–9. PMID: 10963527.

9. Podda M, De Simone B, Ceresoli M, Virdis F, Favi F, Wiik Larsen J, Coccolini F, Sartelli M, Pararas N, Beka SG, Bonavina L, Bova R, Pisanu A, Abu-Zidan F, Balogh Z, Chiara O, Wani I, Stahel P, Di Saverio S, Scalea T, Soreide K, Sakakushev B, Amico F, Martino C, Hecker A, de'Angelis N, Chirica M, Galante J, Kirkpatrick A, Pikoulis E, Kluger Y, Bensard D, Ansaloni L, Fraga G, Civil I, Tebala GD, Di Carlo I, Cui Y, Coimbra R, Agnoletti V, Sall I, Tan E, Picetti E, Litvin A, Damaskos D, Inaba K, Leung J, Maier R, Biffl W, Leppaniemi A, Moore

E, Gurusamy K, Catena F. Follow-up strategies for patients with splenic trauma managed non-operatively: the 2022 World Society of Emergency Surgery consensus document. World J Emerg Surg. 2022;17(1):52. https://doi.org/10.1186/s13017-022-00457-5. PMID: 36224617; PMCID: PMC9560023.

10. Shatz DV, Schinsky MF, Pais LB, et al. Immune re-sponses of splenectomized trauma patients to the 23-valent pneumococcal polysaccharide vaccine at 1versus 7 versus 14 days after sple-nectomy. J Trauma. 1998;44:760–6.

11. Shatz DV, Romero-Steiner S, Ellie C, et al. Antibodyresponses at 14 and 28 days post-splenectomy intrauma patients receiving the 23-valent pneumococ-cal vaccine. J Trauma. 2002;52:194–200.

12. Siriratsivawong K, Zenati M, Watson GA, Harbrecht BG. Nonoperative management of blunt splenic trauma in the elderly: does age play a role? Am Surg. 2007;73(6):585–9; discussion 590. PMID: 17658096.

13. Stassen NA, Bhullar I, Cheng JD, Crandall ML, Friese RS, Guillamondegui OD, Jawa RS, Maung AA, Rohs TJ Jr, Sangosanya A, Schuster KM, Seamon MJ, Tchorz KM, Zarzuar BL, Kerwin AJ, Eastern Association for the Surgery of Trauma. Selective nonoperative manage-ment of blunt splenic injury: an Eastern Association for the Surgery of Trauma practice man-agement guideline. J Trauma Acute Care Surg. 2012;73(5 Suppl 4):S294–300. https://doi.org/10.1097/TA.0b013e3182702afc. PMID: 23114484.

Chapter 39
Stomach and Small Bowel Injuries

Sevara Akramova

Introduction

Stomach and small intestinal injuries may occur from both blunt and penetrating mechanisms. In blunt trauma, it is relatively uncommon to see hollow viscus injury, especially stomach injury, given the high force required to cause rupture of all layers. Small intestine injury is a little more common [1]. In penetrating trauma to the anterior abdomen, however, injury to the stomach and small intestine are relatively common [2]. If untreated, these injuries can cause life-threatening sepsis, so a high index of suspicion to facilitate early detection and prompt treatment, is essential.

Mechanism of Injury

Blunt Injury

A significant force of impact is necessary to cause stomach rupture from blunt trauma, due to the stomach's thick walls. However, perforation most often results when the patient already has a very distended stomach, usually shortly after ingesting a large meal. Small intestine injuries may occur in conjunction with mesenteric tears and defects, commonly called "bucket handle" injuries. Compared to lacerations or hematomas without devascularization, these lesions are the highest grade of blunt mesenteric injury (Fig. 39.1).

S. Akramova (✉)
Department of Surgery, University Medical Center, TTUHSC, Lubbock, TX, USA
e-mail: Sevara.Akramova@ttuhsc.edu

© The Author(s), under exclusive license to Springer Nature Switzerland AG 2025
T. S. Brahmbhatt, D. R. Scantling (eds.), *Trauma Surgery Clerkship*, Contemporary Surgical Clerkships,
https://doi.org/10.1007/978-3-032-01412-2_39

Fig. 39.1 Bucket handle
injury

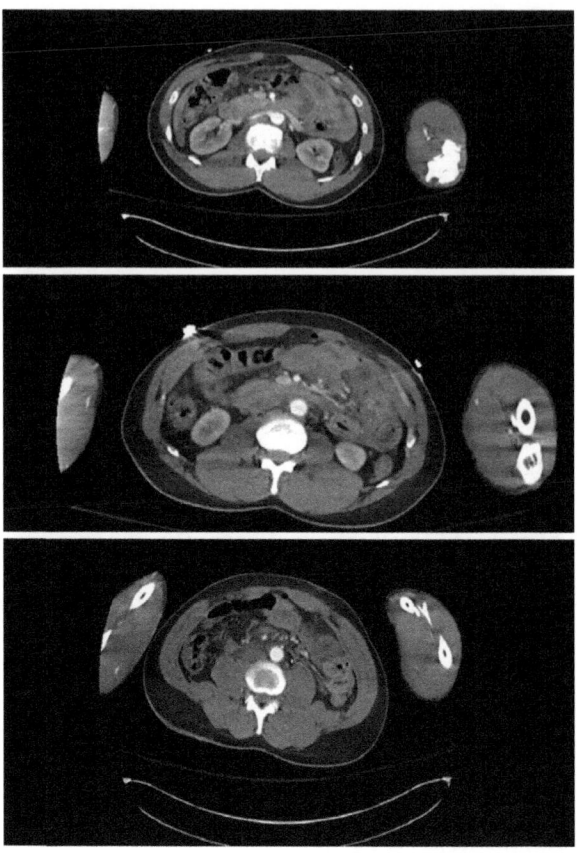

Penetrating Injury

Stab wounds, accidental impalements and gun shots to the anterior abdominal wall
are not uncommon in many regions; any of these mechanisms may result in small
intestine (more common) or gastric injury.

Stomach Injuries

- Often rare due to its anatomically protected location, and thick wall.
- The anterior wall is the area most frequently impacted.

Duodenal Injuries

- The most frequent location for duodenal damage is the second part of the duodenum.
- Duodenal injuries are rarely isolated and there are a number of adjacent critical structures, which tend to be injured.
- The liver is the most affected adjacent organ, accounting for 17% of associated injuries, the pancreas (12%), small bowel (12%), colon (12%), and stomach (12%) were also affected (9%), in an analysis of 1153 duodenal injuries among 3047 linked injuries [3].

Jejunum and Ileum Injuries

- In blunt trauma, intestinal rupture is often associated with mesenteric devascularization—bucket handle injuries.
- In penetrating trauma, it is not uncommon to see "through-and-through" injuries of anterior and posterior walls of the intestine. It is essential that both entry and exit points be actively sought, to avoid missed injuries.

General Management and Indications for Laparotomy

A history of penetrating abdominal injury should spur concern for visceral perforation, including of the small intestine and stomach.

In motor vehicle collisions, a history of seatbelt use, or direct trauma to the abdomen, should raise the possibility of visceral injury. Full abdominal examination should be performed, including specific attention to signs of bruising over the anterior abdominal wall. Peritonitis is a classic indication of hollow visceral injury should prompt surgical exploration. After initial evaluation and resuscitation patients with suspected or identified injuries should undergo immediate surgery.

A seatbelt sign (Fig. 39.2) is a classic indication that mesenteric injury may have occurred and should increase the index of suspicion.

FAST ultrasound examination should be performed, as with any abdominal trauma evaluation.

Fig. 39.2 Seatbelt sign

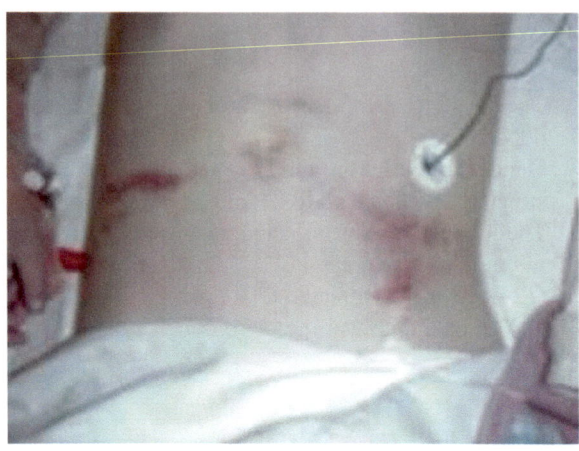

Imaging

Trauma patients with a mechanism for possible abdominal injury should undergo a Focused Ultrasound Assessment (FAST) as part of their primary survey. Fluid visualized in the abdomen should prompt suspicion for possible visceral injury, although this is more commonly an indication of bleeding.

Suspicion for small intestine or stomach injury may prompt several next steps:

- Diagnostic Peritoneal Aspirate/Lavage (DPL) is a traditional method to determine likelihood of visceral injury but is now very uncommon given improved imaging modalities.

Diagnostic Laparoscopy has largely supplanted DPL in many centers, due to the ability to directly visualize the abdominal contents.

- CT scan of the abdomen and pelvis, particularly with oral contrast, has 97% sensitivity and 95% specificity for hollow organ injuries and may be considered in a stable patient [4–6].

After initial evaluation and resuscitation patients with suspected or identified injuries should undergo immediate surgery.

A trauma laparotomy is divided into four stages with the latter two most relevant to bowel and gastric injury.

- Bleeding control.
- Contamination control.
- Injury diagnosis.
- Reconstruction.

There are various sites that might conceal injuries and should be thoroughly examined. The stomach's greater and lesser curvature, as well as the proximal posterior gastric wall. The stomach must be mobilized to identify gastric injuries; exposure is obtained by decompressing the stomach with insertion of nasogastric tube.

Once hemorrhage is addressed, rapid control of gastric or bowel perforations is performed. A running suture repair is ultimately utilized to achieve hemostasis and control gastrointestinal spill.

Alternatively, atraumatic (Allis or Babcock) clamps or stapling devices, or closure with heavy suture or even umbilical tape, may be utilized.

To view the gastric fundus, cardia, and esophagogastric junction, the short gastric vessels may need to be divided and ligated. During division of the gastrohepatic ligament, injury to the vagus nerve or its branches, as well as the anomalous left hepatic artery, must be avoided.

By opening the avascular section of the gastrocolic ligament along the larger curvature of the stomach, and entering the lesser sac, the posterior wall of the stomach can be viewed. To avoid injury to the transverse mesocolon and middle colic artery, enter this area at the upper or mid-section of the greater curvature of the stomach, through the avascular region of the gastrocolic omentum.

It is important to examine it all the way to the diaphragm, to avoid missing an injury high on the posterior wall. A narrow Deaver retractor can be useful for this purpose.

Small Bowel

The small intestine is examined for injury by eviscerating it to the right and carefully inspecting its entire length.

The degree of the damage determines the treatment (Fig. 39.3).

- Grade I: intramural hematoma treated by inversion with one- or two-layer closure, or left alone.
- Grade II: full thickness perforations and less than 50% of the circumference, treated with debridement to healthy edges and primary closure.
- Grade III: resection and anastomosis. There may be an option for primary repair if at least 30% of circumference is maintained.
- Grade IV: complete transection, which requires resection with anastomosis.

Existing literature suggests that both hand-sewn and stapled anastomoses provide equivalent results. Stapled anastomoses are usually quicker; however, in cases where there is significant intestinal distention, there is limited literature suggesting that hand-sewn anastomosis, by virtue of being able to adjust to discrepancies in intestinal thickness, might be preferable [7]. Irrespective of the method utilized, intestinal anastomotic healing is dependent on a healthy blood supply, a tension-free suture or staple line, an adequate lumen, a watertight closure, and no distal obstruction.

Fig. 39.3 Bucket handle
injury

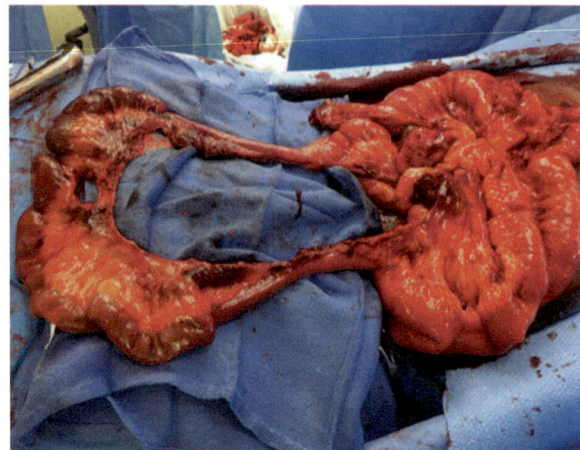

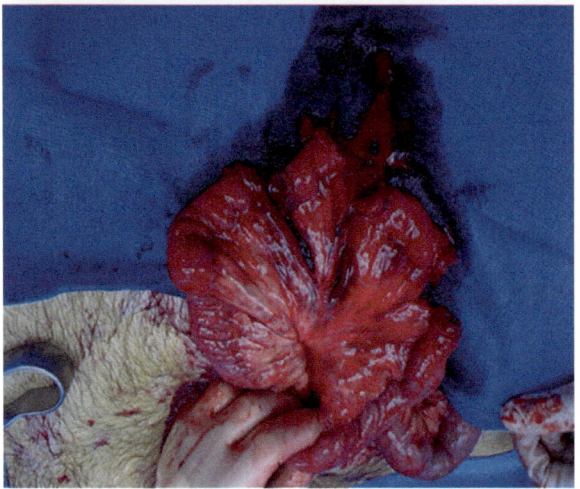

Depending on the hemodynamic stability of the patient, it may be necessary to perform a damage control operation, where the visceral perforations are temporarily closed using staple or suture, to stop spillage of intestinal contents, and the patient returned to intensive care unit for further resuscitation prior to definitive repair or anastomosis. If this option is chosen, either Whipstitch closure (preferred) or a vacuum device may be used for temporary abdominal coverage [8].

References

1. Iaselli F, Mazzei MA, Firetto C, D'Elia D, Squitieri NC, Biondetti PR, Danza FM, Scaglione M. Bowel and mesenteric injuries from blunt abdominal trauma: a review. Radiol Med. 2015;120(1):21–32. https://doi.org/10.1007/s11547-014-0487-8. PMID: 25572542.

2. Mukhopadhyay M. Intestinal injury from blunt abdominal trauma: a study of 47 cases. Oman Med J. 2009;24(4):256–9. https://doi.org/10.5001/omj.2009.52. PMID: 22216378; PMCID: PMC3243872.
3. Asensio JA, Feliciano DV, Britt LD, Kerstein MD. Management of duodenal injuries. Curr Probl Surg. 1993;30(11):1023–93. https://doi.org/10.1016/0011-3840(93)90063-m. PMID: 8222749.
4. Burlew CC, Moore EE, Cuschieri J, Jurkovich GJ, Codner P, Crowell K, Nirula R, Haan J, Rowell SE, Kato CM, WTA Study Group, et al. Sew it up! A Western Trauma Association multi-institutional study of enteric injury management in the postinjury open abdomen. J Trauma. 2011;70(2):273–7.
5. Hamidi MI, Aldaoud KM, Qtaish I. The role of computed tomography in blunt abdominal trauma. Sultan Qaboos Univ Med J. 2007;7(1):41–6. PMID: 21654944; PMCID: PMC3086417.
6. Goodman CS, Hur JY, Adajar MA, Coulam CH. How well does CT predict the need for laparotomy in hemodynamically stable patients with penetrating abdominal injury? A review and meta-analysis. AJR Am J Roentgenol. 2009;193(2):432–7.
7. Fitzgerald JEF, Larvin M. Chapter 15: Management of abdominal trauma. In: Baker Q, Aldoori M, editors. Clinical surgery: a practical guide. CRC Press; 2009. p. 192–204. ISBN 9781444109627.
8. Collins R, Dhanasekara CS, Morris E, Marschke B, Dissanaike S. Simple suture whipstitch closure is a reasonable option for many patients requiring temporary abdominal closure for blunt or penetrating trauma. Trauma Surg Acute Care Open. 2022;7(1):e000980. https://doi.org/10.1136/tsaco-2022-000980. PMID: 36304556; PMCID: PMC9594533.

Chapter 40
Duodenum and Pancreas Injury

Camille Dirago and Dane R. Scantling

Introduction

- Injuries to the duodenum and pancreas present unique challenges due to their intimate anatomic positioning among several critical organs, vessels, and structures
- Their largely retroperitoneal positioning contributes to delays in detection of injury and affords the organs some degree of protection in cases of abdominal trauma, limiting experience in management of these injuries for most trainees
- Contemporary management is dictated by the hemodynamic status of the patient, clinical presentation, and grade of injury

Epidemiology/Pathophysiology

Trauma to the duodenum is most often penetrating in nature and accounts for <1% of all trauma and <5% of abdominal trauma. Trauma to the pancreas also accounts for <1% of all trauma and <11% of abdominal trauma, with blunt trauma being the most common etiology. Associated injuries to surrounding structures are highly common in both.

C. Dirago
Department of Surgery, University of Massachusetts Memorial Medical Center, Worcester, MA, USA
e-mail: Camille.Dirago@umassmemorial.org

D. R. Scantling (✉)
Division of Acute Care Surgery, Boston Medical Center/Boston University Chobanian and Avedisian School of Medicine, Boston, MA, USA
e-mail: Dane.Scantling@BMC.org

T. S. Brahmbhatt, D. R. Scantling (eds.), *Trauma Surgery Clerkship*, Contemporary Surgical Clerkships,
https://doi.org/10.1007/978-3-032-01412-2_40

Anatomy and Surrounding Structures

- *Duodenum*

  - Typically divided into four sections: superior, descending, transverse, and ascending (D1, D2, D3, and D4, respectively)
  - The duodenum is mainly a retroperitoneal structure with the exception of the anterior wall of the first (superior) portion
  - The duodenum is in close proximity to/contact with the vertebral column, psoas muscles, the aorta, the inferior vena cava (IVC), right kidney, liver, pancreas, stomach, and transverse colon

- *Pancreas*

  - Typically divided into four sections: head, neck, body, and tail
  - The head is in close contact with the C-loop of the duodenum
  - The neck lies over the SMA and SMV
  - The body lies over the vertebral column and aorta
  - The tail is intimately associated with the hilum of the spleen, the left kidney, and the splenic flexure of the colon

- The blood supply for both the pancreas and the duodenum is the gastroduodenal and splenic arteries and the SMA

Initial Evaluation and Management

- *Classification*

  - Initial evaluation and classification of extent and severity of injury is guided by the American Association for the Surgery of Trauma (AAST) Organ Injury Scale for Duodenum and Pancreas

- *Initial Management*

  - Hemodynamically unstable patients with a positive FAST (blunt trauma), unstable patients after penetrating trauma, or those with generalized peritonitis should undergo immediate laparotomy
  - Stable patients (with or without a positive FAST) may undergo CT scan to assess for presence intra-abdominal injury

    - The presence of free fluid or stranding on imaging suggests injury and warrants further workup
    - The presence of free air, localized thickened bowel, evisceration, penetrating trauma, or peritonitis warrants immediate exploratory laparotomy

- *Operative Management*

- Surgical management of pancreatic and duodenal injuries is determined by AAST classification, injury location, and patient stability
- Staged pancreatoduodenectomy may be indicated in the case of destruction of the duodenal-pancreatic complex. Pancreaticojejunostomy and pancreatico-gastrostomy have been demonstrated to be equally effective techniques in these cases
- *Duodenal Injury*

  - AAST I: No operative management indicated unless hematoma or laceration does not resolve within 14 days
  - AAST II and III: Primary operative repair
  - AAST V: Damage control with staged approach to reconstruction or pancreatoduodenectomy
  - Consider ancillary procedures (i.e., pyloric exclusion +/− gastrojejunostomy) in grades III–V

- *Pancreatic Injury*

  - AAST I and II: Endoscopic or percutaneous intervention
  - AAST III: If proximal lesion, same as I and II; if distal lesion, distal pancreatectomy
  - AAST IV–V: Damage control with staged approach to reconstruction; consider Whipple procedure or pancreatoduodenectomy

Complications

- Complications of nonoperative management

  - Pseudocyst formation is the most common adverse outcome following nonoperative management of blunt pancreatic injury and can be diagnosed on CT and treated with internal draining
  - In penetrating trauma, pancreatic leaks are managed with resection (if identified early) or percutaneous drainage (if not). This often results in a pancreatic fistula and the need for internal stenting by ERCP to facilitate anatomic drainage; pancreatic fistulas occur 10%–35% of the time after major pancreatic injury. High drain output with elevated drain amylase (nonspecific) or lipase (specific) is confirmatory
  - Pancreatic enzyme leakage can be a major complication that causes breakdown of nearby anastomoses and catastrophic bleeding from repaired vascular injuries
  - While penetrating duodenal trauma is always managed operatively, repair failure can lead to very high output enterocutaneous fistulas, wound breakdown, and significant malnutrition without feeding access. Failed nonoperative management of blunt duodenal injury can result in free perforation, enterocutaneous fistula formation, sepsis, and death

Duodenum injury scale

Grade*	Type of injury	Description of injury	ICD-9	AIS-90
I	Hematoma	Involving single portion of duodenum	863.21	2
	Laceration	Partial thickness, no perforation	863.21	3
II	Hematoma	Involving more than one portion	863.21	2
	Laceration	Disruption <50% of circumference	863.31	4
III	Laceration	Disruption 50%-75% of circumference of D2	863.31	4
		Disruption 50%-100% of circumference of D1,D3,D4	863.31	4
IV	Laceration	Disruption >75% of circumference of D2	863.31	5
		Involving ampulla or distal common bile duct		5
V	Laceration	Massive disruption of duodenopancreatic complex	863.31	5
	Vascular	Devascularization of duodenum	863.31	5

*Advance one grade for multiple injuries up to grade III. D1-first position of duodenum; D2-second portion of duodenum; D3-third portion of duodenum; D4-fourth portion of duodenum

Pancreas Injury Scale

Grade*	Type of Injury	Description of Injury	ICD-9	AIS-90
I	Hematoma	Minor contusion without duct injury	863.81-863.84	2
	Laceration	Superficial laceration without duct injury		2
II	Hematoma	Major contusion without duct injury or tissue loss	863.81-863.84	2
	Laceration	Major laceration without duct injury or tissue loss		3
III	Laceration	Distal transection or parenchymal injury with duct injury	863.92/863.94	3
IV	Laceration	Proximal? transection or parenchymal injury involving ampulla	863.91	4
V	Laceration	Massive disruption of pancreatic head	863.91	5

*Advance one grade for multiple injuries up to grade III. *863.51,863.91 - head; 863.99,862.92-body;863.83,863.93-tail. ªProximal pancreas is to the patients' right of the superior mesenteric vein.

Fig. 40.1 The American Association for the Surgery of Trauma (AAST) Organ Injury Scales for Duodenum and Pancreas are presented here. (Adapted from Moore et al. [1])

- Mortality
    - Mortality is often attributable to associated injuries
    - Duodenal injury is associated with mortality rates of 6%–25%
    - Pancreatic injury is associated with mortality rates of 40%–66%

Take-Home Points for Patient Care

- Duodenal and pancreatic injury are uncommon findings in blunt and penetrating trauma, making experience managing their presentation rare in surgical training. Both injuries confer major morbidity and a high risk of death
- The retroperitoneal positioning of these structures can delay diagnosis of serious injury in hemodynamically stable patients
- Close anatomical associations of these structures make complications and related injuries highly common
- AAST organ injury grading scale drives operative management decisions
- While rare, pancreatic and duodenal injuries have high mortality rates relative to other types of abdominal trauma

Reference

1. Moore EE, Cogbill TH, Malangoni MA, et al. Organ injury scaling II: pancreas, duodenum, small bowel, colon, and rectum. J Trauma. 1990;30:1427–9.

Chapter 41
Colon Injury

Shari N. Reid-Gruner and Michael D. Cline

Introduction

- Historically, given high mortality associated with colon injury, management with colostomy was mandatory
- However, as available data emerged challenging this mandate, a selective management approach has seen decreased morbidity and mortality
- Contemporary management is dictated by the extent of injury, location, and the hemodynamic and physiologic status of the patient

Epidemiology/Pathophysiology

The majority of colon injuries are due to a penetrating mechanism (i.e., gunshot or stab wound), while blunt mechanisms account for less than 1% of injuries. Colon injury due to blunt trauma is the result of pressurization of a hollow viscus and/or mesenteric avulsion and devascularization.

Anatomy and Embryology

- *Anatomic Relations*

S. N. Reid-Gruner (✉) · M. D. Cline
Thomas Jefferson University Hospital, Philadelphia, PA, USA
e-mail: shari.reid@jefferson.edu

© The Author(s), under exclusive license to Springer Nature
Switzerland AG 2025
T. S. Brahmbhatt, D. R. Scantling (eds.), *Trauma Surgery Clerkship*,
Contemporary Surgical Clerkships,
https://doi.org/10.1007/978-3-032-01412-2_41

- – Right and left colon are partially retroperitoneal
- – Transverse and sigmoid colon are intraperitoneal

- *Midgut*

    - – Colonic contributions include the cecum, appendix, right ascending colon, and proximal two-thirds of the transverse colon
    - – Arterial blood supply via the superior mesenteric artery (SMA), which gives rise to the middle colic, right colic, and ileocolic arteries
    - – Venous drainage via the superior mesenteric vein (SMV), which merges with the splenic vein at the portal vein confluence

- *Hindgut*

    - – Colonic contributions include the distal one-third of the transverse, left (descending), and sigmoid colons
    - – Arterial blood supply via the inferior mesenteric artery (IMA), which gives rise to the left colic, sigmoid, and superior rectal arteries
    - – Venous drainage via the inferior mesenteric vein (IMV), which merges with the splenic vein lateral to the ligament of Treitz and posterior to the pancreas

- *Anastomotic Arcades*

    - – Marginal artery of Drummond connects the SMA and IMA at the mesenteric border of the colon
    - – Arc of Riolan connects the proximal SMA and IMA

Initial Evaluation and Management

- Initial evaluation is dictated by Advanced Trauma Life Support (ATLS) principles

    - – Tachycardia and hypotension may be seen in hemorrhagic shock due to a concomitant vascular injury
    - – Generalized peritonitis may be present with intraperitoneal hollow viscus perforation, although retroperitoneal perforation may not manifest with peritonitis
    - – Digital rectal examination (DRE) demonstrating blood has a high specificity for colorectal injury, but is limited by poor sensitivity

- Hemodynamically unstable patients or those with generalized peritonitis should undergo immediate laparotomy
- Hemodynamically stable patients without generalized peritonitis may be further evaluated with contrast-enhanced (IV +/− rectal) CT (CECT) of the abdomen and pelvis

- CECT has a sensitivity and specificity of >90% for full-thickness colon injury
- Radiographic findings include pneumoperitoneum, unexplained peritoneal fluid, thickened colonic wall or pericolonic fat stranding, and extravasation of rectal contrast, although absence of extravasation of rectal contrast does not rule out an injury

Classification

- The AAST Organ Injury Scaling for Colon (see Table 41.1) classify traumatic injury among five grades according to the extent of hematoma or laceration.

Operative Management

- General considerations
  - Pericolic hematomas due to penetrating injury must be explored, while those due to blunt injury may be selectively explored
  - Missed injuries are most commonly at the mesenteric border as well as at difficult to mobilize regions (i.e., splenic flexure)
  - Proximal and distal manual compression followed by gently milking of the bowel contents toward the suspected injury may assist in its identification
  - Primary repair refers to direct closure of a defect (single or double-layer closure with absorbable or nonabsorbable suture) or segmental resection and primary anastomosis

Table 41.1 AAST Colon Injury Scale [1]

Grade[a]	Type of injury	Description of injury
I	Hematoma	Contusion or hematoma without devascularization
	Laceration	Patrial-thickness laceration without perforation
II	Laceration	Laceration <50% of circumference
III	Laceration	Laceration ≥50% of circumference without transection
IV	Laceration	Transection of the colon
V	Laceration	Transection of the colon with segmental tissue loss
	Vascular	Devascularized segment

Moore et al. [2]
[a]Advance one grade for multiple injuries up to grade III

- Nondestructive (<50% of bowel wall injured without devascularization) [3, 4]

    - Debridement and primary repair with absorbable or nonabsorbable suture or segmental resection and anastomosis
- Destructive (>50% of bowel wall or devascularization) [3, 4]

    - Segmental resection and anastomosis
    - Although consideration of resection and end colostomy in patients at high risk for abdominal complications (severe fecal contamination, greater than or equal to 4 units of blood transfusions within 24 h, inappropriate antibiotic prophylaxis) is reasonable, data suggest that primary repair is equivalent in regard to abdominal complications, even following damage control surgery. [5–7]

Complications

- Intra-abdominal septic complications

    - Abscess
    - Anastomotic dehiscence
    - Fascial dehiscence
- Stoma complications

    - Necrosis, retraction, prolapse, parastomal abscess, and parastomal hernia
- Wound infection

    - Skin should be left open to decrease the incidence of fascial dehiscence and necrotizing fasciitis; delayed primary closure may be considered
- Mortality

    - Early death is typically due to exsanguination from concomitant injuries
    - Late morality is a result of sepsis and multisystem organ failure

Take-Home Points for Patient Care

- Initial evaluation and management are dictated by ATLS
- Patients with generalized peritonitis or hemodynamic instability should undergo immediate laparotomy
- Hemodynamically stable patients without generalized peritonitis may undergo CECT to further delineate intra-abdominal injury
- Operative management of colon injury is dictated by whether the injury is destructive or nondestructive
- Contemporary data suggests that primary repair is safe, even in those patients at high risk for abdominal complications

References

1. AAST Injury Scoring Scale [Internet]. Chicago: The American Association for the Surgery of Trauma; cited 2022 November 30. Available from: https://www.aast.org/resources-detail/injury-scoring-scale.
2. Moore EE, et al. Organ injury scaling, II: pancreas, duodenum, small bowel, colon, and rectum. J Trauma. 1990;30(11):1427–9. PMID: 2231822.
3. Mattox K. Trauma. 7th ed. New York: McGraw Hill Medical; 2013.
4. Asensio J. Current therapy of trauma and surgical critical care. 2nd ed. Philadelphia: Elsevier Inc.; 2016.
5. Cullinane DC, Jawa RS, Como JJ, Moore AE, Morris DS, Cheriyan J, Guillamondegui OD, Goldberg SR, Petrey L, Schaefer GP, Khwaja KA, Rowell SE, Barbosa RR, Bass GA, Kasotakis G, Robinson BRH. Management of penetrating intraperitoneal colon injuries: a meta-analysis and practice management guideline from the Eastern Association for the Surgery of Trauma. J Trauma Acute Care Surg. 2019;86(3):505–15. https://doi.org/10.1097/TA.0000000000002146.
6. Demetriades D, Murray JA, Chan L, Ordoñez C, Bowley D, Nagy KK, Cornwell EE 3rd, Velmahos GC, Muñoz N, Hatzitheofilou C, Schwab CW, Rodriguez A, Cornejo C, Davis KA, Namias N, Wisner DH, Ivatury RR, Moore EE, Acosta JA, Maull KI, Thomason MH, Spain DA, Committee on Multicenter Clinical Trials, American Association for the Surgery of Trauma. Penetrating colon injuries requiring resection: diversion or primary anastomosis? An AAST prospective multicenter study. J Trauma. 2001;50(5):765–75. https://doi.org/10.1097/00005373-200105000-00001. PMID: 11371831.
7. Miller PR, Chang MC, Hoth JJ, Holmes JH 4th, Meredith JW. Colonic resection in the setting of damage control laparotomy: is delayed anastomosis safe? Am Surg. 2007;73(6):606–9. https://doi.org/10.1177/000313480707300613; discussion 609–10. PMID: 17658099.

Chapter 42
Abdominal Vascular Injuries

Maha H. Haqqani and Jeffrey J. Siracuse

Introduction

- Abdominal vascular injury, while rare, has the potential to be lethal [1].
- Patients who sustain major abdominal vascular trauma are at risk of profound hemorrhagic shock and rapid clinical deterioration.
- Many patients with injuries to the great vessels (aorta, inferior vena cava) do not survive to hospital presentation [2–4].
- Those who do survive are at risk of early death secondary to exsanguination, or late death due to multisystem organ failure in the setting of profound coagulopathy and acidosis [1, 2, 5].
- Recent years, particularly with advances in endovascular therapy, have seen lower mortality associated with blunt, but not penetrating, abdominal vascular injuries [5].

M. H. Haqqani (✉) · J. J. Siracuse
Division of Vascular and Endovascular Surgery, Boston Medical Center, Boston University Chobanian and Avedisian School of Medicine, Boston, MA, USA
e-mail: Jeffrey.Siracuse@bmc.org

T. S. Brahmbhatt, D. R. Scantling (eds.), *Trauma Surgery Clerkship*, Contemporary Surgical Clerkships, https://doi.org/10.1007/978-3-032-01412-2_42

Epidemiology

Statistics

Incidence

- Vascular trauma accounts for approximately 1.6–5.9% of all civilian trauma, with abdominal vascular injuries accounting for 8–25% of all vascular trauma [6–8].
- Abdominal vascular trauma is less common in pediatric and geriatric populations [6].
- Males are more likely to suffer from abdominal vascular trauma than females, accounting for 70–80% of adults with such injuries [6–8].
- Males are more likely to have penetrating trauma than females (48% vs. 17%) [9].
- Black patients are more likely to suffer from penetrating trauma, with 77% of black patients having a penetrating mechanism as opposed to 20% of white patients [9].
- Black patients are almost twice as likely to die from major abdominal and pelvic vascular injuries than white patients [9].

Causes

- Blunt abdominal vascular injury is more common than penetrating (57% vs. 40%) [9].
- The majority of blunt abdominal vascular trauma is secondary to traffic accidents, particularly involving motor vehicles and motorcycles [10].
- While blunt trauma has historically been the leading cause of abdominal vascular injury, penetrating trauma in the United States continues to rise.
- The incidence of penetrating trauma is higher in male than female sex [6].
- Approximately 10% of all firearm injuries involve a vascular injury, with about a third of those involving vessels in the abdomen or pelvis [11].

Morbidity and Mortality

- Major abdominal vascular injury is the number one cause of noncompressible torso hemorrhage [6, 12].
- Most commonly injured vessels include the iliac arteries (17.7%), the inferior vena cava or IVC (10.3%), the abdominal aorta (8.6%), and renal arteries (7.1%) [9].
- Overall mortality rates for abdominal vascular trauma range from 20% to 60% [1].

- Blunt trauma is associated with greater mortality than penetrating abdominal vascular trauma [6].
- Injuries to the IVC are associated with the highest mortality, with 30–50% of patients dying before hospital presentation [13, 14].

General Presentation

- Abdominal vascular injuries rarely present in isolation, with approximately 33–50% of patients having a concomitant hollow viscus or liver injury [6].
- Blunt abdominal vascular trauma is also often associated with concomitant neurologic, thoracic, or orthopedic injuries.
- Only one in ten cases of blunt abdominal aortic injuries (BAI) occurs in isolation, and approximately half have an associated lumbar spine or pelvic fracture [15, 16].
- Patients with major abdominal vascular trauma often present with hemodynamic instability secondary to massive intraperitoneal or retroperitoneal hemorrhage, although many may present initially tachycardia as the only indicator of shock.
- A high index of suspicion should be held for major abdominal vascular trauma in hemodynamically unstable patients with signs of abdominal or pelvic trauma and peritonitis [6].
- A proportion of patients may present in cardiopulmonary arrest and require a resuscitative anterolateral thoracotomy, with poor associated survival rates and overall outcomes [1, 2].
- However, hemodynamic stability does not exclude the presence of major abdominal vascular injury, as hemorrhage may be contained by retroperitoneal tamponade [6, 17].

Anatomy

Arterial

- The abdominal aorta begins at the level of the diaphragm and bifurcates into the right and left common iliac arteries at the level of the L4 vertebra (Fig. 42.1).
- The common iliac arteries further branch into the external and internal iliac arteries. The external iliac arteries go on to become the common femoral arteries and provide the blood supply for the extremities, while the internal iliac arteries provide the bloody supply to the pelvis.
- The three major mesenteric branches of the abdominal aorta are the celiac axis (or celiac trunk), the superior mesenteric artery (SMA), and the inferior mesenteric artery (IMA), with the latter typically branching off below the level of the

Fig. 42.1 Abdominal aorta and its major branches [18]

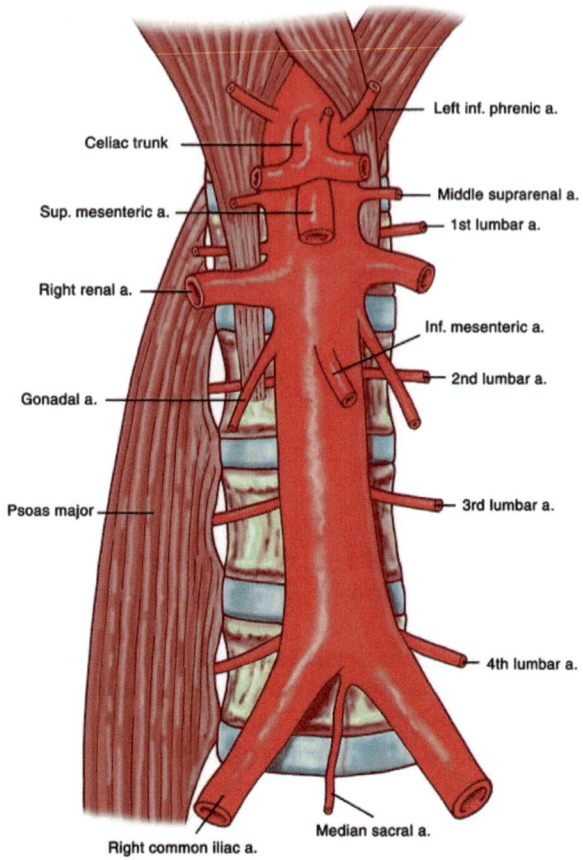

Celiac trunk

Sup. mesenteric a.

Right renal a.

Gonadal a.

Psoas major

Left inf. phrenic a.

Middle suprarenal a.

1st lumbar a.

Inf. mesenteric a.

2nd lumbar a.

3rd lumbar a.

4th lumbar a.

Median sacral a.

Right common iliac a.

renal arteries. Injury to one or more of these arteries and their branching vessels carries the risk of bowel ischemia.

Venous

- The external and internal iliac veins on both the right and left combine to form the common iliac veins, which drain blood from the pelvis.
- The right and left common iliac veins form the IVC at the level of the L5 vertebra.
- The IVC is classified into multiple zones based on its relationship to the liver and the kidneys, as shown in Fig. 42.2.
- The renal veins drain directly into the IVC.
- Veins from the gastrointestinal tract, pancreas, spleen, and gallbladder drain into the portal vein and not directly into systemic circulation.

Fig. 42.2 The major branches draining into the IVC [19]

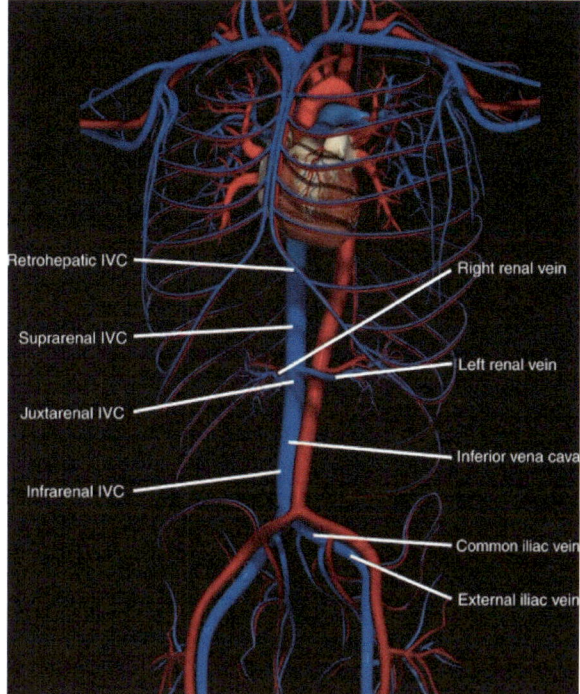

History

- In cases of trauma, there is often insufficient time to obtain a thorough history of present illness and past medical history.
- Nonetheless, information from Emergency Medical Services (EMS) providers about the scene of the incident can be helpful, particularly in cases of blunt trauma, in guiding providers toward formulating a differential diagnosis about possible injuries.
- Velocity of vehicles involved, rollover, height of a fall, or major bleeding at the scene or en route can alter index of suspicion for major vascular injuries. However, this information should not serve to bias clinical judgment during the initial trauma resuscitation.
- Any information on prior surgical history is also relevant as it may affect potential operative approach or other intraoperative considerations in the event that the patient needs emergent intervention.

Physical Exam

- The primary and secondary surveys during initial trauma evaluation are critical in evaluating for potential abdominal vascular injuries.
- Patients with abdominal vascular trauma are likely to present with tachycardia, hypotension, abdominal tenderness, and/or distension.
- A "seatbelt sign" (as shown in Fig. 42.3) is associated with mesenteric injuries and lumbar spine fractures, particularly Chance fractures, but less commonly can also indicate a BAI.
- Bilateral femoral pulses should be examined to evaluate for aortic and/or iliac artery injuries [6].
- Distracting injuries such as extremity and spinal fractures can confound the abdominal exam; a high index of suspicion for chest, abdominal, or pelvic vascular injury should remain in those who present with hemodynamic instability following blunt trauma.
- In cases of penetrating trauma, location of stab or ballistic wounds on the patient's body can provide important information on potential injuries.
- When possible, paper clips should be applied onto penetrating wounds to allow identification on cross-sectional imaging and help determine trajectory.

Types of Injury

Blunt

Dissection

- Arterial dissection occurs when a tear in the intima, the innermost layer of the arterial wall, allows blood to flow between the intimal and medial layers, causing a false lumen.
- Dissections have the potential to be flow limiting and cause ischemia to organs perfused by the involved vessel and its branches.

Fig. 42.3 Abdominal seatbelt sign following a motor vehicle collision [20]

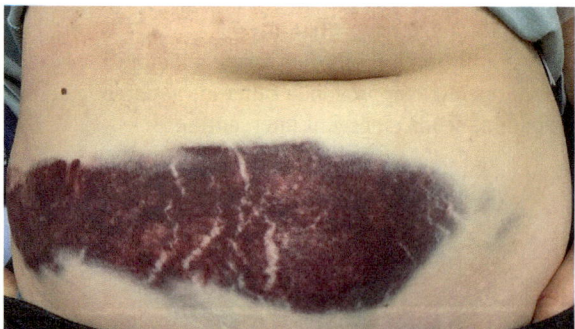

- Dissection of the abdominal aorta is rare but can occur with major trauma, and is often complicated by thrombosis, with mortality rates approaching 75% with conservative management and 18–37% with operative management [21].
- Blunt dissection of mesenteric arteries such as the celiac trunk and SMA can also occur and in recent years have been effectively treated with angiography and stenting, although long-term data on outcomes of endovascular management is limited [22].

Blunt Aortic Injury (BAI)

- BAI is classified into four types based on severity. These are as follows:
  - Grade 1: intimal tear
  - Grade 2: intramural hematoma
  - Grade 3: pseudoaneurysm
  - Grade 4: free rupture [23]
- Grade 1 and 2 BAI are typically able to be managed nonoperatively.
- In recent years, advances in endovascular therapy have allowed Grade 3 BAI to be largely managed with an endovascular approach [15, 24].
- Unfortunately, patients with Grade 4 BAI are highly unlikely to survive to hospital presentation due to early exsanguination.

Avulsion

- Avulsion injuries of mesenteric vessels occur in about 1–5% of all blunt abdominal trauma cases [25].
- Mesenteric avulsion can compromise blood supply and lead to intestinal ischemia and perforation [25].
- Signs include abdominal wall bruising, ecchymosis, melena, and less commonly, shock and hemodynamic instability.
- Missed injury rates at the time of initial evaluation can be as high as 58% [25, 26].

Retroperitoneal Hematoma

- Traumatic retroperitoneal hematomas are most often caused by blunt trauma and venous bleeding into the retroperitoneal space [27].
- The retroperitoneum is divided into three zones, each of which contains certain important vascular structures:
  - Zone I: between the psoas muscles; contains the abdominal aorta, IVC, duodenum, and pancreas.

- – Zone II: lateral to the psoas muscles on each side; contains kidneys (including part of the renal artery and vein), adrenal glands, ureters, and portions of the colon.
- – Zone III: the pelvic zone; contains the iliac vessels and all their pelvic branches [27].

- All Zone I hematomas from penetrating trauma should be operatively explored.
- Most blunt Zone I hematomas also warrant operative exploration due to likelihood of major vascular injury, unless preoperative imaging argues against evidence of ongoing bleeding.
- Zone II and III hematomas from blunt trauma can be observed if non-expanding.
- Expanding Zone II hematomas typically warrant operative exploration, while expanding Zone III hematomas require preperitoneal pelvic packing and/or angioembolization of bleeding vessels [6].

Penetrating

Firearm

- Ballistic or firearm injuries carry high-intensity kinetic energy and can have an unpredictable course, with the potential to damage multiple intra-abdominal structures including solid organs, hollow viscera, and vasculature [28].
- The mainstay of treatment for ballistic wounds with vascular injury is operative management.

Non-firearm

- Stab and pierce wounds from knives or other sharp objects deliver focal kinetic energy and tissue damage along their tract, as opposed to more widespread damage associated with ballistic wounds.
- Other sources of non-firearm penetrating trauma include pieces of glass, metal, or other shards, with or without an associated blunt mechanism.
- Back and flank stab wounds carry a greater risk of injury to retroperitoneal structures including the abdominal aorta, IVC, and kidneys [29].

Imaging

Focused Assessment with Sonography for Trauma (FAST)

- The FAST exam is a useful adjunct for identifying significant intra-abdominal bleeding, but it is neither particularly sensitive nor specific for abdominal vascular trauma.
- Sensitivity is only about 40% in cases of blunt trauma without hypovolemic shock, and even in the hands of skilled ultrasound operators, false negative rates are close to 10% even in the presence of abdominal vascular trauma [30].
- Specificity can be as low as 18% following gunshot wounds.

Computed Tomography (CT) Angiography

- CT angiography (CTA) is the diagnostic imaging modality of choice for vascular injuries.
- Sensitivity and specificity of CTA for identifying blunt aortic injury are 86–100% and 40–100%, respectively [30].
- Multiphase contrast imaging including arterial, venous, and delayed phases can help differentiate between arterial and venous bleeding [6].
- CTA can provide information on location, nature, and severity of major abdominal vascular injuries (Fig. 42.4).
- This information can help guide intervention and may save the patient the morbidity of a large laparotomy.
- CTA should always be considered in the absence of profound hemodynamic instability necessitating emergent operative intervention.

To Image or Not to Image?

The Hemodynamically Unstable Patient

- In cases of hemodynamic instability following blunt or penetrating trauma and concern for intra-abdominal bleeding, the patient should be taken expeditiously to the operating room for a laparotomy.
- Delaying operative intervention to obtain further imaging in this scenario is inappropriate and may compromise patient safety and outcomes.

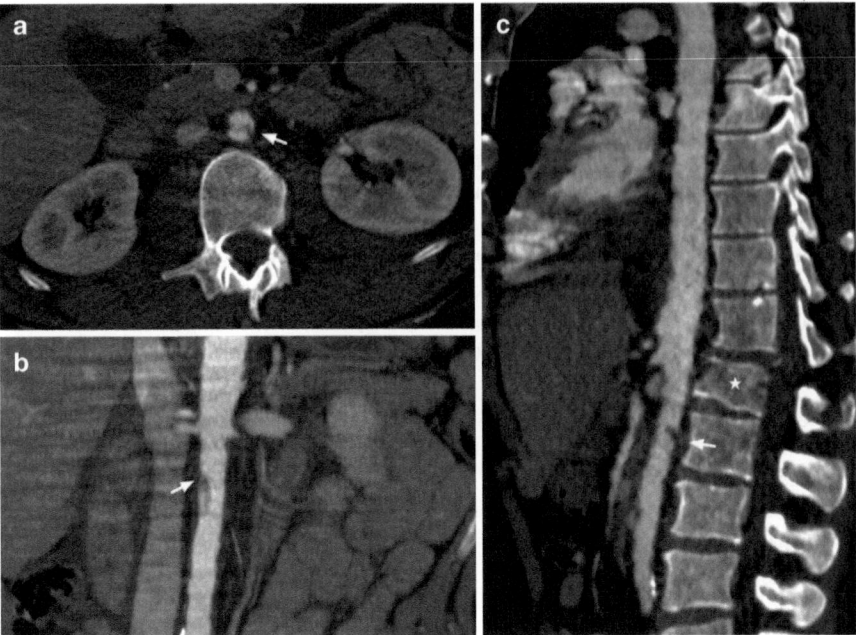

Fig. 42.4 CTA showing BAI with a dissection flap (white arrows) following a motorcycle collision [31]

The Stable Patient or the "Responder"

- In the hemodynamically stable patient with a positive FAST, or a patient who presents with hypotension and/or tachycardia but responds well to transfusion of blood products, CT angiography should be obtained when readily available.
- Surgeon discretion and clinical judgment play a major role in deciding when to obtain cross-sectional imaging versus proceeding directly to the OR.

Treatment

Observation

- Nonoperative management with observation is an option for hemodynamically stable patients with low-grade injuries, as well as carefully selected patients with intimal tears and pseudoaneurysms of major vessels [6].
- Patients undergoing nonoperative management should be monitored carefully with serial abdominal exams, labs to determine their serum hemoglobin and hematocrit, and in some cases interval imaging to evaluate progression of disease.

- Any hemodynamic or clinical change warrants a low threshold for repeat CT imaging and consideration of open or endovascular intervention.

Endovascular

Stent Graft

- Stent grafts, or covered stents, are composed of a metal stent lined with a prosthetic material. They allow preservation of flow across the main body of the involved vessel.
- Endovascular repair for blunt vascular injuries is associated with lower blood loss, decreased operating time, hospital length of stay, and in-hospital mortality [32].
- Endovascular repair of BAI is on the rise, and stent grafts are routinely used for endovascular aortic repair (EVAR) [24].
- Blunt mesenteric and renal artery injuries can also be managed with stent grafts or, less often, bare metal stents [22].

Coil Embolization

- An alternative to stent grafts is coil embolization, which is typically used to control life-threatening bleeding or to exclude blood flow to a pseudoaneurysm at risk for rupture.
- Coils are made of steel or platinum, and are looped in various shapes and sizes, promoting clot formation and thrombogenicity [33].
- Coil embolization can be highly effective for controlling bleeding vessels in the pelvis, especially in conjunction with repair of orthopedic injuries.

Open

Repair

- Laparotomy is indicated in cases of hemodynamic instability following blunt or penetrating abdominal trauma, with the goal of quickly identifying and addressing the most life-threatening injuries, including major vascular injuries.
- Small injuries to large vessels such as the aorta, IVC, and iliac vessels, and to the celiac axis and SMA, can be repaired primarily with nonabsorbable, monofilament suture such as Prolene [1].

- If the defect is large enough that primary repair could significantly narrow the vessel lumen, patch angioplasty can be performed with synthetic material or autologous vein [1].
- In some instances, the patient's condition may not allow for a complex repair and may necessitate temporizing interventions such as intravascular shunts, or in cases of venous injury, ligation.
- If performing ligation of the IVC or iliac vein(s), prophylactic four-compartment lower extremity fasciotomies should be considered due to the risk of compartment syndrome [6].
- Fasciotomies should also be considered for combined arterial and venous abdominal or pelvic vascular injuries.

Bypass

- In cases of significant tissue loss or segmental damage, an interposition or bypass graft from the proximal undamaged segment to the distal segment is performed using autologous vein or a Dacron or polytetrafluoroethylene (PTFE) graft [1].
- Mesenteric vessels should be attempted to be repaired via a vein patch, interposition graft, or even reimplantation, particularly in the case of the SMA [6].
- Significant injuries to the celiac axis may be managed with ligation provided adequate collaterals exist [6].
- Renal arteries should be primarily repaired when possible, but may need complex reconstruction with interposition graft. In cases of hemodynamic instability and life-threatening hemorrhage, renal artery ligation and nephrectomy may be indicated [1].

Complications

Intraoperative

- The most common intraoperative complication is exsanguination and cardiopulmonary arrest from massive uncontrolled hemorrhage.
- Intraoperative graft thrombosis is also a potential complication and may require reexploration of a newly created bypass.
- When operating on major vessels such as the abdominal aorta and iliac arteries, distal embolization of plaque or thrombus to the extremities is possible, and distal pulses or Doppler signals should always be checked once perfusion to the extremities is restored following removal of vascular clamps.

Postoperative

- Postoperative complications following open repair include thrombosis of the repair or bypass graft and suture line dehiscence.
- Postoperative infections are particularly an issue with penetrating traumatic injuries as well as with orthopedic hardware or with gross contamination from nearby bowel injuries [34].
- Specific complications following endovascular therapy include stent graft thrombosis, in-stent stenosis, and in case of EVAR, endoleaks (caused by a lack of complete seal to exclude the pseudoaneurysm or injured portion).
- Major abdominal venous injuries also carry a significant risk of venous thromboembolism (VTE) in the postoperative period [14].

Prognosis

Outcomes

- Mortality associated with abdominal vascular injury remains high, with an overall mortality rate of 29% [35].
- Injuries to the abdominal aorta, IVC, and portal vein carry particularly high mortality, at 68%, 42%, and 67%, respectively [35].
- Mortality due to abdominal vascular trauma from a single stab wound is lower than that from multiple stab wounds or firearms [6].
- Even following initial damage control operation or repair of abdominal vascular injuries, patients may spend weeks to months in the hospital recovering from their injuries, and often require both physical and psychological rehabilitation.
- Overall, data on long-term outcomes following repair of major abdominal vascular injuries is limited, partly due to challenges with follow-up and surveillance in the trauma patient population.

Surveillance

- There is a lack of clear guidelines on surveillance of bypass grafts and mesenteric stents in the trauma population.
- Endovascular aortic repairs (EVAR) should undergo a CTA within 30 days of intervention to evaluate for an endoleak. If negative, annual duplex ultrasound of the abdominal aorta can be performed for ongoing surveillance [36].
- Patients with major abdominal venous injuries requiring ligation do not necessarily need additional surveillance for lower extremity edema or deep vein thrombosis (DVT) beyond a physical exam [37].

References

1. Kobayashi LM, Costantini TW, Hamel MG, Dierksheide JE, Coimbra R. Abdominal vascular trauma. Trauma Surg Acute Care Open. 2016;1:e000015. https://doi.org/10.1136/tsaco-2016-000015.
2. Asensio JA, Chahwan S, Hanpeter D, et al. Operative management and outcome of 302 abdominal vascular injuries. Am J Surg. 2000;180:528–34.
3. Giannakopoulos TG, Avgerinos ED. Management of peripheral and truncal venous injuries. Front Surg. 2017;4:46. https://doi.org/10.3389/fsurg.2017.00046.
4. Huerta S, Bui TD, Nguyen TH, Banimahd FN, Porral D, Dolich MO. Predictors of mortality and management of patients with traumatic inferior vena cava injuries. Am Surg. 2006;72:290–6.
5. Branco BC, Musonza T, Long MA, Chung J, Todd SR, Wall MJ, Mills JL, Gilani R. Survival trends after inferior vena cava and aortic injuries in the United States. J Vasc Surg. 2018;68:1880–8.
6. Kobayashi L, Coimbra R, Goes AMO, et al. American Association for the Surgery of Trauma–World Society of Emergency Surgery guidelines on diagnosis and management of abdominal vascular injuries. J Trauma Acute Care Surg. 2020;89:1197–211.
7. Barmparas G, Inaba K, Talving P, David J-S, Lam L, Plurad D, Green D, Demetriades D. Pediatric vs adult vascular trauma: a national trauma databank review. J Pediatr Surg. 2010;45:1404–12. https://doi.org/10.1016/j.jpedsurg.2009.09.017.
8. DuBose JJ, Savage SA, Fabian TC, et al. The American Association for the Surgery of Trauma PROspective Observational Vascular Injury Treatment (PROOVIT) registry. J Trauma Acute Care Surg. 2015;78:215–23. https://doi.org/10.1097/TA.0000000000000520.
9. Talbot E, Evans S, Hellenthal N, Monie D, Campbell P, Cooper S. Abdominal and pelvic vascular injury: a National Trauma Data Bank study. Am Surg. 2019;85:292–3.
10. Barbati ME, Hildebrand F, Andruszkow H, Lefering R, Jacobs MJ, Jalaie H, Gombert A. Prevalence and outcome of abdominal vascular injury in severe trauma patients based on a TraumaRegister DGU international registry analysis. Sci Rep. 2021;11:20247–9. https://doi.org/10.1038/s41598-021-99635-9.
11. Siracuse JJ, Cheng TW, Farber A, James T, Zuo Y, Kalish JA, Jones DW, Kalesan B. Vascular repair after firearm injury is associated with increased morbidity and mortality. J Vasc Surg. 2019;69:1524–1531.e1. https://doi.org/10.1016/j.jvs.2018.07.081.
12. Chang R, Fox EE, Greene TJ, et al. Multicenter retrospective study of noncompressible torso hemorrhage. J Trauma Acute Care Surg. 2017;83:11–8. https://doi.org/10.1097/TA.0000000000001530.
13. Matsumoto S, Jung K, Smith A, Coimbra R. Management of IVC injury: repair or ligation? A propensity score matching analysis using the National Trauma Data Bank. J Am Coll Surg. 2018;226:752–759.e2. https://doi.org/10.1016/j.jamcollsurg.2018.01.043.
14. Haqqani MH, Levin SR, Kalish JA, Farber A, Brahmbhatt TS, Richman AP, Siracuse JJ, Jones DW. High mortality and venous thromboembolism risk following major penetrating abdominal venous injuries. Ann Vasc Surg. 2021;71:457. https://doi.org/10.1016/j.avsg.2021.06.002.
15. de Mestral C, Dueck AD, Gomez D, Haas B, Nathens AB. Associated injuries, management, and outcomes of blunt abdominal aortic injury. J Vasc Surg. 2012;56:656–60. https://doi.org/10.1016/j.jvs.2012.02.027.
16. Mellnick VM, McDowell C, Lubner M, Bhalla S, Menias CO. CT features of blunt abdominal aortic injury. Emerg Radiol. 2012;19(4):301–7. https://doi.org/10.1007/s10140-012-1030-7.
17. Magee GA, Cho J, Matsushima K, Strumwasser A, Inaba K, Jazaeri O, Fox CJ, Demetriades D. Isolated iliac vascular injuries and outcome of repair versus ligation of isolated iliac vein injury. J Vasc Surg. 2018;67:254–61. https://doi.org/10.1016/j.jvs.2017.07.107.
18. Devarajan J, Subramaniam B. Applied anatomy of the aorta. In: Subramaniam K, Park KW, Subramaniam B, editors. Anesthesia and perioperative care for aortic surgery. New York: Springer New York; 2011. p. 1–15. https://doi.org/10.1007/978-0-387-85922-4_1.

19. Sandhu H, Charlton-Ouw K. Abdominal vein injuries. In: Dua A, Desai S, Holcomb J, editors. Clinical review of vascular trauma. Berlin, Heidelberg: Springer; 2014. p. 201–11. https://doi.org/10.1007/978-3-642-39100-2_17.
20. Redmond CE, Gibney B, Nicolaou S. The abdominal seatbelt sign. Abdom Radiol. 2020;45:2934–6. https://doi.org/10.1007/s00261-020-02445-2.
21. Berthet J, Marty-Ané C, Veerapen R, Picard E, Mary H, Alric P. Dissection of the abdominal aorta in blunt trauma: endovascular or conventional surgical management? J Vasc Surg. 2003;38:997–1003. S074152140300613X [pii].
22. Safaya A, Carroll FX, Laskowski IA. Blunt mesenteric vascular injuries: endovascular management and midterm outcomes. EJVES Vasc Forum. 2021;53:9–13. https://doi.org/10.1016/j.ejvsvf.2021.08.001.
23. Azizzadeh A, Keyhani K, Miller CC, Coogan SM, Safi HJ, Estrera AL. Blunt traumatic aortic injury: initial experience with endovascular repair. J Vasc Surg. 2009;49:1403–8. https://doi.org/10.1016/j.jvs.2009.02.234.
24. Branco BC, DuBose JJ, Zhan LX, Hughes JD, Goshima KR, Rhee P, Mills JL. Trends and outcomes of endovascular therapy in the management of civilian vascular injuries. J Vasc Surg. 2014;60:1297–307. https://doi.org/10.1016/j.jvs.2014.05.028.
25. Kordzadeh A, Melchionda V, Rhodes KM, Fletcher EO, Panayiotopolous YP. Blunt abdominal trauma and mesenteric avulsion: a systematic review. Eur J Trauma Emerg Surg. 2015;42:311–5. https://doi.org/10.1007/s00068-015-0514-z.
26. Kordzadeh A, Devanesan A, Parkinson T, Rahim K, Panayiotopoulos Y. Subtle mesenteric avulsion in a traumatic abdominal wall hernia: a case report. Int J Surg Case Rep. 2012;3:417–9. https://doi.org/10.1016/j.ijscr.2012.04.020.
27. Mondie C, Maguire N, Rentea R. Retroperitoneal hematoma. In: StatPearls. Treasure Island: StatPearls Publishing; 2022.
28. Forbes J, Burns B. Abdominal gunshot wounds. In: StatPearls. Treasure Island: StatPearls Publishing; 2022.
29. Shanmuganathan K, Mirvis SE, Chiu WC, Killeen KL, Hogan GJ, Scalea TM. Penetrating torso trauma: triple-contrast helical CT in peritoneal violation and organ injury—a prospective study in 200 patients. Radiology. 2004;231:775–84. https://doi.org/10.1148/radiol.2313030126.
30. Patterson BO, Holt PJ, Cleanthis M, Tai N, Carrell T, Loosemore TM. Imaging vascular trauma. Br J Surg. 2011;99:494–505. https://doi.org/10.1002/bjs.7763.
31. Prado E, Chamorro EM, Marín A, Fuentes CG, Zhou ZC. CT features of blunt abdominal aortic injury: an infrequent but life-threatening event. Emerg Radiol. 2021;29:187–95. https://doi.org/10.1007/s10140-021-01964-9.
32. Biagioni RB, Burihan MC, Nasser F, Biagioni LC, Ingrund JC. Endovascular treatment of penetrating arterial trauma with stent grafts. Vasa. 2018;47:125–30. https://doi.org/10.1024/0301-1526/a000672.
33. Lopera J. Embolization in trauma: principles and techniques. Semin Interv Radiol. 2010;27:014–28. https://doi.org/10.1055/s-0030-1247885.
34. Feliciano DV. Approach to major abdominal vascular injury. J Vasc Surg. 1988;7:730–6. https://doi.org/10.1016/0741-5214(88)90032-8.
35. Paul JS, Webb TP, Aprahamian C, Weigelt JA. Intraabdominal vascular injury: are we getting any better? J Trauma Inj Infect Crit Care. 2010;69:1393–7. https://doi.org/10.1097/TA.0b013e3181e49045.
36. Smith T, Quencer KB. Best practice guidelines: imaging surveillance after endovascular aneurysm repair. Am J Roentgenol. 2020;214:1165–74. https://doi.org/10.2214/AJR.19.22197.
37. Sullivan PS, Dente CJ, Patel S, et al. Outcome of ligation of the inferior vena cava in the modern era. Am J Surg. 2010;199:500–6. https://doi.org/10.1016/j.amjsurg.2009.05.013.

Chapter 43
Renal Injury

David T. Lubkin and Bryan A. Cotton

Anatomy

- The kidneys are located bilaterally in the retroperitoneum and are protected by the lower ribs.
- An envelope of connective tissue surrounds the kidney. The anterior renal fascia is also known as Gerota's fascia, and the posterior renal fascia is also known as Zuckerkandl's fascia [1].
- Arterial blood is supplied by the bilateral renal arteries, which branch from the aorta at the level of L1–L2.
- Venous drainage occurs through the bilateral renal veins, which drain directly into the inferior vena cava (IVC) at the level of L1–L2. The left renal vein is substantially longer than the right renal vein, and the adrenal and gonadal veins drain into the renal vein on the left but do not on the right.
- Urine is drained from nephrons into the renal calyces, which coalesce into the renal pelvis at the renal hilum. Urine is then drained from the kidney via the ureter.
- At the renal hilum in standard anatomy, the vein is anterior to the artery and the artery is anterior to the pelvis.

D. T. Lubkin
Department of Surgery, McGovern Medical School at The University of Texas Health Science Center at Houston, Houston, TX, USA
e-mail: David.E.Lubkin@uth.tmc.edu

B. A. Cotton (✉)
Department of Surgery and The Center for Translational Injury Research, McGovern Medical School at The University of Texas Health Science Center at Houston, Houston, TX, USA
e-mail: Bryan.A.Cotton@uth.tmc.edu

© The Author(s), under exclusive license to Springer Nature Switzerland AG 2025
T. S. Brahmbhatt, D. R. Scantling (eds.), *Trauma Surgery Clerkship*, Contemporary Surgical Clerkships, https://doi.org/10.1007/978-3-032-01412-2_43

Epidemiology

- A blunt mechanism of injury is more common than penetrating, with blunt comprising 65% of renal injuries and penetrating comprising 35% of injuries [2].
- Motor vehicle collision is the most common blunt mechanism (63%) while gunshot wound is the most common penetrating mechanism (65%) [3].
- Young males are the most commonly affected patient population.
- Concomitant damage to other intra-abdominal structures is common with both blunt and penetrating mechanisms.

Diagnosis

- Initial evaluation of every trauma patient occurs in a standardized fashion beginning with the primary and secondary survey. Chest X-ray and pelvis X-ray should be performed for high energy blunt mechanisms and may assist in determination of trajectory in penetrating mechanisms. FAST exam should be performed to evaluate for intra-abdominal bleeding.
- In the hemodynamically unstable patient with suspected intra-abdominal bleeding, no further workup should be performed. Resuscitation with blood products should be initiated and the patient should be taken immediately to the operating room where diagnosis can be made definitively intraoperatively.
- In the hemodynamically stable patient without other clear indication for immediate surgery, additional trauma workup should be pursued. Penetrating injuries to the flank and blunt trauma directly overlying the kidneys may increase suspicion for renal injury. Gross or microscopic hematuria may also suggest kidney injury, though it is neither sensitive nor specific. Generally, definitive diagnosis of renal injury is made on contrast-enhanced CT scan. CT scan should include a delayed phase to optimally assess the urinary collecting system and ureter.

Injury Grading

- The American Association for the Surgery of Trauma (AAST) grading system is the most commonly used for grading the severity of renal injuries [4]:
  - Grade I
    - Subcapsular hematoma or contusion, without laceration
  - Grade II
    - Superficial laceration ≤1 cm depth not involving the collecting system (no evidence of urine extravasation)

- Perirenal hematoma confined within the perirenal fascia
- Grade III
  - Laceration >1 cm not involving the collecting system (no evidence of urine extravasation)
  - Vascular injury or active bleeding confined within the perirenal fascia
- Grade IV
  - Laceration involving the collecting system with urinary extravasation
  - Laceration of the renal pelvis and/or complete ureteropelvic disruption
  - Vascular injury to segmental renal artery or vein
  - Segmental infarctions without associated active bleeding
  - Active bleeding extending beyond the perirenal fascia
- Grade V
  - Shattered kidney
  - Avulsion of renal hilum or laceration of the main renal artery or vein: devascularization of a kidney due to hilar injury
  - Devascularized kidney with active bleeding

Management

- >90% of blunt renal injuries can be successfully managed nonoperatively [3].
- Nonoperative management for low grade blunt renal injuries (grade I–III) identified on CT scan in hemodynamically stable patients is widely practiced. Angioembolization should be considered for renal parenchymal injuries with active extravasation seen on CT scan.
- Nonoperative management of blunt grade IV and V injuries is more controversial but is appropriate in some instances [5]. Angioembolization should be considered if there is evidence of active bleeding, pseudoaneurysm, or arteriovenous fistula. Short interval follow-up CT imaging can be considered for high-grade injuries managed nonoperatively to evaluate for complications such as enlarging urinoma and vascular malformations.
- Enlarging or infected urinoma can be managed with ureteral stenting with possible percutaneous drainage and percutaneous nephrostomy tube placement.
- In select cases, it is appropriate to manage penetrating renal injuries nonoperatively. However, operative exploration is often required to evaluate for damage to other intra-abdominal structures.
- In blunt trauma, Zone II retroperitoneal hematomas (renal hilum and lateral) should not be explored unless pulsatile or rapidly enlarging as exploration leads to increased rate of unnecessary nephrectomy [6, 7].
- In penetrating trauma, Zone II retroperitoneal hematomas should be routinely explored.

- Rapid intraoperative kidney exposure can be obtained using right or left medial visceral rotation, respectively. Bleeding parenchymal injuries can be addressed using a combination of direct pressure, packing, coagulation, topical hemostatic agents, and direct repair. If there is rapid bleeding, clamping the renal hilum will slow the rate of blood loss. Unsalvageable renal injuries are managed with nephrectomy. Key steps of a nephrectomy are ligation of the renal artery, renal vein, and the ureter. Under some circumstances, renal vascular injuries may be amenable to repair but nephrectomy may be necessary if the patient's overall clinical status does not allow time for vascular reconstruction.
- Before nephrectomy, evaluation of the contralateral kidney should be performed to ensure the patient will still have one functional kidney. This can be done on CT scan if the patient received preoperative imaging. If the patient was taken directly to the operating room, intraoperative pyelogram can be performed. However, pyelogram can be time consuming and many feel that rapid assessment via palpation of the contralateral kidney to ensure it is of normal size and consistency is sufficient to demonstrate a functional kidney.

Prognosis

- Most patients will recover from a low-grade renal injury without complications or interventions and without any long-term change in renal function.
- After nephrectomy, most patients with previously normal renal function will have a slight rise in their baseline creatinine, but will continue to have adequate long-term renal function. Patients who undergo bilateral nephrectomy or nephrectomy of a solitary functional kidney will require lifelong dialysis.
- High-grade injuries managed without nephrectomy are at increased risk of complications requiring additional procedures as described above. Delayed complications such as post-renal injury hypertension or delayed vascular complications have been reported but are rare.

References

1. Chesbrough RM, Burkhard TK, Martinez AJ, Burks DD. Gerota versus Zuckerkandl: the renal fascia revisited. Radiology. 1989;173(3):845–6.
2. Voelzke B. Management of blunt and penetrating renal trauma. In: Bulger EM, Richie JP, Collins KA, editors. UpToDate. Waltham: UpToDate; 2022. Accessed on 9 Oct 2022.
3. Voelzke BB, Leddy L. The epidemiology of renal trauma. Transl Androl Urol. 2014;3(2):143–9.
4. Kozar RA, Crandall M, Shanmuganathan K, Zarzaur BL, Coburn M, Cribari C, et al. Organ injury scaling 2018 update: spleen, liver, and kidney. J Trauma Acute Care Surg. 2018;85(6):1119–22.

5. Brewer ME Jr, Strnad BT, Daley BJ, Currier RP, Klein FA, Mobley JD, et al. Percutaneous embolization for the management of grade 5 renal trauma in hemodynamically unstable patients: initial experience. J Urol. 2009;181(4):1737–41.
6. Morey AF, Brandes S, Dugi DD 3rd, Armstrong JH, Breyer BN, Broghammer JA, et al. Urotrauma: AUA guideline. J Urol. 2014;192(2):327–35.
7. Wessells H, Suh D, Porter JR, Rivara F, MacKenzie EJ, Jurkovich GJ, et al. Renal injury and operative management in the United States: results of a population-based study. J Trauma. 2003;54(3):423–30.

Chapter 44
Ureteral and Bladder Injury

Jeffrey Santos, Theresa L. Chin, and Jeffry Nahmias

Overview

- Traumatic injury to the lower genitourinary tract (ureter, bladder, and urethra) is relatively uncommon, occurring in approximately 10% of patients sustaining abdominal and pelvic trauma.
- Delayed recognition and treatment are associated with increased morbidity and mortality.
- Treatment options (e.g., primary repair or advanced reconstruction) depend on the location (i.e., upper vs. middle vs. lower third of the ureter or extraperitoneal vs. intraperitoneal bladder), timing of diagnosis, and severity of injury.

Epidemiology

Traumatic injury to the ureter is uncommon because it is relatively well protected within the retroperitoneum. In fact, the incidence is less than 4% for penetrating trauma and under 1% for blunt trauma [1]. Most ureter injuries occur due to iatrogenic non-urologic surgery due to its close anatomical relationship with several

J. Santos (✉)
Department of Surgery, University of California, Irvine, Orange, CA, USA
e-mail: jwsantos@hs.uci.edu

T. L. Chin
Division of Emergency General Surgery, University of California, Irvine, Orange, CA, USA
e-mail: chintl1@hs.uci.edu

J. Nahmias
Division of Trauma, Burns, Critical Care & Acute Care Surgery, University of California, Irvine, Orange, CA, USA
e-mail: jnahmias@hs.uci.edu

411

T. S. Brahmbhatt, D. R. Scantling (eds.), *Trauma Surgery Clerkship*, Contemporary Surgical Clerkships,
https://doi.org/10.1007/978-3-032-01412-2_44

structures (i.e., gynecologic and colorectal structures). Traumatic bladder injury occurs in less than 10% of abdominal and pelvic trauma and is often associated with additional traumatic injuries, most significantly pelvic fractures in blunt trauma [2, 3]. Traumatic urethral injury occurs in ~10% of pelvic fractures and is more common in males compared to females due to a shorter, more mobile urethra [4, 5].

Pathophysiology

Pathophysiology of the injury to the ureter, bladder, and urethra varies by anatomical location. If the surrounding structures are injured, the ureter, bladder, and urethra are more vulnerable to concurrent injury. Thus, proficient knowledge in the anatomical relationships assists in the understanding of the nature of the injury.

Ureter

The ureter is a retroperitoneal structure about 25 cm in length that funnels urine from the kidney to the bladder via vermiculation or peristalsis. It is divided into the proximal ureter starting at the ureteropelvic junction (UPJ) of the kidney until it crosses the sacroiliac joint where it becomes the middle ureter until it reaches the iliac vessels. Finally, the distal or pelvic ureter starts at the iliac vessels and ends at the trigone of the bladder. The ureter has many anatomical relationships with adjacent structures. The left UPJ is posterior to the pancreas and the ligament of Treitz and the proximal ureter rests on the psoas muscle as it courses caudad with the inferior mesenteric artery and sigmoidal vessels positioned anteriorly. The right UPJ is posterior to the duodenum and lateral to the inferior vena cava prior to the ureter coursing distally along the psoas muscle with the right colic and ileocolic vessels positioned anteriorly. In males, the ureter courses anterior to the iliac vessels and posterior to the gonadal vessels. In females, the ureter travels posterior to the ovaries and broad ligament, medial to the anterior vessels, and lateral to the uterus. The ureter receives its blood supply in segmental fashion, which must be considered when undergoing repair. Skeletonizing the ureter can lead to ischemia due to the segmental blood supply. The proximal ureter (near kidney) is supplied directly from the renal artery, the middle ureter from branches off the common iliac arteries, abdominal aorta, and gonadal arteries, and the distal ureter from branches off the internal iliac artery. The ureter is innervated by a ureteric plexus formed by T12–L2 nerve roots and pain may be referred to these dermatomes when the ureter is injured.

Signs and symptoms of urinary obstruction or urinary leakage can indicate ureteral injury or complications. Urinary obstruction can cause hydronephrosis and hydroureter, which can cause acute kidney injury and ultimately, renal failure. Stricture formation from fibrosis narrows the lumen and causes signs of urinary obstruction and can occur from ureteral injury alone or from ureteral repair.

Moreover, urinary leakage can result in abdominal pain or peritonitis, ileus, and/or urinoma (fluid collection of urine), which may become infected, leading to sepsis.

In blunt trauma, the ureter is subject to direct force sustained by the entire body, such as a crush or deceleration mechanism, leading to ureteral injury. In children, an avulsion injury to the UPJ is more common from increased spine mobility and resulting spinal hyperextension. On the contrary, penetrating trauma to the retroperitoneum can result in direct injury to the ureter.

Bladder

An empty bladder is protected within the bony pelvis with its base adjacent to the vagina in females and rectum in males. Bilateral ureters drain into the bladder at the ureteral orifices in the trigone. The anterior bladder is separated from the transversalis fascia by adipose tissue and this retropubic space is known as the space of Retzius. The anterior portion of the bladder is not covered by peritoneum. In males, the superior portion of the bladder is covered by peritoneum, which reflects posteriorly and covers the rectum forming the rectovesical pouch. In females, the superior portion of the bladder is mostly covered by peritoneum reflected from the uterus forming the vesicouterine pouch.

The bladder has four major layers (urothelium, lamina propria, muscularis propria, and serosa), and the muscularis propria, also called the detrusor muscles, has smooth muscle making up the inner longitudinal, outer longitudinal, and circular layers, allowing the bladder to relax for filling and contract to empty. The blood supply comes from the superior and inferior vesical artery branches off the internal iliac artery. The bladder is innervated by sympathetic (T10–L2) and parasympathetic (S2–S4) nerves from the pelvic plexus.

Signs of bladder injury include hematuria, inability to urinate, and abdominal/pelvic pain. Intraperitoneal bladder injury resulting in urine leak can present with abdominal pain or peritonitis, ileus, and/or urinoma, which may become infected leading to sepsis. Extraperitoneal bladder injury may cause pelvic or suprapubic pain, or gross hematuria. Having a high index of suspicion can lead to timely diagnosis of bladder injury, reducing complications.

Injury to the bladder most commonly occurs in blunt trauma (motor vehicle collision, falls, direct trauma to the lower abdomen) and is often accompanied by pelvic fracture. As the bladder fills and expands outside of the bony pelvis superiorly, it exposes itself to injury. Bladder injuries associated with pelvic fractures can be a direct bladder puncture from fragmented bone or the transmission of extreme force, resulting in rupture. Penetrating trauma directly injures the bladder. Injury to the bladder can be intraperitoneal (IP) or extraperitoneal (EP) depending on the injury's location related to the bladder's peritoneal covering and connection to the peritoneal cavity versus true pelvis. This distinction is crucial to management, which will be discussed later in this chapter.

Chronic urinary dysfunction (i.e., incontinence or urgency) can result from injury to the plexus innervating the bladder and/or reducing the size of the bladder during surgical repair.

Urethra

The urethra connects the inferior bladder to the external urethral meatus. In males, it is 18–20 cm in length and is separated into the posterior and anterior urethra. The posterior urethra (also called prostatic or membranous urethra) courses from the inferior bladder through the prostate and becomes the anterior urethra (also called bulbar or penile urethra) once it penetrates through the urogenital diaphragm. The bulbar urethra is fixed in place by the puboprostatic ligament. Blood supply comes from the urethral artery, which branches off the pudendal artery. Additionally, the dorsal penile artery supplies blood through the circumflex branches. The internal urethra sphincter has sympathetic innervation from the pelvic plexus to prevent retrograde ejaculation and parasympathetic innervation comes from S2 to S4 nerve roots. On the contrary, the female urethra is ~4 cm in length and is fixed anteriorly by the suspensory ligament of the clitoris and inferiorly to the pubis by the posterior pubourethral ligaments. Blood supply comes from the vaginal artery and inferior vesicle artery. Parasympathetic innervation also comes from S2 to S4 nerve roots.

In males, signs of urethral injury include blood at the meatus, inability to urinate, genital swelling or ecchymosis, and high-riding prostate on digital rectal exam. In females, blood at the urethral opening (which can be confused with vaginal bleeding), inability to urinate, pain with urination, hematuria, genital swelling or ecchymosis. Urethral injury can lead to infection, urethral stricture formation, and/or erectile dysfunction.

Straddle mechanisms (stretch injury) from direct force to the perineum (i.e., motorcycle or bicycle collisions) cause compression of the urethra between external force and the pubic bone typically resulting in injury to the bulbous urethra in males. The bulbous urethra is the most fixed portion making it more susceptible to injury. Pelvic fractures at the inferomedial pelvic ramus and pubic diastasis increase the risk for posterior urethral injury due to its proximity. Urethral injuries in females are less common from direct force due to the shorter length and the pubic bone that protects the female urethra.

Stricture formation is common after urethral injury and may result after surgical repair due to fibrosis and narrowing of the lumen. Urethral strictures can present with inability to urinate, urinary tract infection, and signs of urinary obstruction.

Current management practice (Table 44.1)

- Imaging and laboratory findings associated with lower genitourinary injury:

    - Urinalysis with significant red blood cells (RBCs) in the urine
    - Plain radiograph: Pelvic fracture (not specific but increases clinical suspicion)

Table 44.1 Exam findings, diagnostic imaging, and management of lower genitourinary injuries

Injury	Exam findings	Diagnostic imaging	Management
Ureter	No specific findings	CT Urogram or retrograde pyelogram	Primary repair over stent if feasible, otherwise: *Proximal/middle ureter*—Transureteroureterostomy *Distal ureter*—Psoas hitch and/or Boari flap for additional length or ureteral reimplantation *Unstable patient*—Proximal ureter ligation and percutaneous nephrostomy tube
Bladder	Suprapubic pain, hematuria	Cystogram (plain radiograph or computed tomography (CT))	*IP*—Two-layer absorbable suture repair with IUC decompression *EP*—Bladder decompression with IUC and delayed repair if needed
Urethra	Blood at the meatus, perineal bruising or swelling, high-riding prostate	Retrograde urethrogram (RUG)	Urology consultation for possible urethral realignment or repair, or placement of suprapubic tube and delayed surgery

IP intraperitoneal, *IUC* indwelling urinary catheter, *EP* extraperitoneal

- Computerized tomography (CT): Soft tissue stranding around structures (ureter, bladder, urethra), disruption of structures (rupture or transection), fluid around structures (simple fluid or blood), dilation or deviation of ureter

Ureteral Injury

- Diagnostic studies

  - Retrograde pyelogram (RPG) is the most accurate study

    - Performed during cystoscopy
    - Obtained once highly concerned for ureter injury and often just prior to urologic intervention

  - CT Urogram (CT abdomen and pelvis with intravenous (IV) contrast and delayed images)

    - Timing of delayed images allows IV contrast to be excreted through the kidneys and opacifies the ureter
    - Preferred imaging to evaluate ureteral injury in trauma

- Immediate diagnosis (within 72 h) should undergo immediate repair:

  - Partial laceration can undergo primary repair over ureteral stent

- Complete laceration or nonviable ureter can be resected to healthy tissue and primarily repaired over ureteral stent
- If primary repair is not feasible (i.e., length limitation or challenging location of injury):

  • Proximal or middle ureteral injury: transureteroureterostomy (urology consultation for repair is advised)
  • Distal ureteral injury: ureteral reimplantation (ureteroneocystostomy)
  • Additional length may be obtained for repair of a distal injury with a psoas hitch and/or Boari flap procedure
  • Patients who cannot undergo formal repair (from instability or lack of resources/expertise) can be managed with proximal ligation of the ureter and subsequent placement of a percutaneous nephrostomy tube

• Delayed diagnosis (after 72 h):

  - Delay often results in stricture of the ureter and urinoma (collection of urine)
  - Ureteral stricture is treated with ureteral stent placement and/or percutaneous nephrostomy tube
  - Urinoma is drained with a percutaneous drain
  - Definitive repair is often delayed until 6 weeks after injury in cases of delayed diagnosis

Bladder Injury

• Diagnostic studies

  - Retrograde cystography

    • Traditional cystogram: Indwelling urinary catheter (IUC) is placed and bladder is filled with contrast prior to plain radiograph
    • CT cystogram (CT scan instead of radiograph once the bladder is filled with contrast) is now preferred as it is readily available and has increased sensitivity (will not miss a small posterior injury that is obscured on a single radiograph view)
    • EP bladder injuries have contrast extravasation around the base of the bladder restricted to the perivesical space and into the perineum (thighs, penis, scrotum)
    • IP bladder injuries have contrast extravasation into the peritoneum resulting in free fluid in the abdominal cavity

  - Methylene blue or indigo carmine can be administered through an IUC intraoperatively to help identify bladder injury or leak

• Intra-peritoneal (IP) bladder injury:

- IUC is placed before repair
- Primary repair with two layers of absorbable suture
- "Leak" test to ensure the repair is watertight is performed after repair by filling the bladder with methylene blue through the IUC
- Can consider cystogram to evaluate for a leak at 10–14 days after repair prior to removing IUC

- Extraperitoneal (EP) bladder injury:

  - Uncomplicated injuries are managed with bladder drainage via IUC for 10–14 days
  - Retrograde cystography is performed prior to removing IUC
  - Advanced urologic surgical repair is indicated if extraperitoneal bladder injury is not healed by 3 months post-injury
  - Surgical repair of an EP bladder injury is indicated when there is an additional rectal or vaginal injury, a foreign body within the bladder wall, or a need for orthopedic repair requiring hardware implantation

- If there is a concomitant urethral injury, insertion of an IUC through the urethra may require urologic expertise or, alternatively, a suprapubic tube may be placed to decompress the bladder and divert urinary flow

Urethral Injury

- Diagnostic studies

  - Retrograde urethrogram (RUG) is the gold standard

    - RUG procedure: Catheter is placed within urethral meatus and contrast injected through the urethra prior to plain radiograph at an oblique angle to capture the course of the urethra. Extravasation identifies a urethral injury

  - CT imaging can suggest injury to the urethra, but a RUG should be obtained to confirm diagnosis

- Immediate management includes bladder decompression, most often done with placement of a suprapubic tube
- In some cases, an IUC can be placed by a urologist or via urethral realignment under direct visualization using cystoscope (advanced urologic technique)
- Penetrating and open urethral injuries require urgent exploration, debridement, and repair
- If a suprapubic tube is placed, delayed urethroplasty occurs ~3 months after injury
- Urethral strictures are managed with dilation procedures and urethroplasty in refractory cases

Take-Home Points for Patient Care
- Traumatic injuries to the ureter, bladder, and urethra are relatively uncommon and timely diagnosis requires a high index of suspicion.
- Treatment is based on anatomical location, timing of diagnosis, and severity of the injury.
- If recognized early, attempts should be made for immediate repair of injuries to the ureter and bladder.
- Closed urethral injury can be treated with bladder decompression and delayed repair if needed.
- Prognosis is generally good following timely treatment of traumatic lower genitourinary tract injuries, but urinary dysfunction and stricture formation of the ureter and urethra can result in chronic morbidity.

References

1. Shewakramani S, Reed KC. Genitourinary trauma. Emerg Med Clin North Am. 2011;29(3):501–18.
2. Bryk DJ, Zhao LC. Guideline of guidelines: a review of urological trauma guidelines. BJU Int. 2016;117(2):226–34.
3. Pereira BMT, de Campos CCC, Calderan TRA, Reis LO, Fraga GP. Bladder injuries after external trauma: 20 years experience report in a population-based cross-sectional view. World J Urol. 2013;31(4):913–7.
4. Chapple CR. Urethral injury. BJU Int. 2000;86(3):318–26.
5. Patel DN, Fok CS, Webster GD, Anger JT. Female urethral injuries associated with pelvic fracture: a systematic review of the literature. BJU Int. 2017;120(6):766–73.

Chapter 45
Rectal Injury

Carlos Fairen Oro and Joanne Favuzza

Anatomy

- The rectum is a 12–15 cm portion of the colon that extends from the sigmoid colon to the dentate line in the anal canal [1].
- The arterial and venous blood supply to the rectum can be divided into thirds:

    - The upper third is supplied by the superior rectal artery coming from the inferior mesenteric artery and is drained by the superior rectal veins, which drains into the inferior mesenteric vein and portal system.
    - The middle third is supplied by the middle rectal artery coming from the internal iliac arteries and drained by the middle rectal vein and into the internal iliac vein/inferior vena cava system.
    - The lower third is supplied by the inferior rectal artery coming from the internal pudendal artery and drained by the inferior rectal vein and into the internal iliac vein/inferior vena cava system.

Evaluation

- Rectal injuries can be associated with blunt or penetrating trauma.

C. F. Oro
Department of Surgery, Boston Medical Center, Boston, MA, USA
e-mail: Carlos.FairenOro@bmc.org

J. Favuzza (✉)
Division of Colon and Rectal Surgery, Department of Surgery, Boston Medical Center, Boston, MA, USA
e-mail: Favuzza@sphp.com

© The Author(s), under exclusive license to Springer Nature Switzerland AG 2025
T. S. Brahmbhatt, D. R. Scantling (eds.), *Trauma Surgery Clerkship*, Contemporary Surgical Clerkships,
https://doi.org/10.1007/978-3-032-01412-2_45

- Penetrating trauma is the most common type of trauma associated with a rectal injury.
- Rectal injuries can be associated with other injuries including pelvic fractures (35%), major vascular injuries (15%), solid organ injuries (12%), and other bowel injuries (33%).
- Patients may present with abdominal complaints, blood per rectum, or no symptoms at all.
- Patients should be assessed for evidence of initial peritonitis in the setting of intraperitoneal rectal injuries, which may eventually lead to severe abdominal pain along with hypotension, tachycardia, and fevers.
- If initial imaging demonstrates free air, a laparotomy should be performed without delay.
- If the patient is hemodynamically stable then the patient should undergo thorough physical examination including the abdomen and pelvis as well as a *digital rectal exam* (DRE). DRE is performed as part of the secondary survey in trauma patients. Blood encountered on DRE should raise a concern for rectal injury when compatible with the mechanism of injury and should be followed by more accurate diagnostic modalities such as CT or rigid proctoscopy [4].

Computed Tomography (CT) Scan with Intravenous (IV) and Rectal Contrast This is the best diagnostic modality for rectal injuries in terms of sensitivity, specificity, and availability for the hemodynamically stable patient. Although rectal contrast is not routinely given in all abdominopelvic traumas, it is indicated in cases with high suspicion for rectal injury.

- Concerning findings on CT scan for rectal injury include: free pelvic fluid, pneumoperitoneum, contrast extravasation from the rectum into abdomen and/or pelvis, rectal hematoma, and mesenteric fat stranding (Figs. 45.1 and 45.2).

Rigid Proctoscopy This is commonly used intraoperatively to diagnose rectal injuries in patients who are unstable from other injuries and were not candidates to undergo a CT with rectal contrast.

- Common findings on proctoscopy are blood in the rectal vault, rectal wall hematoma, and defect in rectal wall.

Classification

- Rectal injuries are classified depending on the extent of the injury as detailed in the American Association for the Surgery of Trauma (AAST) Rectal Organ Injury Scale for blunt and penetrating trauma (Table 45.1). The degree of injury dictates the treatment needed for rectal injuries.

Fig. 45.1 CT abdomen and pelvis with IV contrast showing free air adjacent to rectum consistent with rectal injury

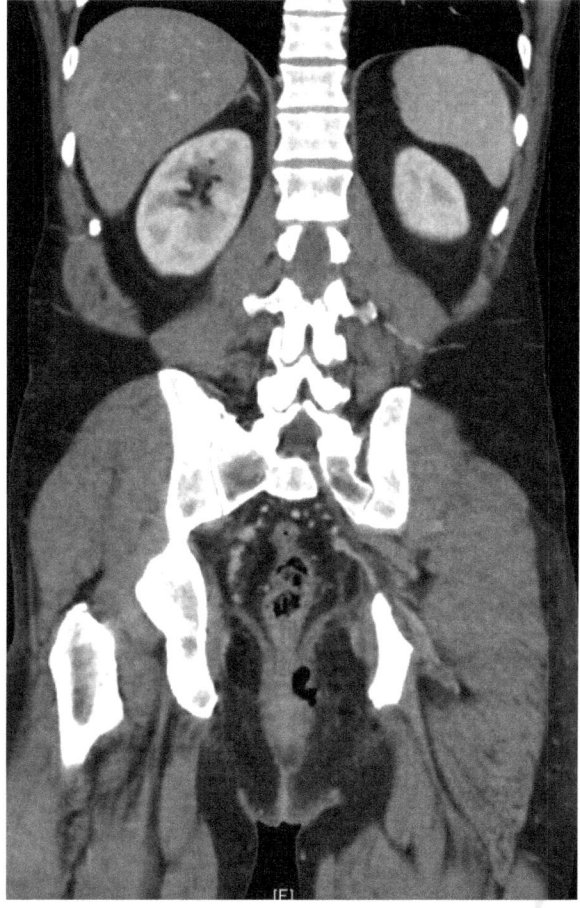

Fig. 45.2 CT abdomen and pelvis with IV contrast showing free air adjacent to rectum consistent with rectal injury (Lung window)

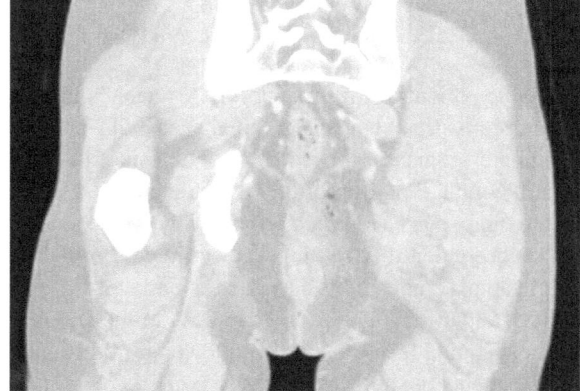

Table 45.1 American Association for the Surgery of Trauma rectum injury scale

Grade	Type of injury	Description of injury
I[a]	Hematoma	Hematoma or contusion without devascularization
	Laceration	Partial thickness laceration
II[a]	Laceration	Laceration injury that includes <50% of the circumference of the rectum
III[a]	Laceration	Laceration injury that includes >50% of the circumference of the rectum
IV	Laceration	Full thickness laceration with extension to the peritoneum
V	Vascular	Devascularized segment

From Moore et al. [3]
[a]Advance one grade for multiple injuries up to grade III

- In addition, the relationship of the rectal injury to the peritoneal reflection is also classified to help determine the likelihood of intraperitoneal contamination and what subsequent treatment is necessary. Intraperitoneal injuries typically occur on the anterior and lateral surfaces of the upper two-thirds of the rectum, whereas extraperitoneal injuries are posterior and in the lower one-third of the rectum.

Management

The first step in the management of rectal injuries is to assess the patient's hemodynamic stability. In a trauma patient presenting with peritonitis, free air or hemodynamic instability, the patient should be immediately expedited to the operating room for laparotomy to identify potential life-threatening injuries.

Once the patient has been stabilized, intraoperative examination of the rectum in combination with digital rectal examination, proctoscopy, and/or colonoscopy can aid in the identification and location of the injuries (Fig. 45.3).

Intraperitoneal Injuries

- Stable patients with intraperitoneal rectal injuries with minimal contamination and early treatment can be managed with primary repair or resection of the injured segment followed by anastomosis [5].
- If the injured portion of the rectum includes less than 25% of its circumference, the injury can be repaired primarily with a two-layer suture repair. Primary repair has been identified to have a lower rate of mortality, infection, and wound complications compared to fecal diversion.
- If the injury involves more than 25% of the circumference, then the injured segment should be resected and followed by anastomosis or fecal diversion [6].
- In patients in shock or requiring more than 4–6 units of packed red blood cells, fecal diversion with closure of the rectal stump should be considered.

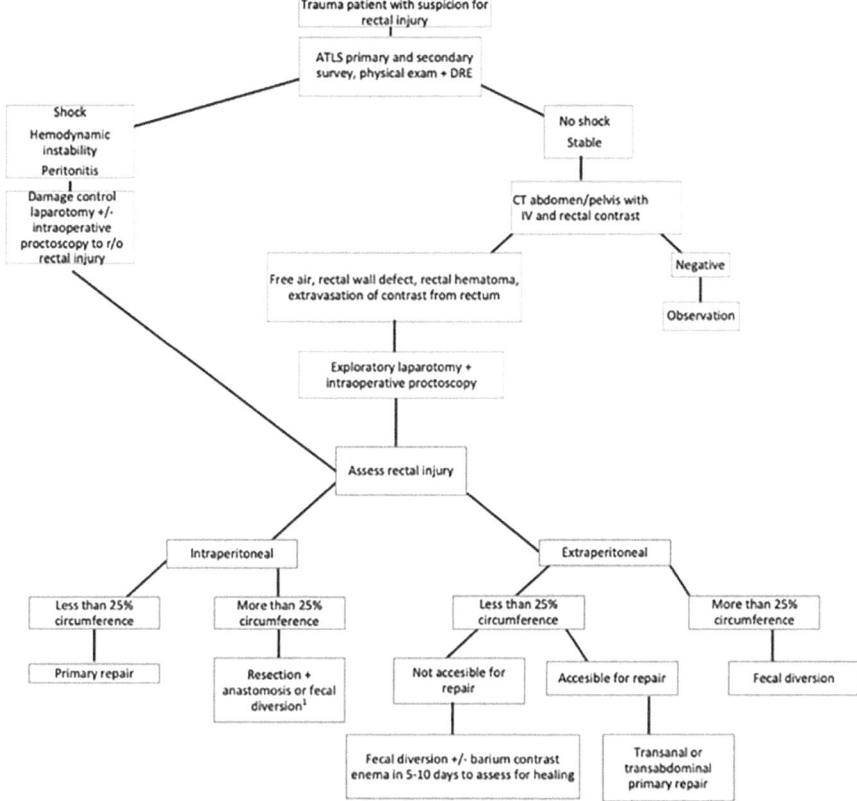

Fig. 45.3 Algorithm of management of rectal injuries. 1. Fecal diversion without primary anastomosis for patients in shock, receiving more than 4–6 units of packed red blood cells or Injury Severity Score >25 [6]

Extraperitoneal Injuries

- Extraperitoneal rectal injuries are more difficult to identify and treat given their location in the pelvis [2].
- Historically, presacral drains and distal rectal washout were used in the treatment and management of all extraperitoneal rectal injuries. However, multiple studies have shown increased rate of infectious complications. Current guidelines recommend against the use of presacral drainage and distal washout techniques for nondestructive rectal injuries [7].
- For destructive injuries of the extraperitoneal rectum that do communicate with the presacral space or where an injury cannot be identified or repaired, careful presacral drainage may be considered.
- Distal rectal washout has fallen out of favor due to lack of protective effect against infection.

- Proximal extraperitoneal rectal injuries that are accessible transabdominally can be primarily repaired if less than 25% of the circumference is affected.
- If more than 25% of the circumference is affected, the patient is in shock or requiring more than 4–6 units of packed red blood cells, fecal diversion is potentially indicated [9].
- Distal extraperitoneal injuries represent a challenge for multiple reasons including the proximity of major vessels, genitourinary tract, and difficulty with exposure or access to such injuries in the pelvis. All these factors make primary repair of these injuries less likely, and distal injuries usually benefit from fecal diversion [8].
- In selected patients, transanal primary repair can be attempted with very distal rectal injuries.

Complications

- Careful management of rectal injuries is necessary to avoid postoperative complications and even sepsis [10].
- Infection is the most common complication in patients with rectal injuries.
- In patients with nondestructive extraperitoneal injuries undergoing primary repair alone, 18.2% will develop infections, while those with primary repair with diversion have a rate of infection of only 8.8%.
- Patients with rectal injuries who develop abscesses can be managed with a combination of intravenous antibiotics and interventional radiology drainage of the abscess. If the abscess is too small for drainage (less than 3 cm), a 10–14-day course of antibiotics will usually suffice.

  – Repeat CT imaging 5–7 days after the initiation of antibiotics can be performed to reevaluate the abscess and assess for resolution.

- Rectal fistulas can also develop between the rectum and the abscess cavity with drainage of feculent material. In these cases, a drain is left in place until it has minimal drainage. A sinogram can be performed to confirm resolution of the fistula at which time the drain can be safely removed.
- In patients that fail antibiotic management and/or drainage of the abscess, additional operative debridement and wide drainage of the infected area may be necessary.
- Patients can also develop necrotizing soft tissue infections of the perineum and retroperitoneum. These patients usually present with pain out of proportion to examination, rapidly spreading erythema of the perineum and crepitus along with laboratory abnormalities such as hyponatremia, elevated C reactive protein, hyperglycemia, leukocytosis, and acute kidney injury. In these cases, early initiation of antibiotics and emergent surgical debridement of the area is warranted.

Conclusions

- Rectal trauma most commonly presents as a result of penetrating trauma and is usually associated with other injuries such as pelvic fractures, vascular, solid organ, or hollow viscus injuries.
- The best diagnostic method is a CT abdomen/pelvis with IV and rectal contrast. Intraoperative proctoscopy can be used to rule out rectal injuries in patients that are not stable to undergo other imaging modalities.
- Rectal injuries are classified as intraperitoneal or extraperitoneal.
- Intraperitoneal injuries can be repaired primarily or with resection of the affected segment with anastomosis or fecal diversion without anastomosis.
- Extraperitoneal injuries amenable for primary repair can be repaired transabdominally or transanally. Otherwise, fecal diversion is the main treatment for extraperitoneal injuries.
- Infection is the most common complication after rectal injury.

References

1. Favuzza J. Rectal foreign bodies. In: Current therapy in colon and rectal surgery. 3rd ed. Elsevier – Health Sciences Division; 2016. p. 118–20.
2. Bosarge PL, Como JJ, Fox N, Falck-Ytter Y, Haut ER, Dorion HA, Patel NJ, Rushing A, Raff LA, McDonald AA, Robinson BR, McGwin G Jr, Gonzalez RP. Management of penetrating extraperitoneal rectal injuries: an Eastern Association for the Surgery of Trauma practice management guideline. J Trauma Acute Care Surg. 2016;80(3):546–51. https://doi.org/10.1097/TA.0000000000000953. PMID: 26713970.
3. Moore EE, Cogbill TH, Malangoni MA, Jurkovich GJ, Champion HR, Gennarelli TA, McAninch JW, Pachter HL, Shackford SR, Trafton PG. Organ injury scaling, II: pancreas, duodenum, small bowel, colon, and rectum. J Trauma. 1990;30(11):1427–9. PMID: 2231822.
4. Esposito TJ, Ingraham A, Luchette FA, Sears BW, Santaniello JM, Davis KA, Poulakidas SJ, Gamelli RL. Reasons to omit digital rectal exam in trauma patients: no fingers, no rectum, no useful additional information. J Trauma. 2005;59(6):1314–9. https://doi.org/10.1097/01.ta.0000198375.83830.62. PMID: 16394903.
5. Nelson R, Singer M. Primary repair for penetrating colon injuries. Cochrane Database Syst Rev. 2003;(3):CD002247. https://doi.org/10.1002/14651858.CD002247. PMID: 12917927.
6. Demetriades D, Murray JA, Chan L, Ordoñez C, Bowley D, Nagy KK, Cornwell EE 3rd, Velmahos GC, Muñoz N, Hatzitheofilou C, Schwab CW, Rodriguez A, Cornejo C, Davis KA, Namias N, Wisner DH, Ivatury RR, Moore EE, Acosta JA, Maull KI, Thomason MH, Spain DA, Committee on Multicenter Clinical Trials, American Association for the Surgery of Trauma. Penetrating colon injuries requiring resection: diversion or primary anastomosis? An AAST prospective multicenter study. J Trauma. 2001;50(5):765–75. https://doi.org/10.1097/00005373-200105000-00001. PMID: 11371831.

7. Gonzalez RP, Falimirski ME, Holevar MR. The role of presacral drainage in the management of penetrating rectal injuries. J Trauma. 1998;45(4):656–61. https://doi.org/10.1097/00005373-199810000-00002. PMID: 9783600.
8. Gonzalez RP, Phelan H 3rd, Hassan M, Ellis CN, Rodning CB. Is fecal diversion necessary for nondestructive penetrating extraperitoneal rectal injuries? J Trauma. 2006;61(4):815–9. https://doi.org/10.1097/01.ta.0000239497.96387.9d. PMID: 17033545.
9. Cameron JL, Cameron AM, Peitzman AB. Current management of rectal injury. In: Current surgical therapy. Philadelphia: Elsevier; 2020. p. 1190–3.
10. Gordon PH, Beck DE, Wexner SD, Rafferty JF. Gordon and Nivatvongs' principles and practice of surgery for the colon, rectum, and anus. New York: Thieme; 2019.

Chapter 46
Upper Extremity Vascular Injury

Brenda Lin and Elizabeth King

Introduction

- Management of peripheral vascular trauma hinges on assessing the extent of injury, control of hemorrhage, reestablishing blood flow, and treatment of reperfusion injury. While these injuries are relatively rare, they may pose an immediate threat to life and limb. Surgical exposures, hemorrhage control techniques, and repair methodology can be nuanced and all will be discussed here.

Epidemiology

- Extremity trauma occurs in approximately 1–2% of all civilian trauma, and vascular injuries occur in ~1% of all extremity injuries
- Peripheral vascular injury accounts for 20–50% of all vascular injuries
- Upper and lower extremity arterial injuries occur with almost equal frequency
- Most commonly injured vessels:

  - Lower extremity: popliteal (blunt), superficial femoral artery (penetrating)
  - Upper extremity: forearm vessels > brachial > axillary/subclavian

B. Lin · E. King (✉)
Division of Vascular and Endovascular Surgery, Department of Surgery, Boston Medical Center, Boston University Chobanian & Avedisian School of Medicine, Boston, MA, USA
e-mail: brenda.lin@bmc.org; elizabeth.king@bmc.org

© The Author(s), under exclusive license to Springer Nature Switzerland AG 2025
T. S. Brahmbhatt, D. R. Scantling (eds.), *Trauma Surgery Clerkship*, Contemporary Surgical Clerkships, https://doi.org/10.1007/978-3-032-01412-2_46

427

- Blunt and penetrating mechanisms occur with nearly equal incidence. Blunt trauma is more frequently seen in the lower extremities and penetrating trauma is more common in the upper extremities.
- Vascular injury secondary to blunt trauma is associated with higher rates of mortality (2–5%) and amputation (7–30%) than penetrating trauma. This is attributed to concomitant injuries and the high-energy mechanism causing associated bony, soft tissue, and nerve injury.
- Amputation is more common in popliteal and forearm level injuries, and in the presence of a significant soft tissue defect.
- Less than 2% of extremity fractures and dislocations are complicated by vascular injuries. However, skeletal trauma may be present in up to 10% of patients with traumatic peripheral vascular injuries.

Anatomy (Figs. 46.1 and 46.2)

Classification

- Peripheral vascular trauma is graded with the AAST Organ Injury Scale
- Mangled Extremity Severity Score (MESS) of ≥7 correlates with primary amputation
- Mangled Extremity Syndrome Index (MESI)

Fig. 46.1 Major vessels in the arm

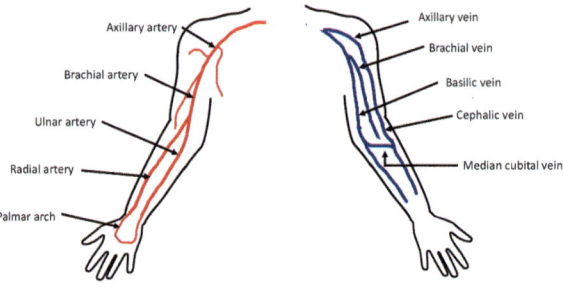

Fig. 46.2 Major arteries of the leg

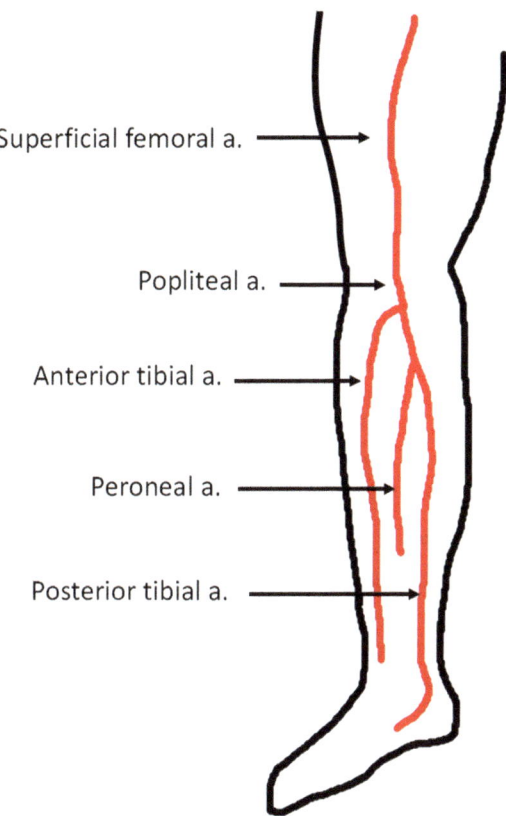

Superficial femoral a.

Popliteal a.

Anterior tibial a.

Peroneal a.

Posterior tibial a.

Table 46.1 Hard and soft signs of vascular injury

Hard signs	Soft signs
Absent pulses	Small, nonpulsatile hematoma
Palpable thrill or audible bruit	Recent hemorrhage from site
Expanding hematoma	Neurologic deficit
Active pulsatile bleeding	Proximity of wound to a named vessel
Distal ischemia (6Ps: pain, pallor, paralysis, paresthesia, poikilothermia)	

Presentation and Evaluation

- Hard and soft signs of vascular injury (Table 46.1)

  - Hard signs of vascular injury require immediate operative exploration and repair while soft signs allow further imaging for evaluation.
  - Hard signs of vascular injury on physical exam have a positive predictive value of ~100%
  - Incidence of arterial injuries in patients with soft signs is 3–25%

- Imaging modalities

  - CT angiography (CTA)—assess arterial injuries, in addition to venous injuries if delayed phase performed. This is particularly helpful for planning reconstruction. Sensitivity and specificity of identifying arterial injury approaches 100%
  - Duplex ultrasound
  - Invasive arteriography)—useful if endovascular control or repair is considered

- Penetrating vs. blunt patterns of vascular extremity injury

  - Ischemia arising from arterial occlusion is more likely following blunt trauma
  - Axillary artery injuries are associated with dislocation of the humeral head and humerus fractures
  - Brachial injuries are associated with supracondylar fractures and elbow dislocation
  - Popliteal injuries associated with knee dislocation

- History: timing of injury, mechanism of injury, duration of tourniquet time, estimated blood loss prior to arrival
- Physical exam:

  - Examine all extremities to establish baseline
  - Note vitals including systolic blood pressure, heart rate and rhythm, and temperature as these can affect the pulse exam
  - Pulse exam—begin with palpation, proceed to Doppler assessment if necessary
  - Sensory and motor exam
  - Ankle-Brachial Index (ABI)/Injured extremity index (IEI)—Doppler-derived arterial pressure distal to injury compared to normal brachial artery/uninjured extremity pressure
  - ABIs may not be reliable in a patient with diabetes due to the non-compressibility of distal vessels
  - ABIs in a healthy individual without diabetes should be >0.9. If <0.9, consider dedicated imaging to assess for potential vascular injury (Fig. 46.3)

Fig. 46.3 Obtaining Doppler-derived arterial pressure

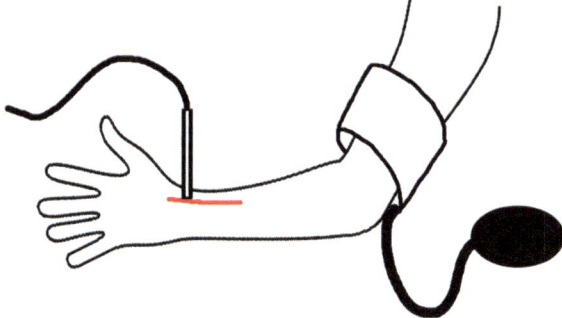

Types of Injuries

- Intimal irregularity or tear: <25% narrowing of the vessel
- Dissection/intramural hematoma (>/=25% narrowing of the vessel) or partial transection
- Occlusion
- Complete transection
- Pseudoaneurysm
- Arteriovenous fistula

Nonoperative Management

- In certain cases of non-flow limiting arterial injuries (intimal flap, dissection, stenosis, spasm, small pseudoaneurysm, and AV fistula), nonoperative management with serial examinations and anticoagulation or antiplatelet agents if flap/dissection, can be considered

Initial Management

If hemorrhage cannot be controlled with direct pressure, place a tourniquet with the goal of expeditious removal

Open Repair

- Widely prep injured extremity and potential harvest sites for autologous conduit
- Establish proximal and distal control, control side branches

- Once hemorrhage is controlled, assess extent of injury
- Systemic anticoagulation used in the absence of contraindications
- Debride injured arterial segment back to normal appearing wall
- Clear any thrombus with use of thromboembolectomy (Fogarty) catheters
- In a stable patient proceed with definitive vascular repair. In unstable patient, polytrauma, or an unclear trauma burden, consider damage control management, such as an intravascular shunt, until the patient stabilizes
- Temporary shunts can be used to restore distal perfusion in a damage control situation, or to allow time for orthopedic fixation, wound debridement, and harvest of autogenous conduit
- Definitive repair

  - Primary repair can be attempted if the injury is small and will not result in stenosis of the lumen
  - Patch angioplasty should be performed if there is concern for stenosis and >50% uninjured arterial wall present
  - A spatulated end-to-end anastomosis can be performed if there is sufficient length for a tension-free repair
  - Interposition grafts are used for reconstruction in the presence of longer defects, preferably with autologous vein; however prosthetic grafts (Polytetrafluoroethylene (PTFE), dacron) can be used in an uninfected field
  - If none of the above are viable options, a surgical bypass with ligation of the intervening segment can be performed with either autologous vein or prosthetic conduit.
  - Repair should be covered with viable soft tissue to prevent anastomotic breakdown and subsequent hemorrhage
  - Consideration should be given to performing prophylactic fasciotomies

- Upon completion of the repair, blood flow should be evaluated via palpation, Doppler, intraoperative duplex, or arteriogram
- In some instances where there is redundant circulation, as in the tibial or forearm vessels, a selective revascularization strategy can be employed

  - Injury to a single vessel can be ligated if there is adequate collateral flow to provide distal perfusion

- Most venous injuries can be ligated given the inherent redundancy of the venous system; however repair of larger, proximal veins should be considered in the stable patient to decrease venous hypertension and potential long-term morbidity

  - Compression and elevation should be used in either case

Open Surgical Exposures

- Upper Extremity
  - Subclavian artery: proximal right subclavian artery exposed through median sternotomy, left subclavian artery access through high anterolateral thoracotomy, mid/distal exposed through combined supra and infraclavicular incisions or via resection of the clavicle Avoid injury to the brachial plexus, vagus and phrenic nerves, and thoracic duct (left side)
  - Axillary artery: infraclavicular incision extended along deltopectoral groove, division of clavipectoral fascia, and pectoralis minor

    - Avoid injury to brachial plexus and axillary vein

  - Brachial artery: incision on medial arm in groove between biceps and triceps. Avoid injury to median nerve
  - Radial and ulnar arteries: can be exposed in the AC fossa via an S-shaped incision

    - When assessing for injury to either of these vessels, perform a Doppler Allen's test to determine if the palmar arch is intact

- Lower Extremity

  - External iliac artery: exposed through a retroperitoneal incision, distal external iliac can be exposed via an inguinal incision
  - Common femoral artery: access via a longitudinal incision beginning at the inguinal ligament, extending distally to expose the bifurcation of the superficial femoral and profunda femoris arteries
  - Mid/distal superficial femoral artery: access via longitudinal incision along medial thigh, depending on level retract sartorius either medially or laterally
  - Popliteal artery: fixed in place due to its association with the adductor tendon, geniculate collaterals, and the gastrocnemius.

    - Given these points of fixation, exposure is best achieved with the patient's leg bent and a medial incision from the proximal popliteal space to the distal popliteal space
    - Divide the medial head of the gastrocnemius and semimembranosus and semitendinosus tendons to expose the popliteal artery, vein, and tibial nerve
    - The soleus can be reflected for additional exposure if needed

  - Posterior tibial/peroneal arteries: exposed through a medial lower leg incision
  - Anterior tibial artery: approached through a lateral lower leg incision

Endovascular Repair

- Most useful when the morbidity difference is greatest between open and endo-vascular procedures, as is the case with more proximal vessels (subclavian, iliac)
- Endovascular balloon occlusion can be used to obtain proximal vascular control
- Definitive management of hemorrhage or occlusion can be achieved using covered stent-grafts to exclude the area of injury
- Endovascular outcomes are best in larger vessels as compared to smaller vessels
- Catheter-directed embolization can be useful for treating smaller bleeding vessels, pseudoaneurysms, or fistulas in patients without hard signs of vascular injury and are hemodynamically stable

Fasciotomies

- Incisions to open the fascial compartments of the extremities and relieve pressure to treat or prevent compartment syndrome
- Increased pressure extremity compartments can come from direct compression due to hematoma, or reperfusion injury following reestablishing of blood flow

  - Reperfusion injury is postulated to occur because of decreased vascular integrity leading to increased interstitial edema, or an increase in the proinflammatory response

- Determination of compartment syndrome requiring decompressive fasciotomies is through a combination of physical exam and measuring compartment pressures
- 6Ps: pain with passive motion, pallor, pulselessness, poikilothermia, paresthesia, and paralysis

  - Of these, pain is usually the earliest symptom to manifest and is often described as "pain out of proportion to exam"
  - Loss of distal pulses is a late sign

- Compartment pressures are measured with a handheld manometer inserted into each compartment. Normal compartment pressures are 0 to 9 mmHg

  - A measurement of ≥25–30 is considered elevated and warrants decompression; however, there is no absolute threshold for diagnosis

- Prophylactic fasciotomies should be considered in patients with >4–6 h of ischemia, combined arterial and venous injuries, crush injuries, high-energy mechanism of injury, injury requiring vascular repair or ligation, and in patients that are unable to be monitored clinically
- Upper extremity (Fig. 46.4)

Fig. 46.4 Forearm (R) fasciotomy incision

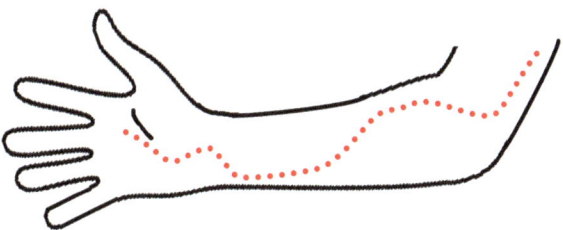

Fig. 46.5 Leg (R) compartments, with fasciotomy incision sites

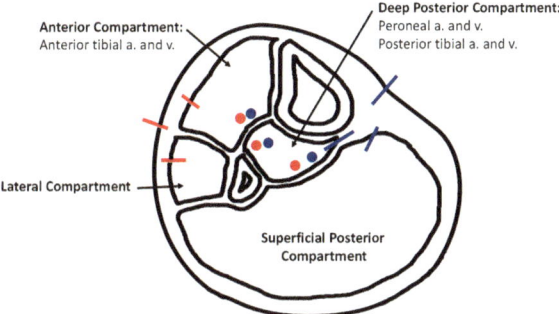

- Incision over medial distal upper arm, extend across AC fossa in S-shape from medial to lateral, extend laterally over extensor wad, curve back to volar aspect, ± carpal tunnel release distally

- Lower leg (Fig. 46.5)

  - Four compartments: anterior, lateral, deep posterior, and superficial posterior
  - Lateral incision: release anterior and lateral compartments, taking care to avoid injury to the peroneal nerve as it runs superficially along the lateral aspect of the tibial head
  - Medial incision: release deep and superficial posterior compartments, taking care to avoid injury to the greater saphenous vein

- Continue to monitor clinically to ensure that no compartments have been missed
- Incisions are left open and delayed closure can be attempted once swelling decreases. Skin grafting may be required for adequate coverage.
- Thigh (less common) (Fig. 46.6)

  - Three compartments: lateral, medial, and posterior
  - A lateral incision is made on the thigh, which is usually enough to release pressure. Sometimes an additional medial incision is required.

Fig. 46.6 Thigh (R)
compartments

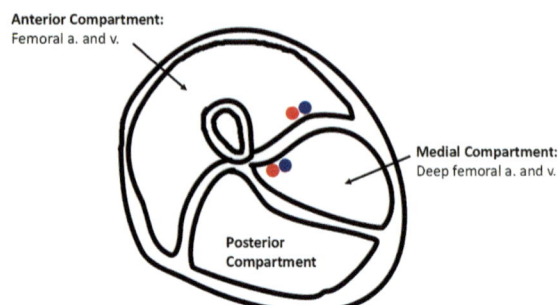

Postoperative Assessment

- Serial monitoring of the pulse exam and motor and sensory function
- Complications: infection, thrombosis, ischemia, hemorrhage, amputation
- Complications within the first 24 h are likely related to technical problems with the repair
- Consideration should be given to the use of antiplatelet agents or anticoagulation depending on the nature of injury and repair, as well as the presence of contraindications due to concomitant injuries
- Interval duplex ultrasound surveillance to monitor patency

References

1. Cronenwett JL, Johnston KW. Rutherford's vascular surgery. 8th ed. Philadelphia: Elsevier; 2014.
2. Feliciano DV, Moore FA, Moore EE, West MA, Davis JW, Cocanour CS, Kozar RA, McIntyre RC. Evaluation and management of peripheral vascular injury. Part 1. Western Trauma Association/critical decisions in trauma. J Trauma. 2011;70(6):1551–6.
3. Fox N, et al. Evaluation and management of penetrating lower extremity arterial trauma: an Eastern Association for the Surgery of Trauma practice management guideline. J Trauma Acute Care Surg. 2012;73:S315–20.
4. Rassmussen TE, Tai NRM. Rich's vascular trauma. 3rd ed. Philadelphia; 2016.

Chapter 47
Orthopedic Trauma, Fractures, and Dislocations

Michael S. Kain and Justin Kleiner

Introduction

Orthopedic trauma involves understanding how the musculoskeletal system affects the overall physiology of the patient. Understanding the basics of fractures and dislocations in the trauma setting will assist one in caring for trauma patients and communicating with the trauma team. Injuries to the axial and appendicular skeleton have significant physiologic impacts on the trauma patient, and identifying injury patterns can provide important information regarding mechanism and associated injuries. Stabilization of skeletal injuries allows for improved physiologic resuscitation of the patient.

- Traumatic injuries to the skeletal system can be separated into the axial skeleton and appendicular skeleton.
- Goals of treatment for orthopedic trauma are focused on stabilizing the patient's skeletal system in order to allow for acute resuscitation, early mobilization, and maximal functional recovery.
- Understanding classification systems is important in order to describe the type of fracture present.
- Understanding the local and systemic physiologic conditions of the orthopedic trauma patient is also critical to trauma care.

M. S. Kain · J. Kleiner (✉)
Department of Orthopaedic Surgery, Boston University, Boston, MA, USA
e-mail: Michael.Kain@bmc.org

© The Author(s), under exclusive license to Springer Nature Switzerland AG 2025
T. S. Brahmbhatt, D. R. Scantling (eds.), *Trauma Surgery Clerkship*, Contemporary Surgical Clerkships, https://doi.org/10.1007/978-3-032-01412-2_47

Epidemiology

- Incidence of trauma and orthopedic injuries [10]
  - High energy in the young
  - Lower energy in the old
  - Incidence and identification of neurologic and vascular injuries
- Understanding the mechanism of injury and the energy involved is important information to obtain so there is a clear understanding of the type of trauma one is managing.
- Younger patients tend to be involved more with high-energy events while older patients are usually involved in lower energy mechanisms.
- The severity of the injuries is usually related to the amount of energy involved.
- Understanding scoring systems can assist the clinician in understanding the severity of injury.

Description of Injuries and Classifications Systems

- Understanding how to recognize, describe, and thus communicate regarding orthopedic injuries in the trauma setting is imperative.
- Classification systems have been developed to evaluate many of these injuries to objectively categorize particular injuries.
- These classification systems help to describe the clinical situation for communication purposes, and good classification systems help to also direct the treatment plan of the patient.

Below are some basic classification systems that are imperative to understand when managing orthopedic trauma patients.

Open Fractures

- Open fractures are classically described using the Gustilo and Anderson Classification system (Table 47.1) to help guide treatment [2].
- This classification helps provide insight into the amount of soft tissue injury around the fracture which is related to an increased risk of infection and non-union.
- The system uses the size of the wound and level of contamination. The system helps guide antibiotic use in the acute trauma period as well as longer term management and there are three grades of open fractures.
- A grade 1 open fracture is a small wound up to one centimeter and has minimal soft tissue and muscle injury.

Table 47.1 The Gustilo-Anderson open fracture classification system

	1	2	3
Skin	Wound Less than 1 cm	Wound 1–10 cm	Wound >10 cm
Contamination	Minimal	Moderate	Severe
Soft tissue damage	Minimal	Moderate	Severe
Vascular injury	No	No	3A. No 3B. No 3C. Yes
Coverage	Primary closure	Primary closure	3A. Primary closure 3B. Soft tissue flap or skin graft required 3C. Soft tissue flap or skin graft required

This classification system provides the clinician with insight into the size of the open wound, the amount of contamination, and the extent of the soft tissue injury around the fracture. Large wounds that are not able to be closed and require soft tissue coverage usually involves plastic surgery and definitive fixation should not be placed until there is a plan to close the wound. The presence of a vascular injury requires close coordination teamwork with the vascular team to coordinate the order in which fixation and revascularization will occur

- A grade 2 open fracture has a wound of 1 to 10 cm in length, minimal contamination, and a minimal to moderate amount of soft tissue stripping. Grade 2 injuries are easily closed after debridement of nonviable tissue.
- Grade 3 injuries are the most severe open fractures and have three subclassifications. These are large wounds greater than 10 cm, and there is some concern of wound closure because there exists severe soft tissue injury and contamination. The subclassifications of grade 3 injuries are described as A, B, C.

  - A grade 3A open fracture will be able to be closed after debridement of nonviable soft tissue and contaminated tissue and will not require additional soft tissue coverage such as muscle flaps.
  - A grade 3B open fracture is one that has gross contamination and severe soft tissue injury that will require soft tissue coverage such as a muscle flap.
  - A grade 3C open fracture involves the presence of a neurologic or vascular injury, the most extreme soft tissue injury one can sustain.

Describing Fractures

- Fracture patterns exist and they provide insight to the clinician as to the type of mechanism that occurred to cause the fracture.
- Fractures occur when forces applied to the bone overwhelm the bone's ability to absorb stress and strain, exceeding the yielding strength of the bone. The direction, or vector, of the force will influence the fracture morphology (Fig. 47.1).

- When the force is directed perpendicular to the long axis of the bone, a straight transverse fracture occurs [10].
- Torsional forces generate a spiral fracture.
- With axial loading or compressive forces, as in a crush injury, there is usually comminution. When there is a combination of forces then oblique fractures are generated.
- In a bending injury, there is a combination of compression and tension forces which will generate a butterfly fragment. One side of the bone is subjected to compressive forces, causing a butterfly fragment on that side, while the other side is subjected to tension forces resulting in a transverse fracture. As the energy increases, there is increased comminution [10].
- Understanding these forces and how to describe fractures will provide insight into the injury pattern, the energy involved, and possible associated fractures.

The forces involved in causing a fracture help to guide the forces and movement required to reduce these fractures by reversing the deforming forces.

Intra-Articular Fractures

- When fractures occur at the ends of the bones, they can enter the joint and are therefore intra-articular fractures involving the weight-bearing surface.
- To help describe these fractures, the Orthopedic Trauma Association/Association of the Study of Internal Fixation (OTA/AO) classification breaks these down into three types of fractures; extra-articular fractures (Type-A), partial articular fractures (Type-B), and complete articular (Type-C) (Fig. 47.2) [4].

Force	Tension	Compression	Bending	Torsion
			Tension side / Compression side	
Fracture Morphology	Transverse	Oblique	Butterfly	Spiral

Fig. 47.1 Fracture pattern is related to the forces placed onto the bone

- These injuries are important to recognize, as early reduction of the joint is necessary to restore joint stability and congruence.
- At times, the soft tissue envelope around the involved joint prevents acute surgical intervention. In these situations, if a cast or splint will not hold the joint reduced, then external fixation can be applied to pull the fracture out to length and stabilize the soft tissues to allow the soft tissue envelop to heal [6].
- Letting the soft tissues heal decreases the risk of infection and later wound breakdown. In particular, intra-articular distal tibia fractures, known as pilon fractures, are susceptible to higher infection rates when operated on acutely. They are typically managed with an external fixation acutely to hold fractures stable and out to length, with a plan for delay open reduction internal fixation.
- Intra-articular injuries involve an injury to the cartilage and restoring the joint allows for restoration of function. These injuries are at increased risk for post-traumatic arthritis and early stabilization along with restoration of the joint will help mobilize the patient acutely and also improve the long-term function of the joint.

Dislocations

- In order to function properly, a joint must be congruent and stable.
- When a joint becomes dislocated, there is a loss of congruence. A joint is completely congruent when the two sides of the joint match perfectly.
- A dislocation occurs when the opposing bones are 100% displaced from each other.

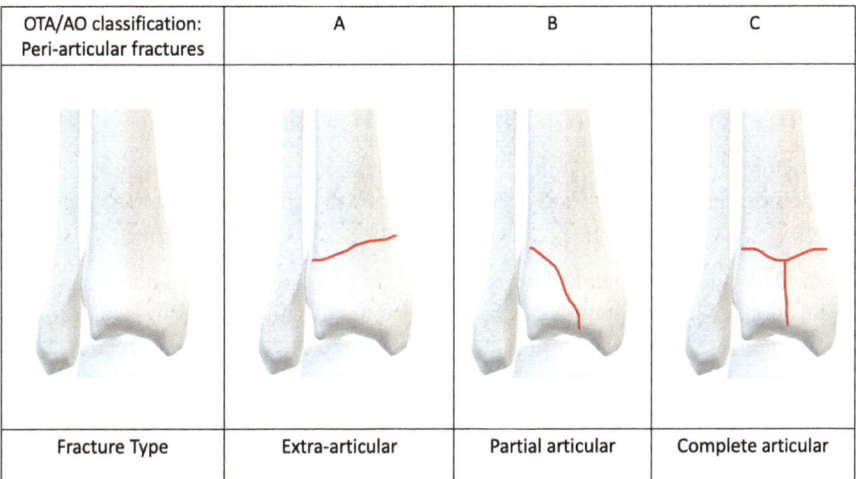

OTA/AO classification: Peri-articular fractures	A	B	C
Fracture Type	Extra-articular	Partial articular	Complete articular

Fig. 47.2 OTA/AO classification of peri-articular fractures

Fig. 47.3 A lateral fracture dislocation of the proximal tibial is show in the AP radiograph. The yellow or medial fragment (**a**) is the portion of the bone that is congruent with the femur and is the reduced piece. The red or lateral fragment is laterally displaced and is the dislocated portion. This is attached to the rest of the lower leg

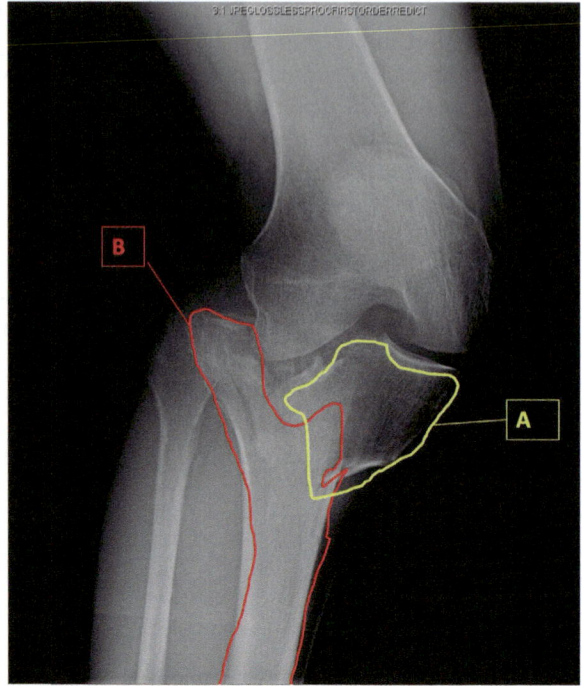

- A subluxation is a partial dislocation where there is some contact between the two sides of the joint, but an incongruent joint still exists.
- Fracture dislocations, including subluxations, occur usually when there is an intra-articular fracture on one side of the joint. In these cases, a portion of the articular surface that is still congruent and reduced is the intact part of the joint, and the dislocated portion is usually the larger fragment.

  - For instance, the proximal tibial fracture dislocations for the knee usually have a small medial condylar fragment that remains congruent. The lateral fragment is then the rest of the dislocated lower leg (Fig. 47.3).

Fracture dislocations require careful examination and are associated with obvious deformities, skin tethering or tenting and most importantly vascular and nerve injuries.

- A good musculoskeletal exam is always important, especially with fracture dislocations, where structures can be stretched to their limits. Neurovascular insults are highly associated with these injuries, particularly around the knee. Understanding the extent of these injuries upon presentation, prior to reduction, and after reduction is imperative when managing these injuries [10].
- Early recognition of these injuries is imperative to optimize the outcome.

Pathophysiology of Orthopedic Trauma

- Fractures occur when a bone is exposed to more force than it is able to structurally absorb.
- The force required to cause a long bone fracture results in both a local and systemic insult.
- Care of orthopedic trauma patients requires management of both the local and systemic effects of trauma.

Systemic Pathophysiology

- Trauma patients sustain a systemic insult which must be recognized and managed.
- Orthopedic trauma patients may present with hemodynamic instability, and there is a significant amount of blood loss associated with long bone or pelvic fractures.
- Pelvic fractures in particular may be associated with significant blood loss that can be life-threatening. Most commonly, pelvic bleeding is venous. Arterial bleeding also occurs and is associated with open book or some anteroposterior compression (APC) pelvic fractures as well as in older patients particularly with peripheral artery calcification [3].
- Any hemodynamic instability requires acute resuscitation. In patients with pelvic fracture and hemodynamic instability, further studies such as CT-angiogram or interventional radiology procedures may be necessary to identify and control bleeding.
- In patients with widening of the pubic symphysis, a pelvic binder may be used to decrease pelvic bleeding.
- In patients with femur fracture, up to 2 liters of blood can be lost into the thigh. Humeral or tibial fractures can result in 500 mL to 1 L of blood loss. Blood loss associated with long bone fractures can be decreased with early stabilization, either with splinting or placement in traction [1].
- The blood loss associated with orthopedic trauma may result in decreased organ perfusion. It is important to ensure that patients are adequately resuscitated.
- In addition to hemodynamic concerns, orthopedic trauma patients are at significant risk of pulmonary complications.
- Long bone fractures can directly affect pulmonary function through fat embolism syndrome. Bone marrow contains a significant amount of fat, and as the fat globules are released into the bloodstream after a fracture, they can occlude small blood vessels [5, 7].
- The risk of fat emboli is reduced with fracture immobilization. However, orthopedic surgical procedures can further increase the risk of acute respiratory distress. Placement of intramedullary nails for fracture fixation, or insertion of cement and prosthetic joints can increase intramedullary pressure, resulting in

increased load of fat emboli and risk of acute respiratory distress, particularly if there is an existing associated injury.

- Adequate hemodynamic resuscitation and recognition of associated pulmonary and thoracic injuries are essential to help manage and mitigate increased risk for pulmonary complications.
- Associated rib fractures or pulmonary contusions may also result in impaired lung function. In addition, prolonged bed rest in trauma patients can result in atelectasis or pneumonia. Any patient with fracture is also at risk for deep venous thrombosis. This can result in pulmonary embolism and can be fatal.
- Pulmonary embolism should be considered in any orthopedic trauma patient with signs such as fever, tachycardia, or increased calf swelling or tenderness.

Local Pathophysiology

- Locally, in the region of fracture, the injury is not isolated to the fractured bone. The surrounding skin, muscle, neurovascular structures, and periosteum are subjected to the same energy that caused the fracture. As a result, the surrounding soft tissue must be evaluated as well.
- First, the integrity of the skin must be assessed. Note any visible deformity and the location of any skin abrasions. Explore any open wounds with high suspicion for open fracture. A continuously oozing wound is a common indicator of an open fracture. In the case of open fracture, the open wound may not necessarily be found in the same location as the fracture. Patients with dislocation or fracture dislocation may have threatened or tented skin. Inspect the patient for any areas of lighter or blanched skin, and test for capillary refill in these areas. An urgent reduction may be necessary in the case of open or threatened skin.
- In the area surrounding the fracture, there is often associated muscle injury. Compartment syndrome must be considered in any orthopedic trauma patient with long bone fracture particularly with fractures involving the tibia and forearm [5].

  - Muscles are contained within distinct fascial compartments. The swelling from orthopedic trauma can result in elevated pressure within one or more muscle compartments. When the pressure in a fascial compartment becomes elevated, commonly defined as within 30 mm Hg of diastolic blood pressure, the muscle and nerves within that compartment will no longer be adequately perfused.
  - This occurs because the capillary beds in the compartment will collapse when compartment pressure is too high. Further, venous outflow may become impaired. Structures within these compartments begin to undergo irreversible damage within hours, and elevated compartment pressures for greater than 6 to 8 hours will result in significant ischemia and permanent impairment.

- A compartment pressure monitor may be used to measure compartment pressures in the affected extremity. However, the diagnosis of compartment syndrome relies primarily on clinical symptoms. Early symptoms of compartment syndrome include severe pain, decreased strength or range of motion, and increased pain with passive stretch of the compartment. Late symptoms include decreased sensation (paraesthesias), pulselessness, and pallor. Compartment syndrome most commonly occurs in areas of the body that are less able to accommodate this swelling, such as the lower leg or forearm.

- In addition to evaluation of the compartments, inspect for any evidence of contusion or bruising. Palpate for any focal areas of fluctuant swelling.

  - This can represent a Morel-Lavallee lesion, a degloving injury of the subcutaneous fat from the underlying muscle and can lead to hematoma or skin necrosis if not recognized [9].
  - These lesions typically form within one month of injury, and most commonly self-resolve within 6 months if uncomplicated.

- Nerves and blood vessels are also at risk of injury in patients with orthopedic injuries, and it is important to perform a detailed neurovascular exam in any affected extremity. These structures are at increased risk in the presence of dislocation, open fracture, penetrating trauma such as stab or gunshot wounds, and multiply injured patients. Patients with pelvic fractures are also at increased risk of vascular injury. This is especially true in patients over 60 years old, as stiffer calcified blood vessels are less able to stretch without rupturing in the setting of trauma [3].

- A vascular exam should include a pulse exam and capillary refill in the fingers or toes. In patients with lower extremity injuries, ankle/brachial index (ABI) may be performed. An ABI <0.9 may indicate arterial injury. Further testing such as a CT-angiogram may be performed for further evaluation [8].

  - Common types of vascular injury include spasm, intimal injuries including dissection, pseudoaneurysm, true aneurism, complete transection, and arteriovenous fistula.

- Orthopedic trauma patients may also present with nerve injuries. Types of nerve injury include a contusion (neuropraxia), crush injury (axonotmesis), or complete transection (neurotmesis).

  - There is increased risk for nerve injury in patients with penetrating trauma, open fractures, high-energy trauma, and multiply injured patients. In the case of closed fracture, nerve injury is most commonly neuropraxia and will typically resolve with observation.
  - Certain closed fracture patterns are also associated with patterns of nerve injury. Radial nerve injury is most common with humerus shaft fracture, particularly spiral fractures of the distal humeral shaft. Median nerve injury or acute carpal tunnel may be present in patients with distal radius fracture.

Acetabular fractures may be associated with sciatic nerve injury. Proximal tibia fractures may be associated with peroneal nerve injury.

- Injury to the bone and periosteum must also be assessed.
- The pattern of fracture indicates the direction of force applied to the bone. Spiral fractures are caused by twisting or rotational force. Transverse fractures are caused by a tension force. Oblique fractures are caused by compression force. Butterfly fragments occur when the bone is subjected to both a bending and axial compression force, and may suggest a higher energy injury. Segmental fractures, where the same long bone is fractured in multiple locations, also suggests higher energy injury [10].
- It is also important to consider injury to the periosteum, as this tissue is responsible for much of the blood supply and nutrition to the bone, and is important for fracture healing.

  - Patients with open fractures, or high-energy patterns, including segmental fracture and comminuted fracture, will often have significant stripping of the periosteum from the bone.

Current Management Practice

- Acute stabilization of appendicular skeletal injuries in the upper and lower extremity requires early stabilization using splints and casts.
- Skeletal traction is used for femur, hip, and pelvic and acetabular fractures to temporality provide stability to injuries that cannot be splinted or casted.
- Traction uses ligamentotaxis to help provide stability and helps hold length. Using approximately 10–20% of body weight for traction is all that is typically needed.
- Open fractures should be debrided and irrigated thoroughly to minimize contamination and reduce infection and nonunion risks.
- External fixation can be performed acutely to hold fractures out to length and stabilize the soft tissues. External fixators can be used temporarily or as definitive fixation.
- Intramedullary fixation is excellent for extra-articular long bone fractures such as the femur and tibia. These rely on endochondral ossification healing and can be placed percutaneously.

Take-Home Points for Patient Care

- Follow ATLS and ABC's of trauma to resuscitate the patient.
- Perform a complete secondary survey to Identify musculoskeletal injuries, as well as associated neurologic or vascular injuries.

- Use proper terminology to communicate injury patterns.
- Understand the physiology of compartment syndrome.

References

1. Cooper N. Hemorrhagic shock. StatPearls; 2022.
2. Gustilo RB. Problems in management of type III (severe) open fractures: a new classification of type III open fractures. J Trauma. 1984;24:742–6.
3. Kazley JM. Team approach: evaluation and management of pelvic ring injuries. JBJS Rev. 2020;
4. Meinberg E. Fracture and dislocation classification compendium. J Orthopaed Trauma. 2018;
5. Olson SA, Glasgow RR. Acute compartment syndrome in lower extremity musculoskeletal trauma. J Am Acad Orthopaed Surg. 2005;
6. Roberts CS. Damage control orthopaedics: evolving concepts in the treatment of patients who have sustained orthopaedic trauma. Instr Course Lect. 2005;
7. Rothberg DL. Fat embolism and fat embolism syndrome. J Am Acad Orthop Surg. 2019;
8. Scalea TM. Western Trauma Association critical decisions in trauma: management of the mangled extremity. J Trauma Acute Care Surg. 2012;
9. Scolaro JA. The Morel-Lavallée lesion: diagnosis and management. J Am Acad Orthop Surg. 2016;
10. Tornetta P. Rockwood and Green's fractures in adults, 9e. Lippincott Williams & Wilkins, a Wolters Kluwer Business; 2019.

Chapter 48
Burns and Inhalation Injury

Christine Wu and Stephanie Nitzschke

Burn Classification

Anatomy

- Skin is composed of two distinct layers:

  - Epidermis (outer layer) serves as a protective barrier
  - Dermis (inner layer) contains blood vessels, nerves, and sweat glands to help maintain thermoregulation

- Local area of injury is divided into three zones:

  - Zone of coagulation—irreversibly damaged, cells are necrotic
  - Zone of stasis—decreased tissue perfusion, cells may survive or undergo coagulative necrosis
  - Zone of hyperemia—area of vasodilation from surrounding inflammation, most viable tissue from which healing begins

- Depth of a burn is classified by the level of skin and tissue involved (Table 48.1)

C. Wu · S. Nitzschke (✉)
Department of Surgery, Brigham and Women's Hospital, Boston, MA, USA
e-mail: cwu12@bwh.harvard.edu; Snitzschke@bwh.harvard.ed

© The Author(s), under exclusive license to Springer Nature Switzerland AG 2025
T. S. Brahmbhatt, D. R. Scantling (eds.), *Trauma Surgery Clerkship*, Contemporary Surgical Clerkships,
https://doi.org/10.1007/978-3-032-01412-2_48

Table 48.1 Burn depth classification

Thickness	Depth	Characteristics
Superficial, 1st degree	Epidermis	Blanching erythema, no blistering, painful
Superficial partial, 2nd degree	Dermis, papillary region	Blanching, blisters, painful, weepy wound bed, intact hair follicles
Deep partial, 2nd degree	Dermis, reticular region	Non-blanching, paler, decreased sensation, loss of hair follicles
Full, 3rd degree	Subcutaneous tissue	Non-blanching, dry, waxy, leathery, insensate
4th degree	Beyond fascia to underlying muscle or bone	Charred appearance

Burn Size

- Burn size is estimated by the percentage of total body surface area (TBSA) involved

    - Rule of 9's to assess TBSA burned, only for second- and third- degree burns in adults—head 9%, each upper extremity 9%, chest 18%, back 18%, each lower extremity 18%, perineum 1% (Fig. 48.1)
    - Can also use the patient's open hand as 1% TBSA to estimate burn size

- In children, TBSA burned is measured differently. Given their larger body surface area relative to body weight, burns of equal TBSA have higher fluid needs and can have a greater physiologic impact

Burn Types

- Flame

    - Direct contact with fire/flame
    - Most common type of burn injury in the USA

- Scald

    - From contact with hot liquids
    - Most common in children <5 years

- Electrical

    - Can present with minimal external injury though significant internal injuries to muscle, nerves, and blood vessels
    - Requires cardiac monitoring
    - Can cause rhabdomyolysis, vascular thrombosis, compartment syndrome

Fig. 48.1 Rule of 9's to assess total body surface area involved in adult burn patients

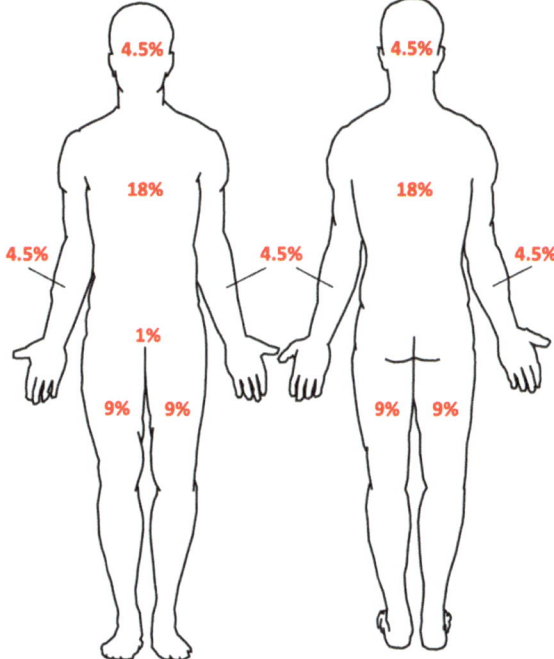

- Chemical

  - Acid burns lead to coagulative necrosis
  - Alkali burns lead to liquefactive necrosis, which extends deeper into tissues
  - Hydrofluoric acid burns can cause severe hypocalcemia as the F^- binds to calcium and magnesium and can cause cardiac arrest, precipitation in the tissues, and ischemia

Evaluation

Initial Assessment

- Start assessment with systematic primary and secondary surveys performed for patients with major trauma to identify life-threatening injuries (starts with securing the airway and evaluation of any other life-threatening traumatic injuries)
- Extinguish and remove burning clothing as soon as possible
- It is important to keep the patient warm with warm fluids and keep the burn wounds covered with dry sterile dressings until they can be transferred to a burn center
- Begin fluid resuscitation on burns >20% TBSA (see section on fluid resuscitation)

Inhalation Injury

- Occurs by direct thermal injury to the upper airway and chemical injury from inhaled toxins to the bronchi and alveoli
- Pertinent history includes mechanism of injury, duration of exposure

  - Greater risk with smoke exposure in an enclosed space

- Signs/symptoms—facial burns, singed facial hair, soot deposits, carbonaceous sputum, swollen facial features, hoarseness, stridor, wheezing
- Diagnosed by fiberoptic bronchoscopy, which can reveal airway soot/charring, edema, erythema, mucosal sloughing, ulceration, and necrosis
- Carboxyhemoglobin level >10% is indicative of carbon monoxide poisoning

  - Signs/symptoms—headache, dizziness, nausea, altered mental status

- Markedly increases mortality when combined with a thermal injury

Management

Airway Management

- Administer 100% oxygen during initial assessment

  - Patients with inhalation injury should receive humidified oxygen
  - Patients with carbon monoxide poisoning should be given 100% oxygen until carboxyhemoglobin levels return to normal

- Have a low threshold for early intubation in the presence of an inhalation injury before rapid progression of pharyngeal edema obstructs the airway completely
- There are no specific therapeutic interventions for inhalation injury other than supportive care

  - Chest physiotherapy, frequent airway suctioning, and early mobilization can prevent atelectasis and development of pneumonia

Burn Shock

- Burn shock is a time-limited shock state that occurs with burns >20% TBSA in the first 24 h after injury (only include second-degree burns or greater in the TBSA calculation. First-degree burns don't count).
- Burns shock causes a release of inflammatory mediators resulting in systemic vasodilation and heat-injured capillary leakage. This leads to rapid, large-volume

intravascular fluid loss, requiring aggressive, though targeted, fluid resuscitation to maintain organ perfusion without causing fluid overload

- Hypermetabolism is a physiologic response in burn patients, and aggressive nutritional support is critical to maximize wound healing and minimize immune deficiency

  - Larger burns will likely need calorie and protein supplementation

Burn Shock

Fluid Resuscitation

- For patients with burns >20% TBSA
- Different formulas have been devised to provide guidelines for the amount of fluid to give:

  - Parkland formula: (4 mL) * (weight in kg) * (% TBSA burn) = volume of fluid given in first 24 h, with half the volume given in the first 8 h and remaining half given in the next 16 h
  - Modified Brooke formula: (2 mL) * (weight in kg) * (% TBSA burn) = volume of fluid given in first 24 h, with half the volume given in the first 8 h and remaining half given in the next 16 h

- Urine output is a marker of resuscitation, with goal 30–50 cc/h for adults, 1 mL/kg/h for children, and 2 mL/kg/h for infants <6 months

  - Fluid rates can be titrated based on hourly urine output

- In general, you should use basic critical care principles to guide resuscitation as the fluid equations from the above formulas tend to give the patient too much fluid. Volume overload can lead to pulmonary edema, conversion of superficial into deep burns, abdominal compartment syndrome, and extremity compartment syndrome, and is associated with worse outcomes

Additional Management

- Initially, burned areas should be cleaned with warm, soapy water, and dressed in antibiotic cream (many options, see below) and clean gauze

  - One of the main goals of burn wound care is to prevent infection. Daily wound care ensures cleanliness and can utilize occlusive dressings to limit exposure to air/bacteria, minimize invasive wound infections, and promote reepithelialization

- There is no role for prophylactic antibiotics
- Early mobilization avoids muscle or tendon contracture and ensures maximal recovery of joint motion and function

Topical Antimicrobial Agents

- Bacitracin

  - Moisturizes the wound
  - Painless with application

- Silver sulfadiazine (Silvadene)

  - Most commonly used for initial wound care
  - Do not use in patients with sulfa allergy
  - Side effects—neutropenia, thrombocytopenia

- Mafenide acetate (Sulfamylon)

  - Good eschar penetration
  - Painful with application to sensate skin
  - Side effects—metabolic acidosis as it is a carbonic anhydrase inhibitor

- Silver nitrate

  - Side effects—electrolyte imbalances (hyponatremia, hypokalemia, hypochloremia, hypocalcemia), methemoglobinemia

Surgical Treatment

- Early surgical excision of compromised tissue and early wound closure primarily by skin grafting allows for quicker wound healing, reduces risks of infectious complications, and mitigates the hypermetabolic response

  - Tangential excision—remove burned tissue by layers until viable tissue encountered

    - Preserves configuration and contour of body parts
    - Greater blood loss

  - Fascial excision—remove all burned tissue down to fascia

    - Reduced blood loss

- Eschar syndrome occurs when there are circumferential full thickness burns to extremities, which limits blood flow to the extremity, or to the chest when there is difficulty ventilating a patient with significant torso burns

- Extremity—medial and lateral incisions to release the burn eschar
- Chest wall—lateral incisions bilaterally at midaxillary line with connecting incision across the chest to relieve the constriction

- Skin grafting promotes durable wound closure. Autografts utilize skin from a donor site to a recipient site in the same individual

  - Full-thickness—less wound contraction, longer time for healing due to thicker tissue and prolonged time for wound to develop new blood supply
  - Split-thickness—easier engraftment as graft is supplied through diffusion through capillaries in the wound bed and neovascularization occurs at postop day 2, greater chance of success, more wound contraction
  - Other sources of skin substitute for temporary wound coverage—allograft (cadaver skin), xenograft (often porcine)
  - Reasons for graft failure—seroma, hematoma, infection, shearing forces

- Surgical excision can lead to massive blood loss. Strategies to minimize blood loss includes the use of dilute epinephrine infiltration or epinephrine-soaked gauze, electrocautery, or tourniquets
- Loss of dermis as the body's thermal regulator results in a high risk of intraoperative hypothermia. Strategies to minimize hypothermia includes the use of warming blankets or fluid warmers, limit the amount of skin surface exposed, maintain room temperature >25 °C

Complications

Burn Wound Infection and Sepsis

- Signs—rapid changes in wound appearance, surrounding erythema, purulent drainage
- Burn wound sepsis is an invasive burn wound infection

  - Signs—systemic signs (fever, tachycardia, hypotension, tachypnea), conversion of partial-thickness injury to full-thickness necrosis

- Definitively diagnose by biopsy of the burn wound
- Most common organisms are *Staphylococcus* and *Pseudomonas*
- Reduce the risk of infection by early surgical excision

Compartment Syndrome

- Caused by high-volume fluid resuscitation
- Can occur in the abdomen or any extremity burned or unburned. Different from eschar syndrome

Pneumonia

- Common cause of morbidity and mortality in burn patients
- Risk factors include endotracheal intubation or inhalation injury. Direct injury to the lungs can result in interstitial edema, ciliary dysfunction, and increased capillary permeability
- Can progress to Acute respiratory distress syndrome (ARDS)

Curling Ulcer

- Acute gastroduodenal stress ulcer is much less common today given improvements with early and routine prophylaxis with proton pump inhibitors and H2 blockers

Burn Center Referral

- Patients with any of the criteria listed should be transferred to a designated burn center:
  - Partial-thickness burns >10% TBSA
  - All full-thickness burns
  - Burns involving the face, hands, feet, genitalia, perineum, or major joints
  - Inhalation injury
  - Electrical or chemical burns
  - Burned patients with preexisting medical disorders that may complicate management, prolong recovery, or affect mortality
  - Patients with burns and concomitant traumas in which the burn injury poses greater immediate risk of morbidity and mortality
  - Burned children in hospitals without qualified personnel or equipment
  - Burned patients who will require special social, emotional, or long-term rehabilitative intervention

References

1. Nitzschke S. Burns & other thermal injuries. In: Current diagnosis and treatment: surgery. 15th ed. New York: McGraw Hill; 2020.
2. Levi B, Vercruysse G. Burns and radiation. In: Trauma. 9th ed. New York: McGraw Hill; 2020.
3. Latenser B. Critical care of the burn patient. In: Principles of critical care. 4th ed. New York: McGraw Hill; 2014.

4. Jeschke MG, Herndon DN. Burns. In: Sabiston textbook of surgery: the biological basis of modern surgical practice. 20th ed. Amsterdam: Elsevier; 2016.
5. Woodson LC, Talon M, Traber DL, Herndon DN. Diagnosis and treatment of inhalation injury. In: Total burn care. 4th ed. Amsterdam: Elsevier; 2012.
6. Greenhalgh DG, Saffle JR, Homes JH, et al. American Burn Association consensus conference to define sepsis and infection in burns. J Burn Care Res. 2007;28:776–90.
7. Chung KK, Wolf SE. Critical care in the severely burned: organ support and management of complications. In: Total burn care. 4th ed. Amsterdam: Elsevier; 2012.

Chapter 49
Care of the Pregnant Trauma Patient

Iman N. Afif and Christina L. Jacovides

Overview

- Trauma occurs in about 1 in 12 pregnancies and is a significant cause of morbidity and mortality for both the pregnant patient and fetus.
- Evaluation and management of the pregnant trauma patient is complicated by alterations in anatomy and physiology and may require close collaboration with obstetricians and neonatologists.
- Fetal assessment should not interfere with or delay the trauma workup and resuscitation of a pregnant patient, but can often be performed in parallel with the trauma evaluation.
- Concerns about fetal radiation exposure may lead to inadequate workup of injuries in the pregnant patient, resulting in missed injuries with potential devastating effects for the pregnant patient and/or fetus.
- For non-obstetric injuries, indications for operative intervention or interventional radiology procedures are the same for pregnant and nonpregnant patients.

I. N. Afif
Department of Surgery, Temple University Hospital, Philadelphia, PA, USA
e-mail: Iman.Afif@tuhs.temple.edu

C. L. Jacovides (✉)
Division of Trauma Surgery and Surgical Critical Care, Department of Surgery, Temple University Hospital, Philadelphia, PA, USA
e-mail: christina.jacovides@tuhs.temple.edu

Background

- *Epidemiology* Trauma occurs in an estimated 6–8% of pregnancies, and it is the most common non-obstetric cause of mortality in pregnancy [10, 12, 13, 15].
- Blunt trauma is the predominant mechanism, with the most common causes being assault, motor vehicle collisions, and falls [12, 13, 15, 16]. Less common causes include penetrating trauma, homicide, suicide, and burns [12].
- Pregnant persons experience violent trauma at almost double the rate of nonpregnant counterparts and are at greater risk of death due to trauma [5, 12]. Domestic violence is estimated to occur in about 8% of pregnancies [12].

Anatomic and Physiologic Changes in Pregnancy

- Pregnancy is accompanied by a multitude of anatomic and physiologic alterations that directly and indirectly impact the body's response to trauma.

Anatomic

- The uterus is situated and well-protected in the pelvis for the first trimester, or until about 12 weeks. During early pregnancy, the uterus is thick-walled and the fetus is small, mobile, and well-protected by the large volume of amniotic fluid. By the 20th week of gestation, the fundal height reaches approximately the level of the umbilicus, and by 34 to 36 weeks, it reaches the costal margin [1].
- When in vertex position, the fetal head and skull are protected within the pelvic brim, although they can be seriously injured in the case of pelvic fracture of the pregnant patient. Pubic symphysis widening to about 4 to 8 mm, as well as widening of the sacroiliac joint spaces in the third trimester are expected during pregnancy and should be considered when interpreting pelvic imaging [1].

Cardiovascular

- Over the course of pregnancy, the pregnant patient's heart rate (HR) increases by about 15 to 20 beats per minute and cardiac output (CO) increases by as much as 50% at term (Table 49.1). A concurrent decrease in systemic vascular resistance (SVR) allows high flow and low resistance perfusion of the uterus and placenta. By the end of pregnancy, the uterus and placenta experience a fourth of the pregnant patient's total CO [7, 12].

Table 49.1 Normal ranges for vital signs and laboratory values in pregnant patients (by trimester), compared to those in nonpregnant patients [3, 7, 8]

Value	1st trimester	2nd trimester	3rd trimester	Nonpregnant
Vital signs				
Heart rate	63–105		68–115	60–100
Systolic BP	92–133	93–136	95–139	
Diastolic BP	55–86	55–85	57–88	
Lab values				
Hematologic				
Hemoglobin (g/dL)	12–14	10–15	9.5–15	12–16
Hematocrit (%)	31–41	30–39	28–40	35–44
Blood gas				
P_{CO2} (mm Hg)	–	–	25–33	38–42
HCO_3^- (mmol/L)	–	–	16–22	22–26

- The increase in CO and decrease in SVR translate into a decrease in the pregnant patient's blood pressure (BP) by about 10 to 12 mm Hg in the second and third trimesters with a return to baseline by the end of pregnancy (Table 49.1) [1, 7, 12, 19].
- Given these changes in HR and BP, care should be taken in interpreting vital signs of pregnant trauma patients (Table 49.1). Moreover, pregnant patients can lose up to 30% of their total blood volume (or about 1200 to 1500 mL) before vital sign abnormalities are present [1, 7].

Pulmonary

- As early as the first trimester, high circulating progesterone levels result in physiologic hyperventilation, e.g., increased respiratory rate and tidal volume. This results in mild respiratory alkalosis—or decrease in plasma carbon dioxide (CO_2) levels—with a compensatory drop in bicarbonate (HCO_3^-) levels (Table 49.1). Because of the physiologic decrease in CO_2, a normal CO_2 level of 35 to 40 mm Hg can be a sign of impending respiratory collapse in pregnant patients [1, 3, 7, 14].
- Oxygen consumption is elevated during pregnancy by as much as 20%; for this reason, it is important to ensure adequate oxygenation of the pregnant trauma patient [1, 7, 14].

Gastrointestinal

- During pregnancy, progesterone reduces lower esophageal sphincter tone and delays gastric emptying, both of which increase the risk of aspiration [1, 7, 14].

Renal

- Renal blood flow and glomerular filtration rate rise during pregnancy, resulting in a decrease in serum creatinine and urea nitrogen levels. As a result, relatively small elevations in creatinine in the setting of acute kidney injury may reflect a significant loss in glomerular filtration rate [1, 7].

Hematologic

- During pregnancy, there is an increase in total blood volume to compensate for blood loss during delivery. Plasma volume expands more than red blood cell volume, therefore, these changes result in relative dilutional anemia (Table 49.1) [7, 12].
- Pregnancy also increases synthesis of coagulation factors and fibrinogen— fibrinogen levels are typically doubled during pregnancy (reference range 400 to 650 mg/mL in pregnancy, versus 150 to 400 mg/mL in nonpregnant patients). Relatively low fibrinogen levels in a pregnant patient (<200 mg/mL) should raise suspicion for a consumptive coagulopathy such as disseminated intravascular coagulopathy (DIC) [3, 15].

Current Practice

First and foremost, the care of pregnant trauma patients should adhere to the standards of care for nonpregnant patients, although some adjustments and additional steps may be appropriate to account for physiologic changes during pregnancy and to evaluate the fetus. Ultimately, the best care for both the fetus and the pregnant patient is to optimize the care of the pregnant patient.

Primary Survey [1, 4]

- Airway—ensure patency of airway

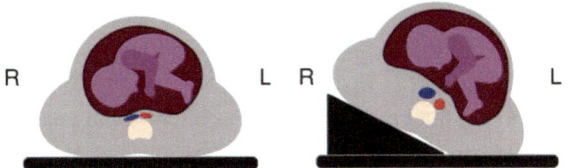

Fig. 49.1 In the second and third trimester, the uterus can cause compression of the aorta and IVC with resulting hypotension. Left lateral tilting of the patient will allow offloading of the aorta and IVC

- Emergent intubation may be complicated in pregnancy due to airway edema and increased aspiration risk.

- Breathing—check for bilateral breath sounds, oxygen saturation, supplemental oxygen if needed

  - Goal SpO2 ≥95% for pregnant patients, PaO_2 >70 mm Hg [14]

- Circulation—check for central and distal pulses, establish two large-bore intravenous catheters, start crystalloids or blood as indicated
- Disability—assess Glasgow Coma Scale (GCS)
- Exposure—fully expose patient to assess for other injuries and apply warm blankets
- Special considerations

  - If chest tube required, consider placing it one to two rib spaces above typical location given diaphragmatic compression by gravid uterus.
  - In second or third trimester, if able, tilt the patient 15 to 30 degrees toward left to offload uterus from inferior vena cava (IVC), if unable to tilt, can manually displace uterus to left (Fig. 49.1).

Adjuncts to Primary Survey

- X-ray examinations [1, 17]

  - Shield uterus when possible if not obscuring the area being imaged (e.g., during chest X-ray).

- Focused Assessment with Sonography in Trauma (FAST) ultrasound

  - Any free fluid should be considered pathologic.

Secondary Survey

- Head-to-toe examination
- Pregnant patients may not have classical signs of peritonitis such as guarding and rebound tenderness due to rectus diastasis and displacement of organs by gravid uterus [14]
- Palpation of uterus [14]

  - Size
  - Tenderness
  - Frequent and/or hypertonic contractions are concerning for placental abruption
  - Palpable fetal parts are concerning for uterine rupture

- Focused history [14]

  - Medical and surgical history
  - Obstetric history

    - Prior pregnancies—mode of delivery, complications
    - Current pregnancy—fetal or placental anomalies, complications

  - Mechanism of injury, severity
  - Symptoms after trauma—vaginal fluid loss or bleeding, contractions, fetal movement

Fetal Assessment [9, 10, 14, 17]

- Should be done after life-threatening injuries to pregnant patient are ruled out and the patient has been stabilized

  - Non-reassuring fetal monitoring (e.g., increase in uterine contractions or fetal heart rate decelerations) can be a red flag for serious parental injuries such as hemorrhage, and may be noted before abnormalities are detected in the pregnant patient's vital signs [15].

- Fetal heart rate

  - Normal 110 to 160 bpm
  - Can obtain using M-mode on ultrasound

- Fetal ultrasound (US)

  - Fetal cardiac activity
  - Fetal viability (can use estimated gestational age and cardiac activity)
  - Estimate gestational age [6, 9, 15]

    - Prenatal records, patient report

- Fundal height (20 weeks at umbilicus, 34 to 36 weeks at costal margin) is the most commonly used means of estimation in emergent situations
- Head circumference, biparietal diameter, abdominal circumference, and femur length can also be assessed by the obstetrical team or trained sonographer

    - Measurements consistent with fetal viability include head circumference ≥200 mm, biparietal diameter ≥55 mm, abdominal circumference ≥180 mm, femur length ≥4 cm [9].

  – Fetal number
  – Placental location (limited evaluation for abruption)
- For viable fetuses, once feasible initiate external fetal monitoring (EFM) and tocodynamometry (TOCO) monitoring

  – Monitor for a minimum of 4 h
  – Extend monitoring to 24 h if any of following are present:

    - ≥6 contractions per hour at any point
    - Nonreactive fetal heart tracing (FHT)
    - Vaginal bleeding ± significant abdominal pain
    - Severe injury or mechanism of injury

Laboratory Tests [6, 14]

- Obtain all routine trauma labs, including complete blood count (CBC), basic metabolic panel, type and screen, coagulation profile including fibrinogen, etc.
- Kleihauer-Betke (KB) test—If abdominal trauma is in an Rh-D negative pregnant patient, obtain to assess degree of fetal–maternal hemorrhage and determine dose of Rho (D) immune globulin.

Imaging

- Computed Tomography (CT) scan—radiation risk to fetus depends on gestational age and dose of radiation [11, 14, 15]

  – Radiation dose to fetus for different imaging modalities (range influenced by gestational age, body habitus of the pregnant patient, parameters of scan):

    - Chest X-ray (2 views): 0.0005 to 0.01 mGy
    - Abdominal X-ray: 0.1 to 3.0 mGy
    - CT head or neck: 1.0 to 10 mGy
    - CT chest: 0.01 to 0.66 mGy

- Abdominal CT: 1.3 to 35 mGy
- Pelvic CT: 10 to 50 mGy

– Doses <50 mGy (<5 rad)—no evidence of increased risk of teratogenicity, growth retardation, or spontaneous abortion
– Doses 50 to 100 mGy (5 to 10 rad)—no known or clinically apparent deleterious effects
– Doses >100 mGy (>10 rad)

  - 3 to 4 weeks gestation—possible spontaneous abortion
  - 5 to 10 weeks gestation—possible malformations, increased likelihood with increased doses
  - 11 to 17 weeks gestation—increased risk of deleterious neurologic or intellectual deficits with increasing doses
  - ≥18 weeks gestation—no evidence of deleterious effects with diagnostic doses

- Magnetic Resonance Imaging (MRI)—limited use in acute trauma setting due to time required for scans

Operative Management and Obstetric Complications of Trauma

- Indications for operative intervention in nonpregnant patients are likewise indications for operative intervention in pregnant patients [14, 15].
- Additional indications for operative intervention in the pregnant trauma patient include:

  – *Placental Abruption* [14, 15]

    - Incidence: up to 7% of trauma cases [15]
    - Symptoms and signs: abdominal pain, uterine tenderness, vaginal bleeding, frequent uterine contractions, hemodynamic instability; may be clinically silent in first 24 h
    - Sequelae: hemorrhage, consumptive coagulopathy, preterm labor, fetal demise (if >50% placental separation)
    - Diagnosis: CT scan and TOCO monitoring most sensitive [15]
    - TOCO may show uterine hypertonicity.
    - Management: trial of vaginal delivery if patient is stable and fetal monitoring is normal, otherwise emergent cesarean delivery

  – *Uterine Rupture* [14]

    - Incidence: Rare (<1% trauma in pregnancy)
    - Risk factors: prior cesarean delivery
    - Can range from serosal tears to full-thickness ruptures

- Symptoms and signs: abdominal pain, distention, irregular uterine contour, palpable fetal parts, hemodynamic instability, abnormal fetal monitoring
  - Sequelae: mortality of the pregnant patient (up to 10%), fetal mortality (almost 100%)
  - Management: emergent midline laparotomy, cesarean delivery, uterine repair versus hysterectomy

- *Preterm Labor* [14]

  - Mechanism: due to increased prostaglandin release from trauma, which can stimulate contractions [15]

    - Relevant factors: direct uterine injury, bleeding, hypoxia
    - Can occur in the setting of placental abruption or preterm premature rupture of membranes (PPROM)

  - Symptoms and signs: regular contractions, cervical dilation

- *Fetal Injury* [14]

  - Incidence: uncommon since fetus is protected by uterus, soft tissue, amniotic fluid
  - Blunt trauma with pelvic fracture can result in injury to fetal skull and brain if fetus in vertex position
  - Evaluation: may be seen on imaging done in workup of parental injuries
  - Management: fetal monitoring, neonatology consult

- *Fetal–Maternal Hemorrhage* [6, 15]

  - Definition: entry of fetal blood cells into the pregnant patient's circulation
  - Can result in fetal anemia identified as fetal tachycardia, fetal heart rate decelerations, or sinusoidal tracing on EFM
  - Management: may use KB test to quantify amount of fetal blood that has entered circulation; Rho (D) immune globulin dosing is based on quantity of fetal blood that enters the pregnant patient's circulation and should be given within 72 h of injury.

Obstetrician Involvement

- Page on-call obstetric (OB) team (or activate OB trauma alert) for all trauma patients who are at least 20 to 24 weeks gestation as soon as prenotification or trauma alert is activated.
- Prepare OB ultrasound, precipitous delivery pack, cesarean delivery pack, mobilize neonatal intensive care unit (NICU) team.

Adjunct Therapies

- Rho (D) immune globulin [15]

  - All Rh-D negative pregnant trauma patients should be given Rho (D) immune globulin since the sensitivity of the KB for fetal–maternal hemorrhage is low.
  - If there is concern for significant fetal–maternal hemorrhage, use KB test to guide Rho (D) immune globulin dosing.

- Betamethasone [15]

  - Consider giving betamethasone to accelerate fetal lung maturation for all pregnant trauma patients between 24 and 37 weeks gestation who require hospital admission, since even minor trauma can result in preterm delivery.

Traumatic Cardiac Arrest in Pregnant Patients

- Cardiac arrest in pregnancy requires rapid recognition and intervention because maternal hemodynamic changes can mask early signs of decompensation. Management follows standard ACLS principles with key modifications, including prioritizing high-quality CPR with manual left uterine displacement to relieve aortocaval compression. If return of spontaneous circulation is not achieved promptly, clinicians must prepare for perimortem cesarean delivery, which can improve both maternal and fetal outcomes when performed within minutes

Take-Away Points

- The well-being of the pregnant patient is the number one priority—the best care for the fetus is achieved by providing the best care for the pregnant patient.

  - Fetal distress may alert you to the presence of serious injury to the pregnant patient.

- Important physiologic differences

  - Due to blood volume expansion, pregnant patients may lose more than 30% of blood volume before physiologic signs of shock are present.
  - Physiologic changes in vital signs and laboratory values during pregnancy should be considered during the course of resuscitation.

- Do not fail to order necessary imaging due to concern for fetal radiation exposure—be conscientious with imaging decisions, but obtain any imaging you would otherwise obtain if the patient were not pregnant.

- Indications for operative management and/or interventional radiology are largely the same as for nonpregnant patients.
- Resuscitative hysterotomy, or perimortem cesarean section, may be indicated if the pregnant patient has a cardiac arrest with failure to obtain ROSC within 4 to 5 min, but should occur in tandem, and not interfere, with other resuscitative efforts.

Conflicts of Interest   None

References

1. Advanced Trauma Life Support. Student course manual. 10th ed. Chicago: American College of Surgeons; 2018.
2. Bennett T-A, Katz VL, Zelop CM. Cardiac arrest and resuscitation unique to pregnancy. Obstet Gynecol Clin. 2016;43:809–19. https://doi.org/10.1016/j.ogc.2016.07.011.
3. Cunningham F. Normal reference ranges for laboratory values in pregnancy [WWW Document]. n.d.. https://www.uptodate.com/contents/normal-reference-ranges-for-laboratory-values-in-pregnancy. Accessed 6.3.23.
4. De Vito M, Capannolo G, Alameddine S, Fiorito R, Lena A, Patrizi L, D'Antonio F, Rizzo G. Trauma in pregnancy clinical practice guidelines: systematic review. J Maternal-Fetal Neonatal Med. 2022;35:9948–55. https://doi.org/10.1080/14767058.2022.2078190.
5. Deshpande NA, Kucirka LM, Smith RN, Oxford CM. Pregnant trauma victims experience nearly 2-fold higher mortality compared to their nonpregnant counterparts. Am J Obstetr Gynecol. 2017;217:590.e1–9. https://doi.org/10.1016/j.ajog.2017.08.004.
6. Fung Kee Fung K, Eason E, Crane J, Armson A, De La Ronde S, Farine D, Keenan-Lindsay L, Leduc L, Reid GJ, Aerde JV, Wilson RD, Davies G, Désilets VA, Summers A, Wyatt P, Young DC. Prevention of Rh alloimmunization. J Obstet Gynaecol Can. 2003;25:765–73. https://doi.org/10.1016/s1701-2163(16)31006-4.
7. Gersh B. Maternal adaptations to pregnancy: cardiovascular and hemodynamic changes [WWW Document]. n.d.. https://www.uptodate.com/contents/maternal-adaptations-to-pregnancy-cardiovascular-and-hemodynamic-changes#. Accessed 6.3.23.
8. Green LJ, Kennedy SH, Mackillop L, Gerry S, Purwar M, Staines Urias E, Cheikh Ismail L, Barros F, Victora C, Carvalho M, Ohuma E, Jaffer Y, Noble JA, Gravett M, Pang R, Lambert A, Bertino E, Papageorghiou AT, Garza C, Bhutta Z, Villar J, Watkinson P. International gestational age-specific centiles for blood pressure in pregnancy from the INTERGROWTH-21st Project in 8 countries: a longitudinal cohort study. PLoS Med. 2021;18:e1003611. https://doi.org/10.1371/journal.pmed.1003611.
9. Hirschfeld N, Bormann E, Koester HA, Klockenbusch W, Steinhard J, Schmitz R, Kubiak K. Update reference charts: fetal biometry between the 15th and 42nd week of gestation. Z Geburtshilfe Neonatol. 2022;226:367–76. https://doi.org/10.1055/a-1933-6723.
10. Huls CK, Detlefs C. Trauma in pregnancy. Semin Perinatol. 2018;42:13–20. https://doi.org/10.1053/j.semperi.2017.11.004.
11. Kruskal J. Diagnostic imaging in pregnant and nursing patients [WWW Document]. n.d.. https://www.uptodate.com/contents/diagnostic-imaging-in-pregnant-and-nursing-patients?search=diagnostic%20imaging%20pregnant&source=search_result&selectedTitle=1~150&usage_type=default&display_rank=1. Accessed 6.3.23.
12. La Rosa M, Loaiza S, Zambrano MA, Escobar MF. Trauma in pregnancy. Clin Obstet Gynecol. 2020;63:447–54. https://doi.org/10.1097/GRF.0000000000000531.

13. Mendez-Figueroa H, Dahlke JD, Vrees RA, Rouse DJ. Trauma in pregnancy: an updated systematic review. Am J Obstetr Gynecol. 2013;209:1–10. https://doi.org/10.1016/j.ajog.2013.01.021.
14. Narvaez J, Vrees R. Trauma in pregnancy: a clinical update for obstetrician-gynecologists. Top Obstet Gynecol. 2021;41:1–7. https://doi.org/10.1097/01.PGO.0000753172.54103.b3.
15. Pearce C, Martin SR. Trauma and considerations unique to pregnancy. Obstetr Gynecol Clin N Am. 2016;43:791–808. https://doi.org/10.1016/j.ogc.2016.07.008.
16. Petrone P, Jiménez-Morillas P, Axelrad A, Marini CP. Traumatic injuries to the pregnant patient: a critical literature review. Eur J Trauma Emerg Surg. 2019;45:383–92. https://doi.org/10.1007/s00068-017-0839-x.
17. Rizzo A, Martin M, Inaba K, Schreiber M, Brasel K, Sava J, Ciesla D, Sperry J, Kozar R, Brown C, Moore E. Pregnancy in trauma – a Western Trauma Association algorithm. J Trauma Acute Care Surg. 2022;93:e139–42. https://doi.org/10.1097/TA.0000000000003740.
18. Rose CH, Faksh A, Traynor KD, Cabrera D, Arendt KW, Brost BC. Challenging the 4- to 5-minute rule: from perimortem cesarean to resuscitative hysterotomy. Am J Obstetr Gynecol. 2015;213:653–653.e1. https://doi.org/10.1016/j.ajog.2015.07.019.
19. Thornburg KL, Jacobson S-L, Giraud GD, Morton MJ. Hemodynamic changes in pregnancy. Semin Perinatol. 2000;24:11–4. https://doi.org/10.1016/S0146-0005(00)80047-6.
20. Vanden Hoek TL, Morrison LJ, Shuster M, Donnino M, Sinz E, Lavonas EJ, Jeejeebhoy FM, Gabrielli A. Part 12: Cardiac arrest in special situations: 2010 American Heart Association Guidelines for Cardiopulmonary Resuscitation and Emergency Cardiovascular Care. Circulation. 2010;122 https://doi.org/10.1161/CIRCULATIONAHA.110.971069.

Chapter 50
Trauma in Children

Christopher S. Muratore and Priyanka V. Chugh

Initial Evaluation and Resuscitation

- It is important to note the differences in pediatric vital signs by age and dosing by weight when assessing a trauma patient. Tools such as the Broselow Tape can be used as a guide but caution should be taken due to underestimating weight and underdosing that can occur with these tools [5].
- The unique characteristics of pediatric anatomy and physiology combined with the recognition of common mechanisms of injury produce distinct injury patterns. Blunt trauma with associated head and brain injury result in apnea, hypoventilation, and hypoxia more often than hypovolemia with hypotension.
- *Airway*

  - Children mostly commonly develop cardiac arrest from respiratory arrest. Thus treatment protocols for pediatric trauma patients emphasize aggressive management of the airway and breathing.
  - Increased risk of obstruction

    - Noisy breathing or stridor can be a sign of partial airway obstruction.
    - Children have larger tongues relative to the rest of their oral cavity as well larger tonsillar and adenoid tissue, increasing the risk of oropharyngeal obstruction with altered mental status.
    - The occiput of a child is more prominent, which leads to more neck flexion while supine and more risk of obstruction. Chin lift and jaw-thrust

C. S. Muratore (✉) · P. V. Chugh
Department of Surgery, Boston, MA, USA

Chobanian & Avedisian School of Medicine, Boston University, Boston, MA, USA
e-mail: christopher.muratore@bmc.org; priyanka.chugh@bmc.org

© The Author(s), under exclusive license to Springer Nature Switzerland AG 2025
T. S. Brahmbhatt, D. R. Scantling (eds.), *Trauma Surgery Clerkship*, Contemporary Surgical Clerkships, https://doi.org/10.1007/978-3-032-01412-2_50

maneuvers combined with bimanual inline spine immobilization can open the airway and help improve aeration [6].

- If the child is unconscious, an oral airway may be gently inserted into the oropharynx to assist aeration and preoxygenation with bag-mask ventilation if available. If orotracheal intubation is required, approximating the diameter of the endotracheal tube (ETT) with the child's smallest finger (pinky) is a simple technique to gauge the size of ETT needed. If orotracheal intubation is unsuccessful or not possible, needle cricothyrotomy, rather than surgical, may need to be performed in children at 12 years of age. This is due to narrower space between tracheal rings and the considerably smaller cricothyroid membrane in a child [7, 8].

- *Breathing*
  - The pediatric chest wall is very compliant, resulting in greater risk of pulmonary contusion without associated rib fracture.
  - Pneumothorax in a pediatric patient can result in tension physiology more commonly than in adults due to greater mobility of the mediastinum [9, 10].

- *Circulation*
- Access for fluids, blood, and medication is critically important in pediatric trauma and this should ideally be obtained through two, large-bore peripheral intravenous catheters. However, if peripheral intravenous access is not able to be achieved, intraosseous access is a better second step than central venous access, as they can be placed reliably and quickly [9, 11].

  - Initial single bolus of crystalloid fluid (20 cc/kg) may be administered first. Resuscitation with greater than one crystalloid fluid bolus has been hypothesized to worsen coagulopathy and has been associated with increased need for transfusion, and increased ICU, hospital, and mechanical ventilation days [12].
  - For blood product transfusion, 10–20 mL/kg of PRBC and 10–20 mL/kg of FFP and platelets should be given [7].
  - Response to crystalloid and or blood product administration is critical to assess the patient as a responder, transient responder or nonresponder with the possibility of requiring massive transfusion protocol at appropriate facilities.

- *Disability*
  - Mental status can also be assessed using the Glasgow Coma Scale just like in adults, however in infants it is important to make modifications for their developmental age. Tools such as the modified Pediatric Glasgow Coma Scale can be used [13].
  - Parents and caregivers can be useful in assessing mental status in the trauma bay by helping to comfort the child and to give information on their baseline mental status [9].

– *Exposure*

- Exposing the patient completely is an important part of the primary survey and evaluating for all traumatic injuries. However, it is important to note that hypothermia is a greater risk in children and infants, which can lead to additional consequences such as coagulopathy. Adjustments to ambient temperature and use of warm blankets and fluids can help minimize this risk [9] (Table 50.1).

Neurologic Injury

– Traumatic brain injury (TBI) represents a large portion of traumatic injuries in the pediatric patients, accounting for over 600,000 emergency department visits yearly [14, 15].
– These injuries range from mild, with no symptoms, to severe with intracranial hemorrhage, edema, or diffuse axonal injury. Even without clinically apparent neurologic deficits, patients can have ongoing concussion symptoms leading to attention and memory deficits, as well as impaired performance in school [14].
– The majority of pediatric head injuries are due to falls or motor vehicle collisions (MVC) with many characterized as minor and will not require imaging. Abusive head trauma is the most common cause of major head injury in children less than 1 year of age.

Table 50.1 Comparison of Glasgow Coma Scale and Adelaide Paediatric Scale

Adult scale		Paediatric scale	
Eyes open			
Spontaneously	4		
To speech	3	As in adult scale	
To pain	2		
None	1		
Best verbal response			
Orientated	5	Orientated	5
Confused	4	Words	4
Inappropriate words	3	Vocal sounds	3
Incomprehensible sounds	2	Cries	2
None	1	None	1
Best motor response			
Obeys commands	5		
Localises pain	4		
Flexion to pain	3	As in adult scale	
Extension to pain	2		
None	1		

- To balance the risk of radiation from head CT and the need to evaluate for intra-cranial processes that might require intervention, prediction rules have been developed to aid in assessment and decision making. The following tool has been developed by the Pediatric Emergency Care Applied Research Network (PECARN) [16]
- The rate of cervical spine injuries in pediatric patients is lower than in adults (1–2% vs. 2–4%). However, due to a disproportionately larger size of the head and weaker cervical muscles, cervical injury in children tends to be at higher spinal levels (C1–C3) and more severe with 60% resulting in permanent disability and 40–50% resulting in death [9, 17].
- Evaluation and stabilization of the cervical spine is additionally more difficult in children due to developmentally appropriate behaviors and communication ability (i.e., inability to communicate tenderness on exam, discomfort with a cervical collar) [17, 18].

  • Guidelines have also been developed for imaging decision making and cervical spine clearance. The following is a tool developed from the Pediatric Cervical Spine Clearance Working Group (PCSCWG) [18].
- Spinal Cord Injury Without Radiographic Abnormality (SCIWORA) is an entity described as clinical findings of spinal cord injury but with normal X-ray and CT imaging, and is seen more commonly in children than adults. This occurs due to deformation of the spine that does not result in bony injury, which is more likely to occur in pediatric trauma due to the greater mobility of their immature spinal column. Many of these patients will have findings of trauma on MRI that were not evident on other forms of imaging [17] (Fig. 50.1).

Imaging for Intra-abdominal or Intrathoracic Injury

There is no evidence to support full-body CT imaging to assess for intrathoracic or intrabdominal injuries in pediatric patients. Quality physical exam with laboratory studies is often revealing, requiring only judicious use of adjunct imaging [9, 19].Most intrathoracic injuries can be captured with routine chest X-ray. Only in complex cases would the addition of cross-sectional imaging change management [10].The Pediatric Surgery Research Collaborative (PedSRC) developed a prediction tool to identify patients for which CT scan can be avoided after blunt abdominal trauma.This tool uses serum aspartate aminotransferase (AST), abnormal abdominal examination, abnormal chest X-ray, report of abdominal pain, and abnormal pancreatic enzymes [19].The Pediatric Emergency Care Applied Research Network (PECARN) tool identifies children with blunt trauma who are at low-risk of intra-abdominal injury requiring intervention, such as laparotomy, angiographic embolization, transfusion, or intravenous fluid for >2 days.This tool utilizes only the physical exam and history findings of "no evidence of abdominal wall trauma or

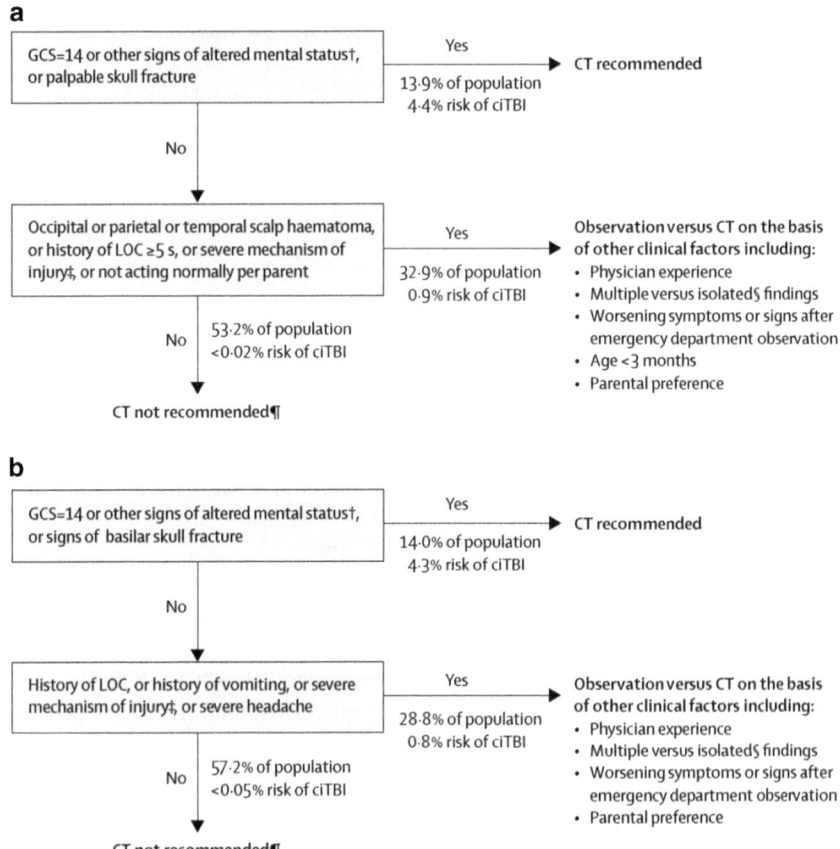

Fig. 50.1 Suggested CT algorithm for children younger than 2 years (**a**) and for those aged 2 years and older (**b**) with GCS scores of 14–15 after head trauma*. GCS = Glasgow Coma Scale. ciTBI = clinically-important traumatic brain injury. LOC = loss of consciousness. *Data are from the combined derivation and validation populations. †Other signs of altered mental status: agitation, somnolence, repetitive questioning, or slow response to verbal communication. ‡Severe mechanism of injury: motor vehicle crash with patient ejection, death of another passenger, or rollover; pedestrian or bicyclist without helmet struck by a motorised vehicle; falls of more than 0.9 m (3 ft) (or more than 1.5 m [5 ft] for panel (**b**); or head struck by a high-impact object. §Patients with certain isolated findings (ie, with no other findings suggestive of traumatic brain injury), such as isolated LOC, isolated headache, isolated vomiting, and certain types of isolated scalp haematomas in infants older than 3 months, have a risk of ciTBI substantially lower than 1%. Risk of ciTBI exceedingly low, generally lower than risk of CT-induced malignancies. Therefore, CT scans are not indicated for most patients in this group. Pediatric GCS (**a**) [13]. (**b**) This is a Springer publication – permission attached. PECARN head trauma. (**a**) [16]. (**b**) Elsevier- permission attached. Ped C spine Working Group. (**a**) [18]. (**b**) Wolters Kluwer Health – permission attached

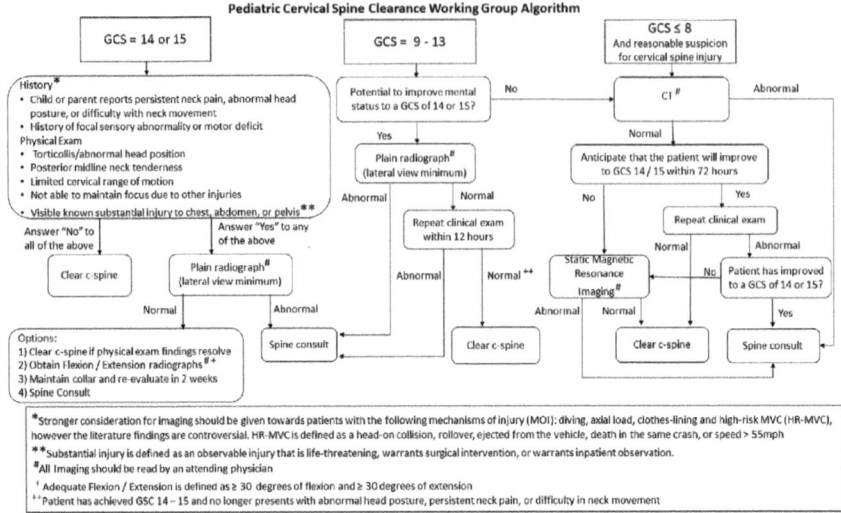

Fig. 50.2 The PCSCWG algorithm. C-spine = cervical spine

seat belt sign, Glasgow Coma Scale score greater than 13, no abdominal tenderness, no evidence of thoracic wall trauma, no complaints of abdominal pain, no decreased breath sounds, and no vomiting." [20]There is ongoing debate regarding the use of ultrasound or Focused Assessment with Sonography in Trauma (FAST) in pediatric patients. Studies have shown that for pediatric patients there is a sensitivity of around 70% with a specificity of 80–95% for free abdominal fluid. Positive findings on ultrasound may be convincing for presence of free fluid and aid in operative decision making; however, a negative ultrasound does not necessarily rule out the presence of intra-abdominal injury [21–24].

- There is evidence that childhood exposure to ionizing radiation is associated with higher rates of malignancy. Increased radiation associated risk has been seen in solid abdominal tumors, brain tumors, and leukemia. Epidemiologic data has shown that for every 10,000 head CT scans that happen before the age of 10, there will be one excess case of leukemia and one excess case of brain cancer in 10 years [25]. Additional evidence shows that the risk increases is cumulative, so for those children that do require CT imaging, the Image Gently campaign was developed to create guidelines to reduce the amount of radiation children are exposed to [26] (Fig. 50.2).

Thoracic Injury

– The most common intrathoracic injuries in pediatric trauma are pulmonary contusions and pneumothorax. This is due in part to the elastic nature of pediatric bones, resulting in depression and rebound of the chest wall, transferring energy to the intrathoracic cavity, rather than the fracturing of ribs like in adults [10].

Solid Organ and Gastrointestinal Injury

– In children, blunt abdominal trauma is more common than penetrating. When a child sustains a blunt trauma, they have a higher likelihood of solid organ or gastrointestinal injury due to less protective intra-abdominal fat and overall smaller torso size [27].
– Certain physical exam findings or mechanisms of injury raise concern for intra-abdominal injury in a child.

   • "Seat belt sign," or abrasions, ecchymosis, or erythema in the pattern of a seatbelt, after MVC should raise concern for gastrointestinal injury, with rates reported up to 25% [28]. While less common, solid organ or vascular injuries such as to the aorta can also occur. Chance fractures, or flexion-distraction injuries of the spine, can also occur due to the immobility of the spine when a child is restrained in a seatbelt. A finding of a Chance fracture should prompt investigation for intra-abdominal injury, particularly intestinal or pancreatic [27, 28].

      – Sports-related injuries with direct trauma to the abdomen and bike injuries with impact of the handlebar are more common in children and can result in intra-abdominal injuries.
      – In penetrating trauma of the torso, it is essential to do a thorough physical exam to evaluate for all wounds. Although penetrating trauma accounts for a small percentage of pediatric injuries, it results in significant morbidity and mortality. Gunshot and stab wounds are the most common causes in children aged 11–19 years, whereas impalement injuries predominate in younger children [27]. Firearm violence has consistently been increasing in the pediatric population and, as of 2019, it is the leading cause of mortality for ages 0–19 in the United States [29].

– Management of abdominal trauma is driven by patient's physical exam, hemodynamic stability, and the organ system involved.

   • The most commonly injured organs in pediatric blunt abdominal trauma are the liver and spleen [27]. The evidence-based management of blunt solid organ trauma in pediatrics has successfully evolved to be largely nonoperative with use of angioembolization as needed and operative intervention only in cases of persistent instability. The American Pediatric Surgical Association (APSA) has developed guidelines for the management of these injuries. [30]

Updated APSA Blunt Liver/Spleen Injury Guidelines 2019

Admission

- **ICU Admission Indicators**
  - Abnormal vital signs after initial volume resuscitation
- **ICU**
  - Activity - Bedrest until vitals normal
  - Labs – q6hour CBC until vitals normal
  - Diet – NPO until vital signs normal and hemoglobin stable
- **Ward**
  - Activity - No restrictions
  - Labs - CBC on admission and/or 6 hours after injury
  - Diet – Regular diet

Procedures

- **Transfusion**
  - Unstable vitals after 20 cc/kg bolus of isotonic IVF
  - Hemoglobin < 7
  - Signs of ongoing or recent bleeding

- **Angioembolization**
  - Signs of ongoing bleeding despite pRBC transfusion
  - Not indicated for contrast blush on admission CT without unstable vitals

- **Operative exploration with Control of Bleeding**
  - Unstable vitals despite pRBC transfusion
  - Consider massive transfusion protocol

Set Free

- Based on clinical condition **NOT** injury severity (grade)
- Tolerating a diet
- Minimal abdominal pain
- Normal vital signs

Aftercare

- **Activity Restriction**
  - Restricting activity to grade plus 2 weeks is safe
  - Shorter restrictions may be safe but there is inadequate data to support decreasing these recommendations
- **Follow up Imaging**
  - Risk of delayed complications following spleen and liver injuries is low
  - Consider imaging for *symptomatic* patients with prior high grade injuries

- Bowel injury can occur in penetrating or blunt trauma. In blunt trauma, it is often due to shearing forces at points of fixation in the abdomen such as at the cecum or Ligament of Treitz [27]. Obvious injuries identified on imaging warrant surgical intervention; however, occult bowel injury can be more subtle and findings may not be identifiable on presentation. A high index of suspicion for bowel injury is required for the evolution of possible delayed intestinal compromise. Injuries such as mesenteric bucket-handle tears, where the mesentery is avulsed from the bowel, can result in devascularization and eventual ischemia or necrosis of a portion of bowel and may not present immediately [31].

Child Maltreatment and Non-Accidental Trauma (NAT)

– The Center for Disease Control (CDC) defines child maltreatment as "all types of abuse and neglect of a child under the age of 18 by a parent, caregiver, or another person in a custodial role (such as a religious leader, a coach, a teacher) that results in harm, the potential for harm, or threat of harm to a child." This is inclusive of physical, sexual, emotional abuse and neglect [32]. At least one in seven children experience abuse and in 2020, about 1750 children died from abuse or neglect [33].
– Certain physical exam findings that are not easily explainable by history or age-appropriate behavior can be signs of NAT and require further investigation [34, 35]. These include:

- • Bruising in nonambulatory children, especially in TEN-4 regions (Torso, Ear, or Neck in children less than 4)
- • Any injury to genitalia
- • Appear defensive, for example, on the outside of an arm as if occurred when holding up an arm in defense
- • Bruising, abrasions, or burns in the pattern of identifiable objects (hangers, cords, cigarette)
- • Burns with an immersion pattern on feet, hands, or buttocks only
- • Circumferential marks on extremity or neck can be associated with petechiae (face or extremity)
- • Oral injuries, in particular tearing of the labial frenulum
- • Increasing head circumference can be a sign of skull fracture with edema or intracranial hemorrhage in a child with bulging fontanelles
- • Retinal hemorrhages

- – Radiographic findings can also be telling, especially if they are inconsistent with reported history of injury [34, 35]. These include:

- • Fractures in nonambulatory children
- • Rib fractures in infants and children, especially posterior fractures
- • Fractures of different ages
- • Femoral, scapular, vertebral, sternal, and long bone corner metaphyseal fractures (also known as classical metaphyseal lesions or CML) without a consistent story, due to the force or torque required to sustain such fractures

- – When NAT is suspected, it is important to rule out other causes of the injury pattern, as well as investigate further for other associated injuries.

- • Serologic tests can be performed to look for signs of coagulopathy or intra-abdominal processes such as liver or pancreas injuries. Urinalysis can evaluate for hematuria or myoglobinuria to look for signs of renal or bladder trauma or rhabdomyolysis from severe muscular injury [35].
- • A skeletal survey with full body radiographs is recommended to be performed on any patient under 2 years of age in which NAT is suspected [35, 36].

- – Evaluating for NAT is a multidisciplinary effort between pediatricians, pediatric surgeons, radiologists, and social workers. States have individual requirements for reporting NAT to governmental agencies such as Child Protective Services [35].

Prevention and Advocacy

- – Trauma is not only a major cause of morbidity and mortality in children, it also has lifelong impacts due to the known physical and mental health impacts of Adverse Childhood Experiences (ACEs).

- ACEs have been associated with chronic disease such as cancer, heart disease, and diabetes, as well as mental health problems and substance use disorders [37].
– The best treatment for traumatic injuries and ACEs is prevention.

  - Previously, motor vehicle collisions had the highest rate of morbidity and mortality in the pediatric population. Public health interventions had success in reducing injury and death from motor vehicle collisions by emphasizing design changes in cars, changing legislation, and individual level improvements in seat belt and car seat usage [38].
  - The rate of firearm-related death in pediatric patients in the United States surpassed motor vehicle collisions in 2019. This is a uniquely significant problem in the United States with >90% of worldwide firearm-related deaths in ages 0–14 occurring in the United States [29].
  - The American Pediatric Surgical Association (APSA) makes several recommendations to improve firearm-related injury and death in the United States. These include enforcing background checks for firearm transactions, removal of barriers to receiving federal funding for firearm research, increasing awareness and resources for safe storage of firearms, and restrictions on civilian access to high-capacity, assault style weapons. As public health interventions had a meaningful reduction in rates of motor vehicle death, it is hypothesized that these interventions may have a similar effect on firearm deaths [38].
  - Primary care providers often utilize screening tools such as the Safe Environment for Every Kid (SEEK) Parent Screening Questionnaire or the WE CARE screening tool to assess risk factors in patient's homes. These assess domestic violence exposure, fire alarms in home, parental stress, housing situations, etc. Using these tools provides an opportunity for provider counseling and connection to resources [39].

– For prevention interventions to truly be impactful, they must take into account the environment in which these injuries are occurring. These social determinants of health contribute to disparities that are seen in rates, type, and intent of trauma [40].

  - Socioeconomic status (SES), race, and ethnicity are associated with these disparities. Pediatric patients from lower socioeconomic neighborhoods have higher rates of trauma overall, including firearm injuries, motor vehicle injuries, and non-accidental trauma. These trends also exist in Black and Hispanic children, though race and SES are linked due to a history of structural racism in the United States [40, 41].
  - Pediatric surgeons have an imperative to understand social determinants of health as they relate to trauma and their patients, to incorporate a lens of social responsibility into their practice, and to advocate for policy or interventions that can make an impact on their patients' lives on a larger scale [41].

References

1. United States Department of Health and Human Services CfDCaP, National Center for Health Statistics. Multiple cause of death by single race 2018–2020. 2020. http://wonder.cdc.gov/ucd-icd10.html
2. Chao SSJ, Ruscher K, Armstrong L, Jeziorczak P, Vogel A, Forrester JA, Forrester JD, Taylor J, Vanover M, Wood L. Injury Prevention. Pediatric surgery NaT. American Pediatric Surgical Association. 2022. https://www.pedsurglibrary.com/apsa/view/Pediatric-Surgery-NaT/829738/all/Injury_Prevention
3. Lee LK, Douglas K, Hemenway D. Crossing lines – a change in the leading cause of death among U.S. children. N Engl J Med. 2022;386(16):1485–7. https://doi.org/10.1056/NEJMp2200169.
4. Myers SR, Branas CC, French B, Nance ML, Carr BG. A national analysis of pediatric trauma care utilization and outcomes in the United States. Pediatr Emerg Care. 2019;35(1):1–7. https://doi.org/10.1097/PEC.0000000000000902.
5. Knight JC, Nazim M, Riggs D, et al. Is the Broselow tape a reliable indicator for use in all pediatric trauma patients?: A look at a rural trauma center. Pediatr Emerg Care. 2011;27(6):479–82. https://doi.org/10.1097/PEC.0b013e31821d8559.
6. Adewale L. Anatomy and assessment of the pediatric airway. Pediat Anesth. 2009;19:1–8. https://doi.org/10.1111/j.1460-9592.2009.03012.x.
7. Kenefake ME, Swarm M, Walthall J. Nuances in pediatric trauma. Emerg Med Clin N Am. 2013;31(3):627–52.
8. Luten RC, Godwin SA. Pediatric airway techniques. Manual Emerg Airway Manag. 2012:293.
9. Vogel AE, Mauricio A, Edwards MJ. Trauma resuscitation and initial evaluation. Pediatric Surgery NaT. American Pediatric Surgical Association. 2022. https://www.pedsurglibrary.com/apsa/view/Pediatric-Surgery-NaT/829085/all/Trauma_Resuscitation_and_Initial_Evaluation
10. Minervini F, Scarci M, Kocher GJ, Kestenholz PB, Bertoglio P. Pediatric chest trauma: a unique challenge. J Visc Surg. 2020;6(8)
11. Dornhofer P, Kellar JZ. Intraosseous vascular access. In: StatPearls [Internet]. StatPearls Publishing; 2021.
12. Polites SF, Moody S, Williams RF, et al. Timing and volume of crystalloid and blood products in pediatric trauma: an Eastern Association for the Surgery of Trauma multicenter prospective observational study. J Trauma Acute Care Surg. 2020;89(1):36–42.
13. Reilly P, Simpson D, Sprod R, Thomas L. Assessing the conscious level in infants and young children: a paediatric version of the Glasgow Coma Scale. Child's Nerv Syst. 1988;4(1):30–3.
14. Gelineau-Morel RN, Zinkus TP, Le Pichon J-B. Pediatric head trauma: a review and update. Pediatr Rev. 2019;40(9):468–81. https://doi.org/10.1542/pir.2018-0257.
15. Juang DG, Katherine W, Ostlie D. Traumatic brain injury. Pediatric Surgery NaT. American Pediatric Surgical Association, 2022. https://www.pedsurglibrary.com/apsa/view/Pediatric-Surgery-NaT/829118/all/Traumatic_Brain_Injury
16. Kuppermann N, Holmes JF, Dayan PS, et al. Identification of children at very low risk of clinically-important brain injuries after head trauma: a prospective cohort study. Lancet. 2009;374(9696):1160–70.
17. McAllister AS, Nagaraj U, Radhakrishnan R. Emergent imaging of pediatric cervical spine trauma. Radiographics. 2019;39(4):1126–42.
18. Herman MJ, Brown KO, Sponseller PD, et al. Pediatric cervical spine clearance: a consensus statement and algorithm from the Pediatric Cervical Spine Clearance Working Group. JBJS. 2019;101(1):e1. https://doi.org/10.2106/jbjs.18.00217.
19. Streck CJ, Vogel AM, Zhang J, et al. Identifying children at very low risk for blunt intra-abdominal injury in whom CT of the abdomen can be avoided safely. J Am Coll Surg. 2017;224(4):449–58. e3
20. Springer E, Frazier SB, Arnold DH, Vukovic AA. External validation of a clinical prediction rule for very low risk pediatric blunt abdominal trauma. Am J Emerg Med. 2019;37(9):1643–8.

21. Wieck MC, Chokshi NK, Mak GZ. The use of FAST in the pediatric trauma setting. In: Difficult decisions in trauma surgery. Springer; 2022. p. 423–30.

22. Netherton S, Milenkovic V, Taylor M, Davis PJ. Diagnostic accuracy of eFAST in the trauma patient: a systematic review and meta-analysis. Can J Emerg Med. 2019;21(6):727–38.

23. Long MK, Vohra MK, Bonnette A, et al. Focused assessment with sonography for trauma in predicting early surgical intervention in hemodynamically unstable children with blunt abdominal trauma. J Am Coll Emerg Phys Open. 2022;3(1):e12650. https://doi.org/10.1002/emp2.12650.

24. Calder BW, Vogel AM, Zhang J, et al. Focused assessment with sonography for trauma in children after blunt abdominal trauma: a multi-institutional analysis. J Trauma Acute Care Surg. 2017;83(2):218–24. https://doi.org/10.1097/ta.0000000000001546.

25. Kutanzi KR, Lumen A, Koturbash I, Miousse IR. Pediatric exposures to ionizing radiation: carcinogenic considerations. Int J Environ Res Public Health. 2016;13(11):1057.

26. Gelfand MJ, Parisi MT, Treves ST. Pediatric radiopharmaceutical administered doses: 2010 North American consensus guidelines. J Nucl Med. 2011;52(2):318–22.

27. Drexel S, Azarow K, Jafri MA. Abdominal trauma evaluation for the pediatric surgeon. Surg Clin. 2017;97(1):59–74.

28. Borgialli DA, Ellison AM, Ehrlich P, et al. Association between the seat belt sign and intra-abdominal injuries in children with Blunt Torso trauma in motor vehicle collisions. Acad Emerg Med. 2014;21(11):1240–8. https://doi.org/10.1111/acem.12506.

29. Andrews AL, Killings X, Oddo ER, Gastineau KA, Hink AB. Pediatric firearm injury mortality epidemiology. Pediatrics. 2022;149:3.

30. Gates RL, Price M, Cameron DB, et al. Non-operative management of solid organ injuries in children: an American Pediatric Surgical Association Outcomes and Evidence Based Practice Committee systematic review. J Pediatr Surg. 2019;54(8):1519–26.

31. Chowdhury A, Burford C, Pangeni A, Shrestha A. Bucket-Handle mesenteric tears: a comprehensive review of their presentation and management. Cureus. 2022;14(9)

32. Leeb RT. Child maltreatment surveillance: Uniform definitions for public health and recommended data elements. Centers for Disease Control and Prevention, National Center for Injury … 2008.

33. U.S. Department of Health & Human Services AfCaF, Administration on Children, Youth and Families, Children's Bureau. Child Maltreatment 2020. U.S. Department of Health & Human Services AfCaF, Administration on Children, Youth and Families, Children's Bureau. 2022. https://www.acf.hhs.gov/cb/data-research/child-maltreatment.

34. Hanson C. Non-accidental trauma. In: Pediatric surgery. Springer; 2022. p. 113–9.

35. Escobar MA, Zeller KA, Sieren LM, Hamilton NA, Miller-Fitzwater AL, Santore M. Child abuse and maltreatment. In: Pediatric surgery NaT. American Pediatric Surgical Association; 2022. https://www.pedsurglibrary.com/apsa/view/Pediatric-Surgery-NaT/829478/all/Child_Abuse_and_Maltreatment.

36. Wood JN, Fakeye O, Mondestin V, Rubin DM, Localio R, Feudtner C. Development of hospital-based guidelines for skeletal survey in young children with bruises. Pediatrics. 2015;135(2):e312–20.

37. Jones CM, Merrick MT, Houry DE. Identifying and preventing adverse childhood experiences: implications for clinical practice. JAMA. 2020;323(1):25–6.

38. Petty JK, Henry MC, Nance ML, Ford HR. Firearm injuries and children: position statement of the American pediatric surgical association. Pediatrics. 2019;144(1)

39. Flynn AB, Fothergill KE, Wilcox HC, et al. Primary care interventions to prevent or treat traumatic stress in childhood: a systematic review. Acad Pediatr. 2015;15(5):480–92.

40. Kotagal M. Social determinants of health as drivers of inequities in pediatric injury. Elsevier. 2022:151221.

41. Janeway M, Wilson S, Sanchez SE, Arora TK, Dechert T. Citizenship and social responsibility in surgery: a review. JAMA Surg. 2022;157(6):532–9. https://doi.org/10.1001/jamasurg.2022.0621.

Chapter 51
Trauma in the Geriatric Population

Shane Mathew and Amanda L. Teichman

Overview

- Geriatric trauma is on the rise in the United States
- The physiology of geriatric patients is significantly different than their younger counterparts
- Injury presentation may be variable and severity worse in this population
- Evaluation of geriatric trauma patients should be comprehensive and standardized to avoid missing possible serious injuries
- Falls are the leading mechanism of injury in this age group followed by motor vehicle collisions
- Early and ongoing goals of care discussions are important in this population

Background [1–5]

The definition of "geriatric" varies across the literature from as young as 55 up to 70, but most commonly is defined as 65 years or older. They are the fastest growing age group in America since 2010, leading to an increase in geriatric trauma admissions across trauma centers and non-trauma centers alike. Data show that patients who make it to a trauma center but do *not* meet trauma activation criteria tend to have worse outcomes, as occult injuries may be missed, or their initial injury is made worse by associated comorbidities. The most recent National Trauma Data

S. Mathew · A. L. Teichman (✉)
Division of Acute Care Surgery, Department of Surgery, Rutgers Robert Wood Johnson Medical School, New Brunswick, NJ, USA
e-mail: sm2552@rwjms.rutgers.edu; ateich13@rwjms.rutgers.edu

© The Author(s), under exclusive license to Springer Nature Switzerland AG 2025
T. S. Brahmbhatt, D. R. Scantling (eds.), *Trauma Surgery Clerkship*, Contemporary Surgical Clerkships, https://doi.org/10.1007/978-3-032-01412-2_51

Bank Report from 2016 demonstrated that falls were the leading cause of mortality and injury to those over the age of 65, making up 44% of cases overall [4]. After injury, 26% of geriatric trauma patients die directly from their injuries, and 60% due to comorbidities or complications, which is higher compared to their younger counterparts [3]. Special care must be taken when evaluating geriatric patients, given the high incidence of confounding comorbid conditions and because "normal" vital signs or laboratory values may be unreliable.

- Physiology of the Geriatric Patient [3, 5, 7, 8]:

  - *Unique Physiologic Characteristics of Geriatric Patients*

    - Comorbid medical conditions
    - Polypharmacy
    - Frailty
    - Reduced vision and hearing
    - Impaired motor and/or cognitive function
    - Decreased muscle mass and/or strength
    - Decreased bone density
    - Decreased joint flexibility

  - *Frailty*

    - Frailty has been studied as a predictor of how well geriatric patients will do, as it is associated with injury after falls.
    - There is no general consensus on how to quantify frailty; therefore, functional status and sarcopenia have been used as surrogates.
    - Sarcopenia has been associated with increased ventilator days and lower likelihood of discharge to home.
    - The Trauma-Specific Frailty Index has been validated as an effective tool to evaluate discharge disposition, improve communication with family, and appropriately mobilize resources in geriatric trauma patients [7].

  - *Delirium*

    - Definition: Global disturbance of consciousness characterized by fluctuating mental status, inattention, and disorganized thinking.
    - Associated with increased mortality and cost of care.
    - The most common cause is medications, especially those used for sedation and analgesia.
    - Medications such as benzodiazepines and narcotics should be limited.
    - The Beers Criteria uses evidence-based recommendations in regard to medication management in the elderly.

  - *Central Nervous System Changes*

    - Cortical atrophy.
    - Plaque buildup in cerebrovascular vessels.
    - Decrease in all five senses.

- Decreased cerebellar function leading to gait instability.
- Polypharmacy has also been implicated in agitation, delirium, and poor outcomes.

  – *Cardiovascular System Changes*

  - Important when evaluating vital signs in elderly trauma patients.
  - Geriatric patients with a heart rate greater than 90 or a systolic blood pressure of less than 110 have higher mortality when compared to their younger counterparts as they are unable to mount a compensatory increase in their heart rate in response to catecholamines.

  – *Pulmonary System Changes*

  - Kyphosis impairs ventilation.
  - Decreased skeletal mass and strength.
  - Weaker diaphragmatic inspiratory effort.
  - Gradual reduction in lung elastic recoil.
  - Reduction in alveolar surface area.
  - Reduced response to hypoxia and hypercapnia.
  - These changes can lead to hypoventilation, atelectasis, pneumonia, and decreased response to acidosis hypercarbia, and hypoxia.

  – *Renal System Changes*

  - Glomerulosclerosis.
  - Intimal thickening of the renal arterioles.
  - Diminished ability to maintain hemostasis during hypo- and hypertensive states leads to a higher risk of acute kidney injury and inability to recover function afterward.
  - Convert to renally dosed medications (when appropriate), avoid hypotension and nephrotoxic agents, and maintain euvolemia.

  – *Gastrointestinal System Changes*

  - Poor nutritional status and malnutrition have been associated with postoperative morbidity, perioperative mortality, increased hospital length of stay, and decreased quality of life.
  - These changes can be mitigated through nutritional and speech/swallow assessments.

- Mechanisms of Injury [3, 5, 9, 10]:

  – *Falls*

  - Leading cause of morbidity and mortality, particularly in those using antithrombotics and with increased frailty.
  - The cost of falls was estimated to be about 30 billion dollars in 2012 [3].
  - More than 85% are from ground level [9].

- Annually, 33% of those over the age of 65 fall, one third go on to be readmitted or die within the same year [9].
- Of patients that fall, 6% will sustain a fracture and anywhere from 10–30% will have polytrauma [5].
- Falls increase the risk of traumatic brain injury (TBI) among this population with injury exacerbated by coagulopathy and anticoagulant usage.
- This population has a higher prevalence of atrial fibrillation and other conditions that need anticoagulants or antithrombotics.
- Data has indicated that between 11% and 20% of geriatric trauma patients take warfarin at the time of admission [3].
- Patients aged 65–69 accounted for 13% of TBI-related geriatric admissions and 65% of TBI-related admissions were due to falls in this age group [9].

- *Motor Vehicle Collisions*

  - Second leading cause of trauma in patients >65.
  - The risk of falls is almost ten times more common than motor vehicle collisions (MVC) [5].
  - Regardless of speed, elderly patients are at a higher risk for injury.
  - In areas such as traffic intersections, geriatric patients are more likely to be involved in accidents.
  - Data indicates that geriatric patients make up about 11.7% of MVCs but result in 23.4% of deaths [10].
  - Due to the prevalence of injury, the Eastern Association of Surgical Trauma recommends the incorporation of reminders for seatbelt usage in vehicles, improved designation of pedestrian crosswalks with traffic lights or stop signs, and ongoing evaluation of elderly drivers for risks of MVC (e.g., alcohol abuse, frailty, significant diabetes, hearing impairments, severe visual impairments, and coronary artery disease).

- *Pedestrian Struck by Vehicle*

  - Third most common mechanism of injury.
  - About one in five pedestrians killed and one in ten pedestrians injured are geriatric patients and majority of these occurred in areas without traffic signs [5].

- *Assault*

  - Fourth most common cause of trauma in the elderly is assault.
  - Elder abuse may be suspected in patients with repeated injuries or suspicious mechanisms of injury (especially in those with dementia, who are unable to report their abuse).
  - Mortality is *five times* higher in geriatric victims of violence than in the younger cohort as they are less likely to tolerate injuries [5].

Current Practice

- Trauma Evaluation in Geriatric Patients

  - The cause of the fall must be thoroughly investigated, as the subsequent workup for a cardiac or neurologic cause, such as syncope, would be different than if it was just mechanical.
  - Primary, Secondary Survey, Tertiary Surveys.
  - Laboratory Tests.

    - CBC, BMP, Coagulation factors, Verify Now ASA/Plavix, etc.

  - Imaging.

    - FAST exam, CT Head, Chest, Abdomen, Pelvis, X-rays to evaluate for orthopedic fractures

- Common Injury Patterns and Management [1, 3, 5, 6]:

  - *Traumatic Brain Injury*

    - High suspicion for injury and low threshold for imaging to properly diagnose intracranial hemorrhage after a TBI.
    - Liberal use of CT is recommended as the risk of missing an injury will increase morbidity and mortality because reversal of anticoagulation and neurosurgical intervention may be delayed.
    - Important to repeat imaging in patients with both confirmed injury and those with suspected injury without imaging confirmation to evaluate for delayed injury or worsening intracranial hemorrhage.
    - Consider reversal anticoagulation to prevent the worsening of hemorrhage in those with significant hemorrhage and/or reduced Glasgow Coma Score (GCS).
    - Heparin.

      - Reversal Agent: Protamine sulfate

    - Warfarin.

      - Reversal Agent: Vitamin K (slower onset), fresh frozen plasma (FFP)/ prothrombin complex concentrate (FFP/PCC are both rapid onset)

    - Dabigatran.

      - Reversal Agent: Idarucizumab or PCC

    - Reversal agents are in various stages of development for novel oral anticoagulant agents, but most also respond to PCC.

  - *Pulmonary and Thoracic Injuries*

    - Pulmonary contusions are the most common thoracic trauma, seen in up to 75% of patients [5].

  – Risk is heightened with associated rib fractures

- Fractures of greater than three ribs increase the risk for pneumonia and mortality [5].
- The risk of pneumonia at five rib fractures is greater than 50% [5].
- Concomitant liver and splenic injuries are correlated with increased rib fractures.
- Important to appropriately manage chest wall pain.

  – Impacts pulmonary function by causing chest wall splinting, decreased recruitment of alveoli, and increases development of atelectasis

- Patients should be educated regarding forceful cough and usage of incentive spirometers, which can be surrogate measures of pain control.
- Multimodal pain regimens, aggressive chest physiotherapy, and early consideration of open reduction and internal fixation of rib fractures in select patients can reduce the risk of respiratory failure and the need for ventilator support.

– *Orthopedic Injuries*

- Femoral neck fractures are the most commonly reported fracture.
- Fractures to the hip, spine, proximal humerus, and wrist are higher in the geriatric population.
- The goal is to return patients to their previous level of function, prevent further functional decline, and maintain their quality of life.
- Patients with fractures after low energy mechanisms, such as ground level falls, should be evaluated for osteopenia.
- Early repair can reduce the risk of major complications and mortality.
- Early mobility after surgery can reduce the risk of pneumonia, bed sores, and pressure sores.
- Pelvic injuries and fractures in the elderly tend to be more morbid than their younger counterparts.
- More likely to have lateral compression fractures, which increases the risk of pelvic hemorrhage.
- The mortality at 1 year after a hip fracture in this age group can be up to 21% [5].

– *Cervical Spine Injuries*

- Increased prevalence of cervical stenosis and degenerative spinal disease increases risk as the rigidity of the spine predisposes this population to increased injury to the odontoid and C2 compared to younger patients who are more likely to injure C4–7, which is the most mobile portion of the cervical spine.
- Neurological deficits, head injury, and high energy mechanism can be clues to providers that the patient may also have a cervical spine injury.

- Canadian C-spine and National Emergency X-Radiography Utilization Study (NEXUS) can guide imaging and subsequent c-collar removal.
- Dysphagia is a common complication after cervical spine injuries and with the use of c-collars.

- *Abdominal Injuries*

  - Regardless of age, most injuries have moved toward nonoperative management when the patient is hemodynamically stable.
  - A study from the University of Southern California showed that in the geriatric population, 50% of geriatric patients who died after abdominal injury had what was considered normal vitals [5].

- Goals of Care [2, 3]:

  - Important to engage the patient, family, and/or surrogate early regarding goals of care to prevent unwanted or unnecessary treatment not in line with the patient's wishes.
  - This can be done by inquiring about advanced directives, do not resuscitate (DNR) orders, health care power of attorney, or living wills.
  - Goals of care should be frequently addressed during admission, and the use of family meetings can keep the treatment team and family on the same page while also preventing miscommunication.
  - Withdrawal of life-sustaining care accounts for 42–54% of trauma deaths, while less than 20% had preexisting advanced directives, highlighting the importance of goals of care discussions [3].
  - Palliative care is another important resource that can be included in the multidisciplinary approach to treating geriatric trauma patients.
  - Geriatric palliative care is defined as "an approach that aims to improve the quality of life of elderly persons facing severe and life-threatening illness near the end of their lives."
  - The use of palliative care can improve pain management and can address emotional issues, such as depression.

Take-Home Points for Patient Care

- Thorough and comprehensive evaluation is a critical component of geriatric trauma care
- Early identification of comorbid conditions, which may potentially contribute to negative outcomes (e.g., medical conditions, frailty, blood thinners, etc.).
- Falls are the most common mechanism of injury in the geriatric population and have a high association with repeat injury, hospital admission, and mortality.
- Recognition that injuries present differently in the elderly and often with increased severity than in younger patients.

- Goals of care planning is an important aspect of comprehensive geriatric trauma care.

References

1. Bonne S, Schuerer DJ. Trauma in the older adult: epidemiology and evolving geriatric trauma principles. Clin Geriatr Med. 2013;29(1):137–50.
2. Voumard R, Rubli Truchard E, Benaroyo L, Borasio GD, Büla C, Jox RJ. Geriatric palliative care: a view of its concept, challenges and strategies. BMC Geriatr. 2018;18(1):1–6.
3. Kozar RA, Arbabi S, Stein DM, Shackford SR, Barraco RD, Biffl WL, Brasel KJ, Cooper Z, Fakhry SM, Livingston D, Moore F. Injury in the aged: geriatric trauma care at the crossroads. J Trauma Acute Care Surg. 2015;78(6):1197.
4. Chang M. National Trauma Data Bank 2016 Annual Report [Internet]. [cited 2022Nov29]. Available from: https://www.facs.org/media/ez1hpdcu/ntdb-annual-report-2016.pdf
5. Brooks SE, Peetz AB. Evidence-based care of geriatric trauma patients. Surg Clin. 2017;97(5):1157–74.
6. Intracranial Hemorrhage [Internet]. Intracranial hemorrhage. Loyola University Chicago; [cited 2022Nov29]. Available from: http://www.stritch.luc.edu/lumen/MedEd/Radio/curriculum/Neurology/IC_hemorrhage_2013.htm
7. Joseph B, Pandit V, Zangbar B, Kulvatunyou N, Tang A, O'Keeffe T, Green DJ, Vercruysse G, Fain MJ, Friese RS, Rhee P. Validating trauma-specific frailty index for geriatric trauma patients: a prospective analysis. J Am Coll Surg. 2014;219(1):10–7.
8. Callaway DW, Wolfe R. Geriatric trauma. Emerg Med Clin N Am. 2007;25(3):837–60.
9. Adams SD, Holcomb JB. Geriatric trauma. Curr Opin Crit Care. 2015;21(6):520–6.
10. Crandall M, Streams J, Duncan T, Mallat A, Greene W, Violano P, Christmas AB, Barraco R. Motor vehicle collision–related injuries in the elderly: an Eastern Association for the Surgery of Trauma evidence-based review of risk factors and prevention. J Trauma Acute Care Surg. 2015;79(1):152–8.

Chapter 52
Rehabilitation Concerns in Trauma

Sumeet V. Jain and Brian K. Yorkgitis

Introduction

- Trauma is a major cause of death and disability in the United States and is the leading cause of morbidity and mortality in those aged 15 to 44.
- As more people survive severe traumatic injuries, rehabilitation services are necessary to maximize recovery and improve quality of life
- Rehabilitation evaluation and treatment begins in the acute hospital setting, and can extend beyond this to include rehabilitation facilities, home services, and outpatient therapies

General Rehabilitation Considerations

- Patient evaluation begins with multidisciplinary rehabilitation team including physical therapists, occupational therapists, speech therapists, rehabilitation physicians, nurses, psychologists, case managers, and social workers.
- Rehabilitation begins in the acute inpatient setting and progresses along a continuum to the outpatient setting depending on a patient's individual needs.

S. V. Jain
Department of Surgery, University of Florida College of Medicine Jacksonville, Jacksonville, USA
e-mail: summet.jain@jax.ufl.edu

B. K. Yorkgitis (✉)
Department of Surgery, Indiana School of Medicine, Indianapolis, IN, USA
e-mail: byorkgit@iu.edu

© The Author(s), under exclusive license to Springer Nature Switzerland AG 2025
T. S. Brahmbhatt, D. R. Scantling (eds.), *Trauma Surgery Clerkship*, Contemporary Surgical Clerkships,
https://doi.org/10.1007/978-3-032-01412-2_52

- Evaluation begins with understanding a patient's injuries, medical stability, and functional limitations [1].
- Cognitive limitations can occur in the setting of traumatic brain injury (TBI) or extended critical illness and can include memory impairment, agitation/aggression, amnesia, and attention deficits [1–4].
- Physical limitations occur in the setting of major orthopedic injuries, spinal cord injury (SCI), and polytrauma and can include weight-bearing restrictions in extremity fractures, paralysis, deconditioning, or other restrictions from other organ systems such as pulmonary dysfunction [1–3].

Complex Orthopedic Injuries

- Patients may have a variety of weight-bearing and mobility restrictions depending on their injury pattern [1–3].
- Immobility can lead to complications such as pressure ulcers and venous thromboembolism [1–3].
- Weight-bearing restrictions of multiple extremities can significantly impede independence [1–3].
- Goals of rehabilitation include increasing mobility and independence within the framework of the restrictions present [1–3].

Amputation

- Amputation has major implications in both physical and psychological health [1–3].
- Goals include independence with transfers and activities of daily life (ADLs) [1–3].
- Many patients may qualify for prosthetic use, and education and fitting for prosthetics is key part of their rehabilitation [1–3].
- Phantom limb pain can be a major source of discomfort, and is managed with neuropathic pain modulators as well as nonpharmacologic therapy [1–3, 5].

Spinal Cord Injury

- Rehabilitation from spinal cord injuries should occur in specialized units focused on the recovery of this patient population [1–3].
- Identification of the American Spinal Injury Association (ASIA) Score helps determine patient needs: [1–3]

- A: complete impairment, no motor or sensory function below injury level
- B: incomplete impairment, no motor function but intact sensation below injury level
- C: incomplete impairment, weak motor function with sensory loss below injury level
- D: incomplete impairment, motor function intact but no sensation below injury level
- E: No impairment, intact motor and sensory function

- Bowel and bladder function may be compromised, requiring straight catheterization and medical management [1–3].
- Goals include maximizing ADLs, such as hygiene and feeding, as well as maximizing mobility with assist devices [1–3].
- Other needs include prevention of major complications such as pulmonary complications, urinary tract infections, and pressure ulcers [1–3].
- Autonomic dysreflexia is a life-threatening complication that occurs in SCI patients due to unchecked sympathetic tone [1–3, 6].

  - Symptoms include hypertension, headache, flushing/sweating, blurry vision, nasal congestion, and sometimes bradycardia, which can then progress to intracranial hemorrhage, seizure, arrhythmias, or myocardial infarction.
  - Typically occurs in patients with injury level T6 or higher, though cases have been described as low as T10.
  - The most common causes are bladder and bowel distension, though other sources of pain and illness, and even compression devices and constrictive clothing have been implicated.

Cervical Spine Injury (CSI)

- At the C1–C4 level, patients may, depending on the nature of the injury, have little to no extremity movement and will require long-term trained caregiver support [1–3].
- Below C5, patients have much higher levels of independence with the use of devices to support ADLs [1–3].
- High cervical SCI patients are at high risk for bradycardia due to lack of sympathetic drive and unopposed vagal tone, care must be taken with maneuvers such as suctioning or turning [1–3].
- Due to lack of diaphragmatic and intercostal muscle tone, patients have significant respiratory complications and may even be ventilator dependent [1–3].
- Patients with complete paralysis may benefit from mechanical assist devices to increase independence, such as voice control software and specialized motorized wheelchairs [1–3].
- Goals of rehabilitation are to allow independence with ADLs with equipment [1–3].

Lower Spinal Cord Injury

- Lower level cord injuries generally have a better prognosis and demonstrate greater independent functioning than higher level injuries [1–3].
- Early activities include transfers, wheelchair use, and occupational therapy for ADLs [1–3].
- Goals of rehabilitation are to increase independence with all ADLs using assist devices [1–3].

Traumatic Brain Injury

- Evaluation and treatment of cognitive disorders after TBI is the focus of rehabilitation, with a multidisciplinary approach involving careful medication management, physical, occupational, and speech therapy, as well as neuropsychologists and rehabilitation physicians [1, 2, 4].
- Patients with severe TBI may develop paroxysmal sympathetic hyperactivity, also known as sympathetic storm, from a disturbance in autonomic regulation [1–4].

  - Symptoms are similar to sepsis, thyroid storm, and delirium tremens and include tachycardia, agitation, hyperpyrexia, rigidity, and diaphoresis.
  - Medications like propranolol, opioids, gabapentin, and bromocriptine are used for management after ruling out other medical causes.

- Many patients after traumatic brain injury can have behavioral control issues such as agitation or aggression [1–4, 7].

  - Some medications can help, such as propranolol and careful use of antipsychotics.
  - Behavioral problems may be secondary to other causes such as delirium, pain, infection, and sleep disturbances, which can be addressed individually.

- In some patients, somnolence may occur instead of agitation, resulting in decreased participation in medical care and rehabilitation [1–3].

  - Dopamine agonists such as amantadine may help increase wakefulness.
  - Proper sleep hygiene and minimizing sedative medications may also help.

- Other cognitive deficits such as anterograde amnesia, attention deficits, and impulse control that must be rehabilitated to allow for discharge to the community [1–3].

Polytrauma

- Patients who suffer severe traumatic injury may present with a combination of multiple injuries, e.g., multiple complex orthopedic injuries and a TBI [1–3].
- These patients are a clinical challenge due to the numerous physical and cognitive limitations that must all be addressed simultaneously [1–3].
- Polytrauma patients may have had extended ICU length of stays with complications such as prolonged respiratory failure, recurrent infections, physical deconditioning, and catabolism [1–3].
- Polytrauma rehabilitation must also address the psychological component of injury, which may range from anxiety disorder to post-traumatic stress disorder [1–3, 8].
- Rehabilitation goals involve increasing independence and functioning to allow safe integration into the community setting for outpatient management [1–3].
- Outpatient rehabilitation of polytrauma patients requires a strong interdisciplinary team and caregiver support [1–3].

References

1. Brown C. Chapter 55: Rehabilitation. In: Halter J, Ouslander JG, Studenski S, High KP, Asthana S, Supiano MA, et al., editors. Hazzard's geriatric medicine and gerontology. 8th ed. McGraw Hill LLC; 2022.
2. Maitin IB, Cruz E. CURRENT diagnosis & treatment: physical medicine and rehabilitation. 1st ed. McGraw-Hill; 2015.
3. Mitra R. Principles of rehabilitation medicine. 1st ed. McGraw-Hill Education; 2019.
4. Niziolek G, Sandsmark DK, Pascual JL. Neurotrauma. Curr Opin Crit Care. 2022;28(6):715–24. https://doi.org/10.1097/MCC.0000000000001005.
5. Nikolajsen L, Jensen TS. Phantom limb pain. Br J Anaesth. 2001;87(1):107–16. https://doi.org/10.1093/bja/87.1.107.
6. Krassioukov A, Warburton DE, Teasell R, Eng JJ, Team SCIRER. A systematic review of the management of autonomic dysreflexia after spinal cord injury. Arch Phys Med Rehabil. 2009;90(4):682–95. https://doi.org/10.1016/j.apmr.2008.10.017.
7. Schwarzbold M, Diaz A, Martins ET, Rufino A, Amante LN, Thais ME, et al. Psychiatric disorders and traumatic brain injury. Neuropsychiatr Dis Treat. 2008;4(4):797–816. https://doi.org/10.2147/ndt.s2653.
8. O'Donnell ML, Creamer M, Pattison P, Atkin C. Psychiatric morbidity following injury. Am J Psychiatry. 2004;161(3):507–14. https://doi.org/10.1176/appi.ajp.161.3.507.

Chapter 53
The Role of Palliative Care in Trauma

Kwang Kim and Edward Chao

Overview

- Palliative care is a philosophy of care to improve quality of life for patients with serious illness and their families. Provides significant benefit across a spectrum of illness and injury, regardless of prognosis [2].
- Palliative care is delivered concurrently and integrated with other curative and life-sustaining therapies.
- Unit of care is the patient *and* family/next of kin focusing on their physical, emotional, spiritual, and psychosocial well-being.

Background

Indications for Palliative Care

- Palliative care is indicated in patients with functional dependency and advanced care needs, in addition to those with life-threating conditions.
- Often associated with advanced age, do-not-resuscitate (DNR) status, traumatic brain injuries (TBI), mechanical ventilation, and ICU admissions [1].
- Mortality for critically injured patients requiring ICU care ranges from 10% to 20% and is often considered an indication for palliative care evaluation. However,

K. Kim · E. Chao (✉)
New York Health and Hospitals/Jacobi, Bronx, NY, USA

Jacobi Medical Center, Albert Einstein College of Medicine, Bronx, NY, USA
e-mail: kkim2@montefiore.org; Edward.Chao@nychhc.org

© The Author(s), under exclusive license to Springer Nature   497
Switzerland AG 2025
T. S. Brahmbhatt, D. R. Scantling (eds.), *Trauma Surgery Clerkship*,
Contemporary Surgical Clerkships,
https://doi.org/10.1007/978-3-032-01412-2_53

palliative care is not just for the dying patients, it can also be helpful for their families, next of kin, and the care providers as well. [1]
– Palliative care may be most beneficial for elderly trauma patients, given their existing frailty and comorbidities, with a concurrent traumatic injury that may permanently compromise their functional status.

Benefits of Palliative Care

– Palliative care alongside trauma care decreases length of stay, cost, and intensity of non-beneficial care at the end of life while improving quality of care, pain, and symptom management, without increasing in-hospital or ICU mortality [1, 3].
– For the geriatric trauma population, palliative care has been associated with decreased hospital length of stay and hospital costs without an impact on mortality, discharge disposition or functional outcomes [4].

Essential Components of Palliative Care

– Interdisciplinary team includes physicians, nurses, social workers, chaplains, case managers, pharmacists, bereavement specialists, behavioral health specialists, and therapists.
– Partnership with palliative care services and the primary trauma or ICU teams ensures optimal patient-centered care [5].
– Effective communication and support regarding prognosis, treatment options, and shared decision-making are critical.
– Early, continuous assessment and treatment of pain, discomfort, and anxiety [1, 6].

  • Addressing and alleviating underlying cause of physical pain
  • Anxiety control
  • Symptom control, especially when withdrawing life-sustaining therapy: relieving pain, dyspnea, and thirst

– Psychosocial, spiritual, religious, and cultural considerations [7].

  • Psychosocial support plan: identification of religious/community leader(s), collaboration with specific individuals, and involvement of key community members
  • Trauma patients often involve young children in family support system—may require additional staff with expertise in children's behavioral health [8]

Current Practice

Breaking Bad News

- Communicating difficult news of a sudden traumatic death (Table 53.1): [9]

  • Start with an early warning to prepare the listener for bad news in a safe space.
  • Provide a brief context and deliver the news of death—MUST use the "D" words (death, dead, died, or dying).
  • Allow for silence and expression of emotions.
  • Validate emotions and share empathy.
  • Prepare family for what they will see and allow family to spend time with the patient.

- Preparing for a family meeting for a critically ill patient:[10]

  • Ensure access to a safe and quiet environment without interruption.
  • Prepare for conversation and involve multidisciplinary team when appropriate.
  • Huddle with team prior to confirm all information and deliver a unified message.
  • Use language interpreters as appropriate and do not ask family members to interpret.
  • Have comfort items available: tissues, water, etc.
  • Have a safe but compassionate proximity to patients and families.

Palliative Care Assessment and Interventions (Table 53.2)

- Initiate palliative care assessment on admission or early within 24 h [11].

  • Identify health care proxy or surrogate decision maker.

Table 53.1 Communicating difficult news of a sudden traumatic death

Preparation	Gather relevant clinical and patient information. Contact appropriate person to communicate bad news and assess their understanding of what has transpired
Early warning	"I'm afraid I have bad news…"
Context	Provide context regarding traumatic incident. MUST use the "D" words (death, dead, died, dying)
Silence	Allow for grievance and expression of emotions. Expressions of grief may vary in different cultures
Validate	Acknowledge emotions and share empathy
Privacy	Allow family to spend time with the deceased in a private setting. Prepare them for what they will see [10]

Table 53.2 Palliative care assessment in trauma

First 24 h	Initial Palliative Care Assessment
	Identify health care proxy
	Obtain preexisting advance directives, living will, and DNR/Do Not Intubate (DNI) orders
	Gather family and social context for decision making
	Assess prognosis
	Screen for further palliative care needs
Within 72 h	Patients with category 1 or 2 positive screen
	Schedule a family meeting
	Have a GOC discussion for alignment of care
	Schedule a follow-up meeting

- Surrogate decision-making rests on the concepts of substituted judgment and best interest standard.
- Decisions are based on the patient's established or probable wishes, even if they might conflict with their own personal wishes.
- Surrogates are often poorly prepared for their role and need support to preserve patient autonomy.

- Identify any preexisting advance directives, living will, or do-not-resuscitate (DNR) orders.
- Understand family and social context.
- Assess prognosis—includes risk of death and expected functional and cognitive recovery.

- Hold a structured family meeting for critically injured patients as soon as possible (ideally within 72 h of admission) and every 3–5 days thereafter [11].

- A prognosis of death, permanent disability, or uncertainty of either is a trigger for palliative care and GOC discussions.
- Advanced care planning discussions initiated at this time and revisited with each major change in status or care plan.
- The first conversation is important for early alignment of care with patient goals and avoidance of further aggressive or futile care.
- Schedule the date and time for the next meeting.

- The "*surprise question*" is a useful tool for prognostication in palliative care screening—"Would you be surprised if this patient were dead in 12 months?" [11]

- Patient with negative screen if the answer is "yes"—i.e., patients who are primarily young or otherwise healthy with non-life-threatening injuries. They require symptom management and identification of a health care proxy.
- Patients with a positive screen fall into two categories:

  - *Category 1*: Answer to the surprise question is "maybe" or "no." Uncertainty regarding long-term functional recovery or survival due to severe traumatic injuries, age, frailty, comorbidities, or a combination of these factors. These patients need advance care planning discussions and clarification of resuscitation goals. Early GOC discussions are needed to establish priorities.

- *Category 2*: Answer to the surprise question is a "definite no." Major life threatening or disabling traumatic injuries, or lesser injuries with serious comorbidities, frailty, or advanced age. They are at high risk of in-hospital death or discharge to dependent care. These patients need early GOC discussion, clarification of treatment preferences, and end of life care with hospice if appropriate.

Goals of Care Conversation

- All patients with a positive palliative care screen need a GOC conversation as soon as possible with the patient and family members including spouse, children, siblings, relatives, and anyone else essential to the patient's decision making.
- The purpose is to ensure all therapy during hospitalization is concordant with the patient's goals [10].

  • The conversation is specifically to guide therapy.
  • The expected trajectory or further expected declines in functional or cognitive status are discussed along with the benefits and burdens of each therapy.
  • Each conversation must clarify the patient's wishes regarding life-sustaining treatment and whether the treatment should be temporary or prolonged.
  • The outcome of GOC discussion should include decisions on cardiopulmonary resuscitation, mechanical ventilation, artificial nutrition and hydration, hemodialysis, and any other life-sustaining therapies.
  • Determined code status and other preferences are documented and communicated to all treatment teams.

- GOC discussions can be guided using the best case/worst case communication tool (Fig. 53.1) [12].

  • The tool is used to integrate all available clinical information and estimate the range of future outcomes.
  • Describe the best-case and worst-case outcomes regarding overall prognosis, neurologic and functional recovery, and quality of life after hospital discharge if applicable.
  • Describe the "most likely" case based on clinicians' best judgment about what the future may bring.
  • With any change in status or a clinical deterioration, update the family with a new "most likely" scenario.

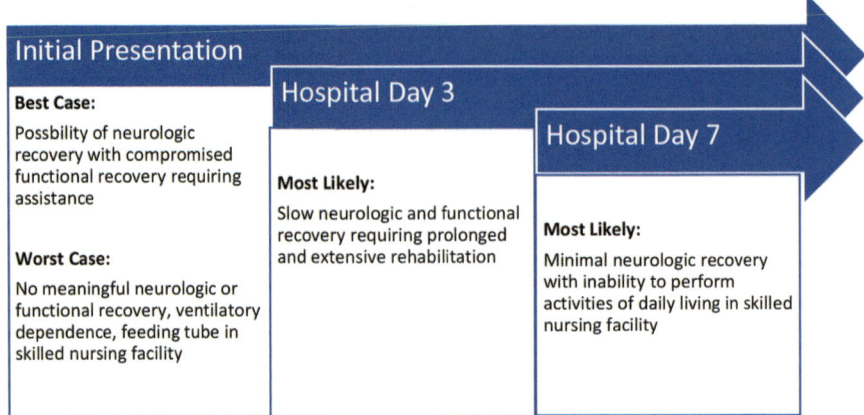

Fig. 53.1 Best case/worst case scenario

End of Life Care

– DNR or DNI orders do not preclude treatment or delivery of care with curative intent.

  • Not all patients with DNR/DNI status are at the end of life, and some still
     choose aggressive therapies that require rescinding of these interventions.
  • Surgical intervention may be appropriate in the right context.
  • A policy of "required reconsideration" of DNR/DNI status around the time of
     surgery is advised.

– Withdrawal of life support does not imply withdrawal of care. [13]

  • Withdrawal of life support is the withdrawal of life-sustaining interventions,
     and the focus shifts to ensuring patient does not experience pain or suffering.
  • A DNR/DNI order needs to be in place.
  • Appropriate preparations are needed for the patient and families, which may
     include generally estimating how rapidly death will occur.
  • Withdrawal of life support must be coordinated:

    – Create a peaceful environment with ample space for the family.
    – Remove all unnecessary equipment, monitoring devices, and restraints.
    – Silence all alarms.
    – Discontinue all medications, feedings, or intravenous lines that are not
       related to comfort.
    – Provide tissues, water, and comfortable chairs for family members.
    – Adjust the bedrails and bed height to enable family–patient contact.
    – Inform the family about the dying process and what might transpire.
    – Allow time for any rituals, especially if death is likely to be imminent fol-
       lowing removal of support.

- Precede the withdrawal of ventilator support with the cessation of neuromuscular blockade and administer appropriate sedative, secretion control, and pain control medications.
- Opioids are first-line treatment of dyspnea. If refractory, titrate benzodiazepines to effect.
- Following declaration of death, allow family and staff to be with the patient.
- Allow involved health care team to debrief and discuss the case.

Take-Home Points for Palliative Patient Care

- Palliative care in trauma and critical care is an essential component of providing high quality care for patients.
- Provides comprehensive care for critically ill and injured patients with poor prognosis or functional recovery.
- Prioritizes appropriate care concordant with patient's wishes and helps determine their wishes via a surrogate when unable to make decisions for themselves.
- Shown to reduce length of stay, unnecessary invasive procedures, cost of hospitalization, without increasing mortality.
- Assessment by primary trauma or critical care teams with early integration of the palliative care team is essential for trauma patients.
- Delivering bad news, initiating palliative care assessment, having GOC discussions, and providing end of life care are all important components of palliative care.

References

1. Mosenthal AC, Weissman DE, Curtis JR, Hays RM, Lustbader DR, Mulkerin C, et al. Integrating palliative care in the surgical and Trauma Intensive Care Unit. Crit Care Med. 2012;40(4):1199–206.
2. Updated May 15 2019, Updated November 14 2022. Palliative care best practices guidelines: Palliative in practice [Internet]. Palliative Care Best Practices Guidelines | Palliative in Practice | Center to Advance Palliative Care. [cited 2022Nov20]. Available from: https://www.capc.org/blog/news-bites-now-available-acs-tqip-palliative-care-best-practices-guidelines/
3. Kupensky D, Hileman BM, Emerick ES, Chance EA. Palliative medicine consultation reduces length of stay, improves symptom management, and clarifies advance directives in the Geriatric Trauma Population. J Trauma Nurs. 2015;22(5):261–5.
4. Aziz HA, Lunde J, Barraco R, Como JJ, Cooper Z, Hayward T, et al. Evidence-based review of Trauma Center care and routine palliative care processes for geriatric trauma patients; a collaboration from the American Association for the surgery of trauma patient assessment committee, the American Association for the surgery of trauma geriatric trauma committee, and the Eastern Association for the surgery of trauma guidelines committee. J Trauma Acute Care Surg. 2019;86(4):737–43.
5. O'Connell K, Maier R. Palliative care in the trauma ICU. Curr Opin Crit Care. 2016;22(6):584–90.

6. Puntillo K, Nelson JE, Weissman D, Curtis R, Weiss S, Frontera J, et al. Palliative care in the ICU: Relief of pain, dyspnea, and thirst – a report from the IPAL-ICU advisory board. Intens Care Med. 2013;40(2):235–48.

7. Wesson JS. Meeting the informational, psychosocial and emotional needs of each ICU patient and family. Intens Crit Care Nurs. 1997;13(2):111–8.

8. McGrath PA. Development of the World Health Organization Guidelines on Cancer Pain Relief and palliative care in children. J Pain Symptom Manag. 1996;12(2):87–92.

9. Dunn GP. Surgical palliative care. Surg Palliative Care. 2019:1–12.

10. Lamba S, Bryczkowski S, Tyrie L, Weissman DE, Mosenthal AC. Death disclosure and delivery of difficult news in trauma #305. J Palliative Med. 2016;19(5):566–7.

11. Weissman DE. Improving generalist palliative care [Internet]. Palliative Care Network of Wisconsin. 2019 [cited 2022Nov20]. Available from: https://www.mypcnow.org/product/improving-generalist-palliative-care/

12. Taylor LJ, Nabozny MJ, Steffens NM, Tucholka JL, Brasel KJ, Johnson SK, et al. A framework to improve surgeon communication in high-stakes surgical decisions. JAMA Surg. 2017;152(6):531.

13. Rubenfeld GD. Principles and practice of withdrawing life-sustaining treatments. Crit Care Clin. 2004;20(3):435–51.

Index

© The Editor(s) (if applicable) and The Author(s), under exclusive license to
Springer Nature Switzerland AG 2025
T. S. Brahmbhatt, D. R. Scantling (eds.), *Trauma Surgery Clerkship*,
Contemporary Surgical Clerkships,
https://doi.org/10.1007/978-3-032-01412-2